MEDICAL SELF-CARE

AND ASSESSMENT

Medical Self-Care

AND

Assessment

By

Brent Q. Hafen, Ph.D.

Professor of Health Sciences
Brigham Young University

With

Molly J. Brog, Ph.D.
and
Kathryn J. Frandsen, Ed.D.

MP

Morton Publishing Company
295 West Hampden, Suite 104
Englewood, Colorado 80110

Printed in the United States of America

ISBN: 0-89582-095-1

To Our Readers:

The authors and publisher of this book do not take responsibility for any possible consequences from any treatment, action, or application of medications or procedures described in this book. The publication of this book does not constitute the practice of medicine, and this book does not attempt to replace your physician or pharmacist. If you are under the care of a physician or have had prior health problems, follow the advice of your physician.

Acknowledgments

Appreciation is expressed to the following for allowing us to use their color photographs:

N. Branson Call, M.D.
Ophthalmic Plastic and
Reconstructive Surgeon
Salt Lake City, Utah

Niles W. Herrod, D.D.S.
Oral and Maxillofacial Surgeon
Provo, Utah

Blayne L. Hirsche, M.D.
Plastic and Reconstructive Surgeon
Provo, Utah

Douglas C. Cox, Ph.D.
Monte L. Bean Life Sciences Museum
Brigham Young University
Provo, Utah

W. Henry Baughman, H.S.D.
Western Kentucky University
Bowling Green, Kentucky

Eugene L. Robertson, M.D.
Plastic and Reconstructive Surgeon
Provo, Utah

James R. Feucht, Ph.D.
Cooperative Extension Service
Colorado State University
Denver, Colorado

SPENCO Medical Corp.
Waco, Texas

Robert W. Wright, Ph.D.
Museum of Natural History
Denver, Colorado

Robert H. Horne, M.D., F.A.C.S.
Murray, Utah

Cliggott Publishing Company
Consultant, Greenwich, Connecticut

Drug Intelligence Publications, Inc.
*Dangerous Plants, Snakes,
Arthropods and Marine Life —
Toxicity and Treatment,*
by Michael D. Ellis, M.s.
Washington, D.C.

Renner Johnston, M.D.
Denver General Hospital
Denver, Colorado

John A. Boswick, Jr., M.D.
University of Colorado Medical Ctr.
Denver, Colorado

Richard E. Albin, M.D., Ph.D.
The Center for Plastic,
Reconstructive, and Maxillofacial
Surgery, P.C.
Denver, Colorado

Paul Wexler, M.D.
Rose Medical Center
Denver, Colorado

Peter Rosen, M.D.
Denver General Hospital
Denver, Colorado

American Academy of Dermatology
and Institute for Dermatologic
Communication and Education

Richard A. Buckingham, Clinical
Professor, Otolaryngology
Abraham Lincoln School of Medicine
University of Illinois
Chicago, Illinois

We also wish to express appreciation to the following:

TIME Magazine
Metropolitan Life Insurance Co.

Other books by Brent Hafen with Morton Publishing Company:

Prehospital Emergency Care and Crisis Intervention
First Aid and Emergency Care Skills Manual
First Responder: A Skills Approach
Faces of Death: Grief, Dying, Euthanasia, Suicide

Contents

CHAPTER 1

INTRODUCTION TO SELF-CARE

WHAT DOES SELF-CARE MEAN?

If you've ever gone to the doctor with symptoms that have turned out to signal the flu or mononucleosis, you know that most of the treatment depended on you—on what you did after you got home. While a doctor's diagnosis is important to rule out the possibility of serious disease, there is much you can do to treat yourself in cases of mild illness, and many ways in which you can take care of common health problems.

If you know how, you can also measure your own vital signs, assess your own symptoms, treat most of your common health problems, and report your own history of illness to a doctor, enabling him or her to make a more accurate diagnosis. All these add up to skills that will enable you to take a more aggressive role in your own health and well-being. Most people are capable of safely caring for a large number of health problems commonly referred to a physician. Self-care proponents argue that from one-third to three-quarters of visits to the doctor's office could be avoided if patients were better prepared.

Self-care, then, means control, responsibility, freedom, expanded options, and improved quality of life. With self-care, "clients are beginning to define their rights, as individuals and families, for developing their own definitions of health, their own priorities, their own options, and their own risk indices. They want to develop their own abilities for living the good and healthful life, for preventing disease, for managing their dis-ease and disease, for assessing and intervening in health and illness, and for using the health care system as often as when they need to."[1]

Other reasons why people are beginning to turn to self-care include:

1. Widespread dissatisfaction with medical care.
2. The fact that personal behavior and environment will help improve health and promote disease reduction.
3. The desire to save money on health expenses.
4. The desire to be able to make better decisions concerning one's own health and the health of one's family, which leads to a certain joy of independence.[2]

Today, medical consumers know more and read more and are better able to evaluate the care that they receive. They are also able to reserve more of the final judgments for their own care. They ask for a great deal more information, which makes them better able to carry out self-care treatments effectively.

In its strictest sense, self-care involves taking over tasks usually relegated to a professional care giver—measuring heart rate and blood pressure, performing home lab tests, or treating influenza. Although we tend to think of these tasks as properly belonging to a doctor or nurse, studies indicate that nonprofessionals can handle them quite well. Patients with a chronic disease have been performing "professional" tasks for years. Diabetics, for instance, test their urine and give themselves insulin injections. Persons with angina (chest pain) medicate themselves with nitroglycerine.

Whatever their doctors' qualms, ordinary people are learning to handle stethoscopes and blood pressure cuffs, administer breast self-examinations and pregnancy tests, and, in some cases, carry out elementary lab tests. Medical devices that were once held at arm's length from the public can now be purchased easily. "Good equipment, in the hands of properly trained lay people, can curtail needless trips to the doctor. The rise of medical costs could be slowed. Skilled use of certain devices could encourage people to see a doctor sooner. A more informed citizenry might follow physician's instructions better."[3] As much as anything, self-care practitioners are learning to heed the messages of their own bodies—and to appreciate the importance of exercise, proper nutrition, relaxation, and habit control in leading healthier lives.

The classic agenda of self-care is perhaps best outlined in the "health activation" program developed by Dr. Keith W. Sehnert. As self-care develops as a new health concept, it is important to remember that any self-care program should be carefully coordinated under the supervision of one's own physician. It is not desirable to give a person half knowledge and half technical skills that could leave him or her with a false sense of what they can do.[4] In addition, Dr. Sehnert not only envisions self-care, but a partnership between the informed patient and the doctor. He states:

> The health partnership I visualize will in time do away with the current and much too frequent adversary setting that intervenes with an optimal doctor-patient relationship. It will alter the common practice of defensive medicine in which the doctor takes multiple X-rays and orders expensive laboratory tests, not for improved diagnosis and medical care, but so that, at some later date, he won't get sued. It will change the typical patient's demand for an expensive prescription when no prescription is needed. The patient will want, indeed, demand, to do as much as he can for himself. And doctors will be—in the historical sense of the word — teachers.[5]

The American Medical Association expresses Dr. Sehnert's idea a little differently. This group speaks of the doctor-patient partnership as a negotiation process: "Negotiation is a process by which two active and equal participants negotiate to obtain their respective goals (which are often at odds). Without appropriate negotiation, the physician cannot help to motivate the patient. Patients will continue to be non-compliant as long as they are treated as inferiors in the process." The key here is "active participation," which is being encouraged by Sehnert and others. Active participation brings about motivation, which, in turn, brings about better health and compliance with treatment procedures when these are necessary for restoring health.

Ideally, Sehnert and other proponents of self-care are trying to educate the public to the concept of total self-care, which embodies the following elements:

1. Monitoring, assessing, and diagnosing illness and abnormal conditions (through such means as breast self-examination, knowing the seven warning signals of cancer, and knowing the symptoms and signs of minor illnesses).
2. Supporting the life processes (by performing such basic hygienic habits as brushing the teeth, washing the hands, and eating).
3. Providing therapeutic and corrective self-care when needed.
4. Preventing disease and maladjustment states (through prevention of risks that cause or predispose a patient to disease).
5. Specifying health needs and care requirements (in other words, formulating options for health care according to the patient's perception).

6. Auditing and controlling treatment programs.
7. Providing self-initiated health care.[6]

INDICATORS OF CRITICAL ILLNESS

A symptom is the first warning sign that something is wrong. A nagging headache, a pain in the stomach, ringing in the ears, a pins-and-needles sensation in the feet—all these are **symptoms.** A symptom is something only you know is there—a symptom cannot be seen by anyone else (or by you, for that matter).

Symptoms are different from **signs.** Signs can be seen—both by you and by a doctor. A rash, a swelling, a bruise, blisters on the throat—all these are **signs,** observable phenomena that accompany **symptoms.** The itching that accompanies a rash is a symptom; the rash itself is a sign. The parched and sore throat that accompany tonsillitis are symptoms; the red throat tissue and the swollen glands are signs.

Figure 1-1
The difference between a sign and a symptom.

SIGN
Visual
Something that you can see.

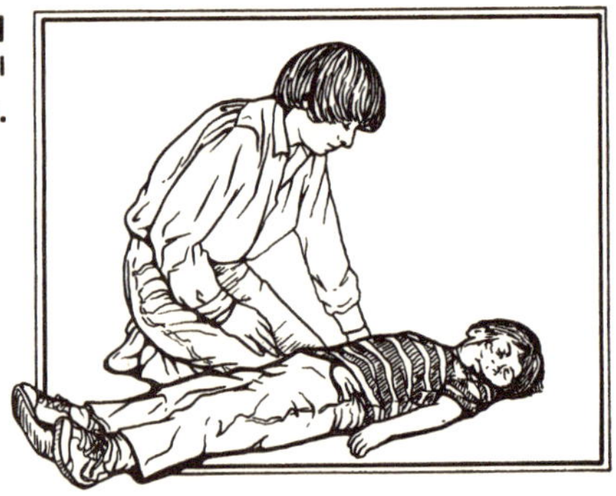

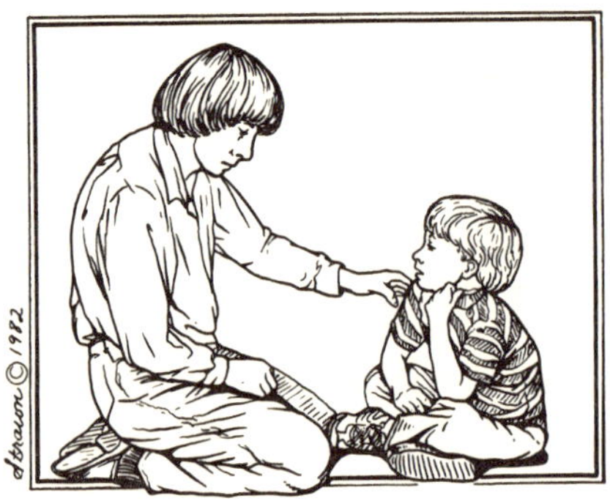

SYMPTOM
Something the person tells about himself, e.g. he feels nauseous or has pain.

In certain cases signs and symptoms indicate illness too critical to be treated without skilled medical help. **If in doubt, always seek help from a competent physician.** Conditions that should be referred to medical help include:[7]

1. Acuteness—the signs and symptoms are so severe that they cannot be endured (for example, chest pains or abdominal pain).
2. Persistence—the signs and symptoms persist for a few days or a week (for example, headaches).
3. Recurrence—the signs and symptoms return without a clear-cut cause (for example, diarrhea or other intestinal upsets).
4. Unusualness—signs and symptoms that raise doubts.

Even though severe or persistent signs and symptoms may indicate that medical attention is needed, a symptom is **not** a diagnosis—it is merely an indication that something is wrong and needs attention. The diagnosis should be left up to the doctor. However, you **can** learn to describe clearly all of your signs and symptoms—which will help the doctor make his or her diagnosis.

INDIVIDUAL RESPONSIBILITY— THE ESSENCE OF SELF-CARE

The most tragic health situation in this country today is that too many people neglect their health, surrendering to someone else (a doctor, a nurse, a folk healer) the responsibility for keeping their body well and functioning. Of course, there are times and situations when you *must* see a doctor. But each one of us is the ideal monitor of our own body. We are most familiar with its peculiarities and are quickest to recognize any changes. **You** are responsible for being in tune with your body, for knowing when self-care is appropriate and when medical help is needed. **You** have the capability of pinpointing your own risk factors—of finding out what habits, life-styles, and things in your background make you susceptible to certain diseases. **You** have the ability to change the things that you can and the intelligence to adapt to the things that you cannot change. **You** are in control of your body and of all the things that affect it.

NOTES

1. Catherine M. Norris, "Self-Care," *American Journal of Nursing,* March 1979, p. 486.
2. Tom Ferguson, "A Conversation with Keith Sehnert, M.D.," *Medical Self-Care: Access to Medical Tools,* Fall 1979, p. 18.
3. John Grossman, "Do-it-Yourself Doctoring," *Family Health,* February 1979, p. 20.
4. "The Self-Care Surge," *Medical World News,* October 3, 1977, pp. 43-54.
5. Lynn Lamberg, "Patient, Help Thyself," *Family Health,* April 1979, pp. 35-38.
6. Norris, p. 488.
7. Leaflet, "When to Call or See Your Physician," American Medical Association.

CHAPTER 2

SELF-DETERMINATION OF VITAL SIGNS

TEMPERATURE

The optimum temperature for cell metabolism and activity is 98.6 degrees Fahrenheit in the human body. Normal temperature is established when there is a balance between heat production and heat loss. Under normal circumstances, heat is produced in the body by ingestion of food and by muscular activity and is lost through conduction, convection, radiation, and evaporation.

Factors That Affect Body Temperature

1. **Biological rhythms.** There is a slight temperature variation (2° F.) in normal people over a twenty-four-hour period. Temperature is generally highest in the late afternoon or from about 8:00 to 11:00 P.M. The lowest body temperature is experienced during sleep from about 4:00 to 6:00 A.M. These temperature variations can probably be explained by an increase or decrease in muscular activity and digestive function.
2. **Hormone secretions.** Oversecretions of the thyroid gland can produce an increase in body temperature. Female hormones such as estrogen

and progesterone and male hormones such as testosterone also influence body temperature.

3. **Environment.** Seasonal changes, clothing, and baths may influence the body temperature to a small degree.
4. **Exercise.** Increased muscular activity will increase the body temperature somewhat.
5. **Eating food.** Ingestion of food and the digestive process can elevate the body temperature slightly after a meal.
6. **Drugs.** Some drugs can either increase or decrease body temperature slightly.
7. **Age.** In babies, the temperature-regulating mechanism is somewhat underdeveloped and imperfect so that the baby's body temperature is influenced by the environment. In the elderly, aging of the body produces a body temperature that is slightly below normal. The following chart will aid you in knowing the average body temperatures for various ages:

Age	Average Fahrenheit Body Temperature
Newborn	97-100 degrees
2 years	100 degrees
3 years	98.9 degrees
7 years	98.6 degrees
12 years	98.6 degrees
Adult	98.6 degrees
Elderly	95 degrees

Reprinted by permission from Kozier, Barbara and Glenora Erb. *Fundamentals of Nursing: Concepts and Procedures.* Menlo Park, California: The Addison-Wesley Publishing Company, Medical/Nursing Division, 1979, p. 241.

8. **Sex.** Women tend to have slightly higher body temperature than men because they have more fat deposition that acts as insulation.

Fevers

When a fever is present, the person may experience the following symptoms and discomforts: aching muscles and joints; hot, dry skin; chilling; flushing; thirst; and malaise. The individual may also have a headache, nausea and vomiting, constipation, or diarrhea.

Fevers usually develop in a certain sequence. The patient first experiences the "cold" fever. The core temperature is increasing and the body is conserving heat. The skin looks blanched and feels cold to the touch. Shivering and goose bumps are present. Next, the patient experiences the "hot" fever. At this point, the fever has peaked. The body radiates heat, feels hot, and is flushed. Next, the fever abates. The vessels in the skin dilate and perspiring occurs.[1]

Types of Fevers

There are several types of fevers. The **continuous** or **sustained fever** persists without normal periods. The fever may vary slightly (no more than 3.6° F.), but it never returns to normal in a twenty-four-hour period. The **intermittent fever** occurs when there is an elevation and return to normal temperature during a twenty-four-hour period. When the temperature varies widely (more than 3.6° F.) during a twenty-four-hour period and never returns to normal, the fever is said to be a **remittent fever.** When an elevated temperature recurs one or more times after a normal temperature that lasts at least one day, the fever is known as a **relapsing fever.** Lastly, when a fever has very marked peaks and troughs, it is said to be **septic.**[2]

Effects of a Prolonged Fever

When the body temperature is elevated for some period, increased perspiration occurs so that water and salt are lost from the body. As a result, the urine and blood become more concentrated. The blood pressure drops because of the decrease in circulatory function. The body needs more oxygen, so the pulse and respiration increase. Brain activity slows. Men produce less sperm for about one to two weeks after a high or prolonged fever. And the metabolism increases so that the body needs more fuel. Usually, a person is not particularly hungry while he or she is running a fever, so the person may lose weight because of the increased demands of metabolism that are not met with a simultaneous increase in fuel. A prolonged fever may cause complications in a pregnant woman and her unborn child.[3]

Taking Temperature

Before taking temperature:

1. Wash your hands.
2. Check the thermometer for breakage; make sure that there are no cracks in the thermometer, especially in the mercury bulb (ingestion of mercury can lead to mercury poisoning).

3. Cleanse the thermometer with a disinfectant (alcohol is a good one), and rinse it under cool running water.
4. If the thermometer reads above 95° F., shake it down, grasp the top end tightly, and shake the thermometer with a snapping motion. Keep your wrist loose, and make sure that you don't hit the thermometer against anything.
5. Make sure that the person has not had hot or cold liquids or been smoking—all of which can alter the temperature. If he or she has, wait for thirty minutes to an hour for the temperature to normalize.
6. Explain what you are going to do so that the person can cooperate.

You need to decide whether to take an oral, rectal, or axillary (armpit) temperature. In taking a temperature, you place the thermometer so that it is surrounded by body tissues that have a good blood supply and that are in a closed space. The most convenient place for taking a temperature is the mouth—but it should not be used if the patient is unconscious, irrational, restless, delirious, or combative; if the mouth is parched or dry; if the mouth is inflamed; if the nose is plugged so that the patient cannot breathe through the mouth; or if the patient is a child or infant who may bite the thermometer accidentally. Taking the rectal temperature is the second best method because the rectum is well supplied with blood vessels and is not affected by the patient taking in hot or cold liquids. The axillary (armpit) temperature is generally inaccurate because the skin in that area is cool from exposure to the air.

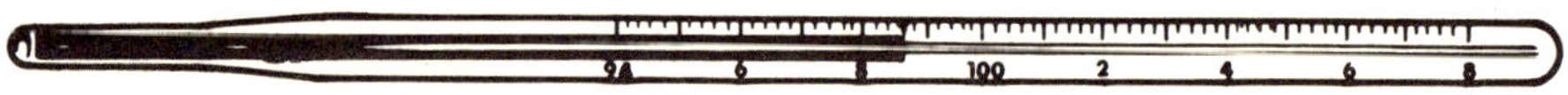

Oral thermometer (used in the mouth)

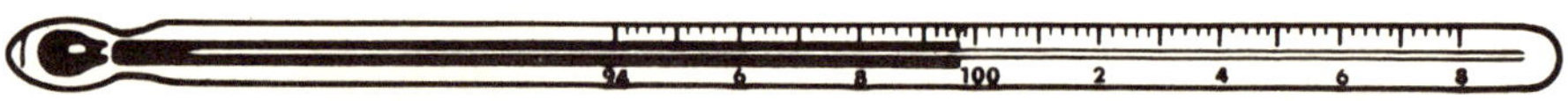

Rectal thermometer (used in the rectum)

Figure 2-1
Oral and rectal thermometers. Before using, be sure to shake the thermometer down to allow the mercury to drop down the stem.

Use these steps in taking a temperature:

Oral

1. Place the mercury end of the thermometer under the tongue; ask the

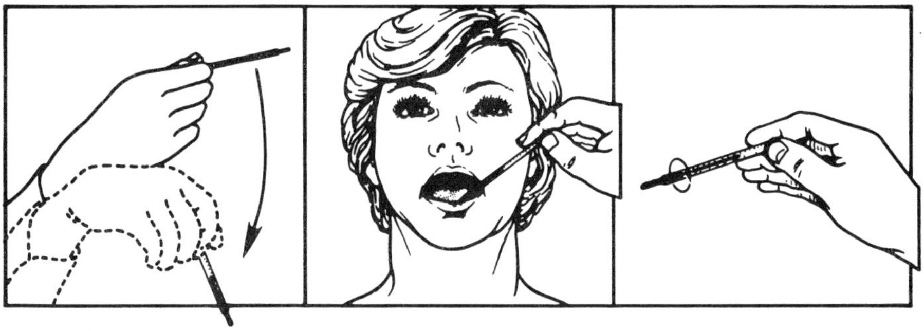

Figure 2-2
(1) Shake the mercury down into the bulb.
(2) Place the bulb under the tongue and have the person close his or her mouth.
(3) The temperature registers at the end of the mercury.

person to keep the mouth tightly closed, but not to bite the thermometer with the teeth. The lips should stay tightly closed. The bulb of mercury should touch the base of the tongue.

2. Leave the thermometer in the person's mouth for three minutes. If the thermometer is left in the mouth for eight to nine minutes, the reading may be more accurate.
3. Remove the thermometer and read it. Normal oral temperature is between 97 and 99° F. (usually expressed as 98.6° F.).

Rectal

The thermometer used to take a rectal temperature has a short, blunt bulb as opposed to the long, slender bulb of the oral thermometer. (Do not use an oral thermometer to take rectal temperature.) To take a rectal temperature:

1. Lubricate the mercury tip of the thermometer with a water-soluble lubricating jelly.

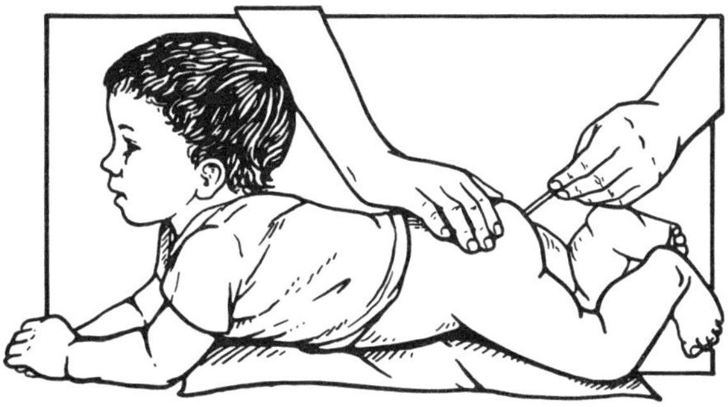

Figure 2-3
Taking a rectal temperature.

2. Insert the thermometer about one-half to one and one-half inches into the rectum, depending upon the size and age of the patient. You would not insert the thermometer one and one-half inches into the rectum of an infant, but one and one-half inches would be an adequate insertion for an adult.
3. Hold the thermometer in place for about three minutes. If the patient is a baby, you should hold him or her in your lap to minimize the danger of the infant rolling over suddenly and breaking the thermometer.
4. Before attempting to read the thermometer, wipe it clean, removing any lubricating jelly and fecal matter (start at the top of the thermometer and wipe toward the bulb). Normal rectal temperature is 97.5 to 99.5° F. (usually expressed as 99.6° F.).

Axillary (Armpit)

Axillary temperature is the least reliable and the most difficult to obtain, and it should only be taken when the other two methods are out of the question. Follow this procedure:

1. Dry the person's armpit thoroughly, then wait for several minutes to take the temperature. The friction from drying the armpit may make the temperature reading higher than it normally would be.
2. Place the bulb of the thermometer (either an oral or rectal type can be used) in the center of the dried armpit, with the opposite end slanting toward the body.
3. Have the person keep his or her arm snugly at the side. Keep the thermometer in place for ten minutes.
4. Normal axillary temperature is 96.5 to 98.5° F. (usually expressed as 97.6° F.).

How to Read a Thermometer

1. Hold the thermometer horizontally so that the numbers are on the bottom and the lines (calibrations) are on the top.
2. Hold the thermometer at eye level, and slowly rotate the thermometer between the thumb and index finger.
3. Watch the area between the lines and the numbers until you see the mercury; notice where the mercury ends.
4. Rotate the thermometer to see which number is closest to the point at which the mercury ends. Count how many lines past the number the mercury extends.

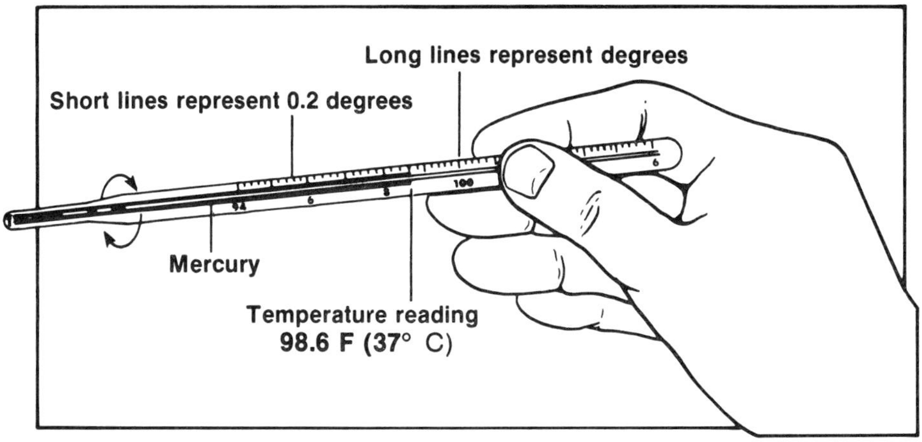

Figure 2-4
How to read a thermometer.

5. The temperature reading is the whole number (100) marked by the long line, plus one-tenth for every short line (if the mercury ends three short lines beyond 100, the temperature is 100.3).

After you have read the thermometer, shake it down again. Rinse it under cold running water, wipe it with rubbing alcohol, and allow it to dry thoroughly before you put it away.

When Is A Fever Dangerous?

You can determine the danger of a fever by using Table 2-1.

If you wish to convert Centigrade (Celsius) to Fahrenheit or vice versa, you may use the following formulas:

$$°F = 9/5\ (°C + 32)$$
$$°C = 5/9\ (°F - 32)$$

Below 97° F., or any temperature that is one full degree below the normal temperature for a given individual, subnormal temperatures of hypothermia exist. This occurs mostly in the elderly, those who are ill-housed, and those who are ill-fed. When the temperature gets below 90° F., immediate medical care is called for.

Although the chart indicates that 98.6° F. is the normal body temperature, normal temperatures may run from 97 to 99.5° F. But note that your temperatures should be consistently the same for it to be considered normal. And remember that your temperature may fluctuate during the day.

When Is a Fever Dangerous?

Table 2-1

Fahrenheit (F)		Centigrade (C)
108°	**Usually fatal**	42.2°
107°	**Critical condition**	41.7°
106°	**Delirium occurs**	41.1°
105°		40.6°
104°	**High fever**	40.0°
103°		39.4°
102°		38.9°
101°	**Moderate fever**	38.3°
100°		37.8°
99°		37.2°
98.6°	**Normal (healthy) temperature**	37.0°
98°	**Subnormal temperature**	36.7°
97°		36.1°
96°		35.6°
95°		35.0°

Ninety-nine and five-tenths to 101° F. indicates a slight rise in the body temperature. Generally, this is no cause for alarm. In children, excitement, apprehension, teething, digestive upsets, and minor respiratory infections may cause the temperature to fall within this range. A cold may cause a slight increase in the temperature of an adult. Medical attention is usually unnecessary unless other symptoms develop and persist.

If a child has a temperature of 101 to 103° F., it is not necessarily an unusual occurrence. Many colds produce a fever of 101 to 103° in children. If such a fever lasts longer than forty-eight hours, however, the child should be taken to a doctor. It is more cause for alarm for an adult to run a fever of 101 to 103°. If symptoms accompany the fever that seem serious, have the person see a doctor.

When the temperature is elevated to 103 to 105° F., always take the person to see a doctor. Children may run this high a fever for serious or relatively trivial conditions, but adults are probably quite seriously ill when the fever is this high.

When the temperature is above 105° F., medical attention should be sought immediately. Until medical help can be obtained, you should sponge the person with tepid (lukewarm) water. Most people who have a temperature of 107° F. for several hours will die, but there are rare instances of people who have survived a 110° fever. When the fever gets this high, the heartbeat is extremely irregular, convulsions may occur, and the liver ceases to function.[4]

Are There Advantages to Having a Fever?

There **are** advantages to having a fever—if it is controlled:

1. Fever may limit the growth of some viruses, a situation that may be beneficial since antibiotics are generally not effective in controlling viruses.
2. Fever helps to mobilize white blood cells, which combat bacterial infections. The increase in white blood cells in turn can help lower the fever.
3. Fever can stimulate the white blood cells to move in and rid the body of infection.[5]

Note also that the body has a built-in mechanism that seems to limit fever. The temperature ceiling for most fevers is usually 104 to 106° F. Any fever of this level **should** be referred to a doctor.

PULSE

The pulse is the alternate contraction and expansion of an artery that corresponds to the contraction and expansion caused by the heartbeat. It is the vibration of a wave of blood as it is forced through the arteries. You can feel the pulse at certain places where arteries lie close to the skin and where they pass over a bone or some other type of solid tissue.

How To Take A Pulse

Radial Pulse

Pulse is taken most easily at the wrist (**radial pulse**) using the following procedure:

1. Place your middle fingertip over the artery on the thumb side of the person's wrist.

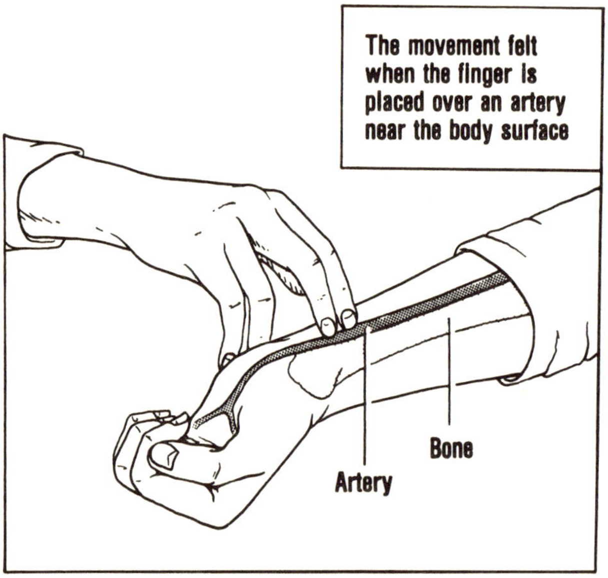

Figure 2-5
Taking the radial pulse.

2. Move your finger around gently until you locate the pulsebeat.
3. Exert enough pressure so that you can feel the pulsebeat, but not so much pressure that you obliterate it.
4. **Never** use your thumb to take a pulse—the thumb has a pulsebeat, and it may conflict with the person's pulsebeat, causing you to get confused and count the wrong beats.
5. When you are able to feel the pulse plainly, count the beats for one minute. It is easiest to take a pulse if you make the first count zero as the second hand of the watch crosses the mark you have set as the beginning of the pulse taking.

Carotid Pulse

Taking the pulse with the radial artery is probably the most used method of taking pulse, but the pulse can also be taken using the carotid artery in the neck. To palpate (feel) the carotid pulse, do the following:

1. Place the index and middle fingers on the Adam's apple, then slide them into the groove between the Adam's apple and the large neck muscle.
2. Move the fingers until you find the pulse.
3. Press firmly enough to feel the pulse but not firmly enough to occlude (obstruct) it.
4. Count the pulsebeats for one minute (fifteen seconds in emergencies).

Figure 2-6
The carotid artery in the neck can also be used to take the pulse. Remember to not press so hard that you obstruct the pulse.

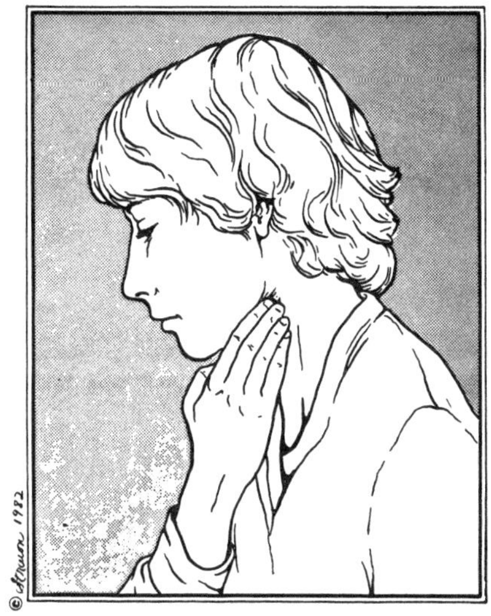

TAKING PULSE ON THE CAROTID ARTERY

> **Count number of beats during 15 seconds. Then multiply by 4.**
>
> **e.g. 18 beats in 15 seconds, so 18 X 4 = 72 beats per minute**

What to Record and Watch For

Record the number of beats per minute. Normal pulse rates are:

Elderly	60-100
Men	60-80
Women	60-80
Children:	
Birth	90-170
1st 6 months	90-160
6-12 months	80-140
1-2 years	80-120
2-6 years	75-115
6-10 years	70-110
10-14 years	65-100
14-18 years	60-100

The classification of pulse in adults is as follows:

60 and below	Slow or subnormal
60-80	Normal (men and women)
80-100	Moderate increase
100-120	Quick
120-140	Rapid
140 and up	Running (hard to count)

Anything that affects the heart and blood vessels will affect the pulse rate. Disease, emotions, and activity will either increase or decrease the pulse rate. For example, pulse rate goes up ten beats per minute for every 1° elevation in body temperature. Physical exertion increases the pulse rate. Just as the temperature may vary over a twenty-four-hour period, so may the pulse rate vary during the day and night. The pulse rate is lowest in the early morning hours. Establish your resting pulse rate by taking the pulse in the morning before you arise. Conversely, the highest pulse rate is in the late afternoon and evening. This variation probably has to do with increased or decreased activity and the functional level of the body.

Also record the force and rhythm of the pulse. The force has to do with the volume of blood that goes through the arteries. So, any change in the amount of blood in the arteries will change the force of the pulse. To test pulse volume, see how difficult it is to shut off the blood flow in the radial pulse by pressing with your fingers. If it is relatively easy to occlude (block) the artery, the pulse is normal. However, if it is difficult to occlude the artery, the pulse may be described as full or bounding. If the pulse is occluded with very minimal effort, the pulse is known as weak, thready, or feeble. For example, if there has been a loss of blood due to accident, injury, or surgery, the pulse will be likely to be occluded very, very easily, which means that it is weak.

Rhythm refers to the steadiness and spacing of the beats. Does the pulse speed up, slow down, or skip beats? Are there strong and weak beats within the same minute in which you are counting the pulse?

There are several irregularities that you may note in taking the pulse. If the pulse rate persists at over 100 beats per minute, this constitutes an irregular condition known as **tachycardia**. Another irregular condition, **bradycardia**, is present when there is a persistent pulse rate of less than fifty beats per minute. (Do not confuse bradycardia with the decreased pulse rate that well-conditioned athletes may have.) If the volume of blood being pumped through the artery differs from beat to beat, the abnormality is known as **bigeminal pulse**. Palpations are irregular and may be felt when the pulse is palpated (felt). Palpations may be described as beats that are pounding, thudding, fluttering, flopping, or skipping.

Some abnormalities of pulse may indicate certain adverse physical conditions. If the pulse is rapid and strong, the patient may be frightened, have heat stroke, have high blood pressure, or be apprehensive. A rapid, weak pulse may indicate that the patient is in shock, has heat exhaustion, is hemorrhaging, or is in diabetic coma. If the pulse is slow and strong, the patient may be having a stroke or may have a concussion. If the pulse is entirely absent, and you have palpated (felt) for a pulse in several different areas of the body, the patient may have had a cardiac arrest, or he may be dead.

RESPIRATION

Respiration is the breathing in of air and the exhaling of gases from the lungs. A respiration, then, is one breath taken in and one let out.

A number of factors can cause the respiration rate to vary: exercise, fever (which elevates the respiration rate approximately four breaths per minute), physical activity, excitement, pain, and injury all cause an increase in the respiration rate. Resting or sleeping reduce the rate.

Normal Respiration

The normal rate of respiration is between fourteen and twenty breaths per minute. There is about one breath for every four heartbeats. The normal resting respiration rate does vary, though, from the elderly to adults to children. The rates are as follows:

Age	Number of Respirations per Minute
Newborn	30-80
One year	20-40
Age 2	20-30
Age 5	20-25
Age 10	17-22
Age 15	15-20
Adult	14-20
Elderly	Increased from the adult level and more shallow

Remember, if the pulse rate goes up, the respiration rate goes up also. If the patient takes only eight respirations per minute or takes over forty respirations per minute, this may indicate the presence of a serious condition.

What to Watch For

In taking respiration, it is more important to record the **kind** of respiration than the number. Note, for instance, the depth of the respiration—how much air is taken in during inhalation. Are the respirations shallow or labored? Note also the characteristics of the respirations. Are they noisy, quiet, or moist? Breathing difficulty may be indicated if the person's chest and abdomen heave while he or she breathes, if he or she has a distressed facial expression, and if there is a bluish tinge to the skin, fingernails, fingers, or toes. If there is no respiration, or if the person is cyanotic (bluish) or ashen gray, the person has probably had a respiratory arrest of some type. If the breathing is rapid and shallow, there may be an obstruction of the respiratory tract, the patient may have heart failure, or he or she may be in physiological shock. If the breathing is deep, gasping, labored, or choking, the patient may be suffering from high blood pressure, hyperventilation, or pain.

Taking Respiration

Respiration should be monitored while the person is in a sitting position—a supine position (lying on the back) makes respiration more difficult. You should observe or count respirations when the person is unaware that you are doing so. If he or she knows that respirations are being counted, the person may breathe abnormally. You might keep your fingers on the pulse as though you are still counting the pulse—and instead count and observe the respirations. Count the respirations for one full minute. Remember that women breathe using the chest muscles, while men and children use the diaphragm and abdominal muscles for breathing.

BLOOD PRESSURE

What Is Blood Pressure?

As blood is pumped through the blood vessels, it presses against the vessel walls. There are two types of blood pressure: **systolic**, which is the highest pressure that the blood places on the vessel walls, and **diastolic**, which is the lowest pressure that the blood places on the vessel walls. Systolic pressure occurs when the heart contracts and the blood is forced out of the heart into the blood vessels. Diastolic pressure, on the other hand, is produced when the heart relaxes after contractions. Often, systolic pressure is called contraction pressure, while diastolic is called relaxation pressure.

There is no sharp dividing line between a normal and abnormal blood pressure. There are general limits, but they are not rigid. High blood pressure has been called the silent disease because only 5 to 10 percent of all cases can be traced to any specific cause.

Blood pressure can be influenced by many factors such as injury, internal bleeding, age, emotional excitement, weight, physical rest, shock, respiration, time of day, stress, food, exercise, position of the body, or disease.

Blood pressure is just like pulse and respiration rates in that it rises during the day and falls during the first hours of sleep. Then, blood pressure rises slightly before you awake. It also rises during and shortly after eating.

The Sphygmomanometer

Blood pressure is taken with a device called a **sphygmomanometer** and a stethoscope. There are three types of sphygmomanometers. The mercury sphygmomanometer has a mercury column in a tube, the aneroid

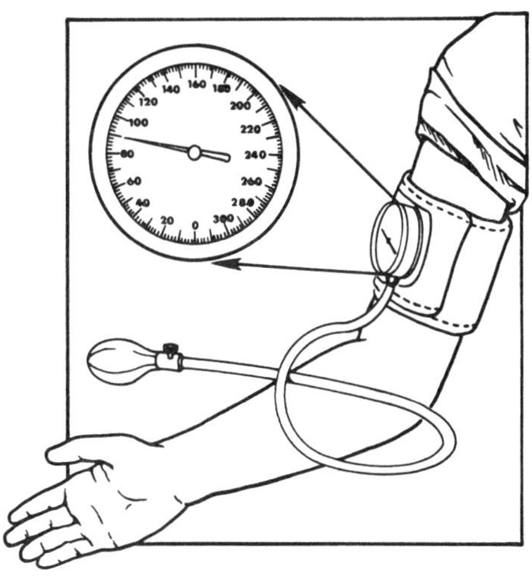

Figure 2-7
Example of an aneroid (gauge) sphygmomanometer. This type of sphygmomanometer is less expensive than those with mercury columns but must be well maintained to retain its accuracy.

sphygmomanometer has a gauge rather than the mercury column, and the electronic aneroid sphygmomanometer has a gauge and a microphone in the cuff so that you do not have to use a stethoscope. Each blood pressure apparatus has a cuff with an inflatable rubber bag, a bulb, rubber tubing, and a valve that opens and closes to admit or let out air.

Mercury sphygmomanometers are more accurate in their readings and retain their accuracy over a longer period of time. One drawback, however, is that if the gauge is broken, the mercury is toxic. On the other hand, the aneroid sphygmomanometer can easily get out of adjustment, especially if it is accidentally dropped. However, the aneroid instrument is less expensive and will maintain its accuracy if properly cared for.

What is Normal Blood Pressure?

Blood pressure is expressed in a fraction-like reading. The systolic pressure is expressed above the line, while diastolic pressure is the number recorded below the line. Normal systolic blood pressure for various ages is listed below:

Age	Average Systolic Blood Pressure
Newborn	75
One month	85
Six months	90
One year	95
Six years	100
Ten years	110
Sixteen years to adult	120

Normal diastolic pressure is between 60 and 90. The World Health Organization defines high blood pressure as a persistent pressure of 140/90 for people under forty years of age, and the American Heart Association indicates that a persistent blood pressure of 160/95 for people over forty years of age is high. Always check with your doctor if you think that you have high blood pressure.

Taking Blood Pressure

Before you begin taking blood pressure, make sure that the blood pressure cuff is the correct size.[6] If the cuff is too narrow for the person, blood pressure will be erroneously high, and if the cuff is too wide, the blood pressure will be mistakenly low for the person.

The person should be in the same position—either supine (lying down), sitting, or standing—every time you take the blood pressure, and the position should be noted each time. Blood pressure should not vary much with changes in position for persons with normal blood pressure but will vary for persons with abnormal blood pressure.

Have the person assume either a sitting, standing, or supine position. His or her arm should be slightly flexed with the whole forearm supported at the heart level. Note that blood pressure can be taken in either arm. In fact, you should initially take blood pressure in both arms. After doing this, the pressure henceforth should be taken in the arm with the highest pressure. And remember that the blood pressure should always be taken in that same arm. You should record the arm on which the pressure is taken each time.

The blood pressure should be taken with the person's arm bare. A tight sleeve may constrict the arm or make it impossible to apply the blood pressure cuff properly.

The cuff should be placed around the person's arm about one inch above the bend in the elbow.

Now, before you actually begin to work with the sphygmomanometer, check the following five items:

1. Be sure that the sphygmomanometer reads zero when there is no pressure in the system.
2. If you are using a mercury sphygmomanometer, be sure that there is sufficient mercury to pump to the top of the column.
3. Check to be sure that the mercury or needle (on the aneroid sphygmomanometer) will stay in place when the valve is closed.
4. Check the valve screw to make sure that it operates smoothly.
5. Inspect your stethoscope for cracks or leaks in the tubing, earpieces, bell, or diaphragm.

You should first feel for the blood pressure. Find the radial pulse. Then inflate the cuff 30 mm Hg beyond the point where the pulse is obliterated. Open the valve and release 2-3 mm Hg per second. When the pulsations of the radial pulse again become palpable, this is the systolic pressure. The diastolic blood pressure occurs when the vibrations in the artery cease. Diastolic pressure is much more difficult to obtain.

Now, you are ready to use the stethoscope to take the blood pressure. Follow this procedure:

1. Position the disc of the stethoscope snugly against the skin where the

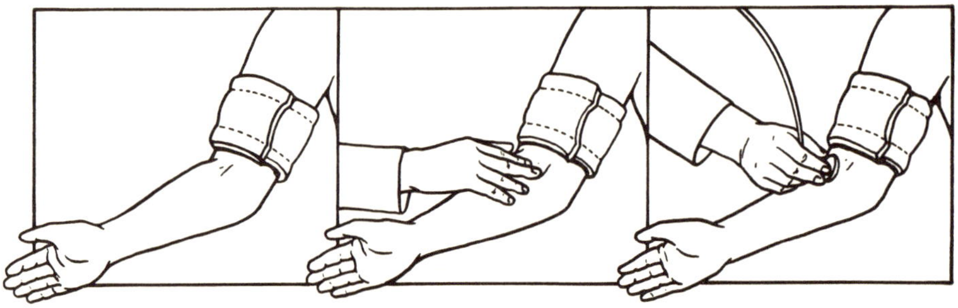

Figue 2-8
How to take blood pressure.

elbow bends—a little to the left of center on the right arm, and a little to the right of center on the left arm. There should be no gaps between the stethoscope and the skin, yet you should not apply any undue pressure. Make sure that the stethoscope is not touching the cuff at any point.

2. Position the earpieces of the stethoscope in your ears (with the earpieces directed forward).
3. Hold the stethoscope disc snugly in position with one hand while you pump the cuff with the other hand.
4. Pump the cuff until the mercury on the scale is about 30 points above the point where you felt the pulse disappear earlier, or about 200 mm Hg.
5. Loosen the valve slightly and permit the pressure to drop slowly. Listen *carefully* for the first sound of a beat—the number on the scale when you hear the first beat is the systolic pressure. (If you think that you missed the first beat or are unsure, tighten the valve again and pump the cuff up; repeat the method, listening carefully.)
6. Continue to deflate the cuff slowly until the last sound of blood is heard. When you hear no more blood flowing, the number on the scale is the diastolic pressure.

—Blood Pressure—Facts and Recommendations—

Remember the following facts about blood pressure:

1. Many people don't know that they have high blood pressure.
2. High blood pressure is a major cause of stroke, heart failure, and kidney failure.

3. High blood pressure cannot be cured, but it can be controlled.
4. Take your high blood pressure medication even though you feel well.
5. Have your blood pressure checked regularly so that you are aware of your progress.
6. Remember—you **can** do something to control your blood pressure. You can comply with your doctor's suggestions of diet, exercise, and smoking habits; you can keep every doctor's appointment; you can take your medication as prescribed; you can tell your doctor about any side effects that may occur as a result of taking the medication; and you can enlist the aid of your family in helping you to control your blood pressure.

LEVEL OF CONSCIOUSNESS

Consciousness is controlled by the brain and the involuntary nervous system. There are four states of consciousness:

1. **Alert.** The person is well aware of what is going on and reacts appropriately to his or her environment. He or she will request what is needed to take care of basic body needs.
2. **Restless.** The person is extremely sensitive to factors in the environment and exaggerates them. For example, he or she may scream when experiencing only moderate pain. The person may want constant attention and may move around in bed (if he or she is confined to bed) continuously and thrash from side to side.
3. **Stuporous.** The person lies quietly in bed, seems to be sleeping, and requests nothing when awakened. After being awakened, he or she returns quickly to a sleeplike state. The person may lose control of bowels and bladder. He or she may be awakened by a vocal stimulus if in a light stupor and may be awakened by pressure if in a deep stupor. The pressure may come in the form of tapping the person lightly on the side of the face or applying pressure over the eyelids.
4. **Coma.** The person appears to be sleeping and cannot be awakened. He or she cannot swallow and may be incontinent (unable to control the flow of urine) or retain urine. Pressure over the eyelids, strong sensations, or calling the person by name will not awaken him or her.

As far as brain function is concerned, in the alert person the brain is functioning adequately. When the person is in a restless condition, the brain is extremely active in attempting to meet the body's needs. Restlessness commonly occurs in the following instances:

1. Anyone who is frightened, worried, or in pain—the brain is hyperactive in preparing for fight or flight.
2. Anyone hemorrhaging—the brain receives a lessened or inadequate blood supply.
3. Anyone with a head injury or a brain tumor—the increased pressure in the brain cuts off the blood supply to a part of the brain.
4. Anyone experiencing a heart attack—the weakened heart does not pump enough blood to the body and brain.
5. Anyone with shock—the blood pressure is so low that the heart is not pumping enough blood to the body and brain.

When the brain cannot correct the conditions that produce restlessness, stupor, coma, or death will follow.

NOTES

1. Barbara Kozier and Glenora Lea Erb, *Fundamentals of Nursing: Concepts and Procedures* (Menlo Park, Calif.: Addison-Wesley Publishing Company, 1979), p. 205.
2. Mary Castle and Jane Watkins, "Fever: Understanding a Sinister Sign," *Nursing 79,* February 1979, p. 27; and Brent Q. Hafen and Keith J. Karren, *First Aid and Emergency Care Workbook* (Denver, Colo.: Morton Publishing, 1980), p. 101.
3. Charles A. Dinarello and Sheldon M. Wolff, "Fever," *Human Nature,* February 1979, pp. 71-72.
4. Michael Stock, *Journal of Practical Nursing,* April 1979, p. 14.
5. Bruno Isaacs, "When to Treat, and When to Leave it Alone," *Family Health,* December 1979, p. 7.
6. Jane Lancour, "How to Avoid Pitfalls in Measuring Blood Pressure," *American Journal of Nursing,* May 1976, pp. 773-775.

CHAPTER 3

SELF-CARE ASSESSMENT

About five this morning you woke up with a sharp pain at the bottom of your spine. The pain was made worse by the slightest movement — it even hurt to cough or laugh. Walking was near to impossible — a sharp pain gutted your leg with every step, followed by an aching in your buttocks.

You called the family doctor, persuaded the receptionist that you needed to be seen *today,* and you took a couple of aspirin and stayed in bed until your appointment at 2:00. Once in the examining room with the doctor, you described your pain. The doctor listened intently, scribbling notes hurriedly on your chart. You were asked lots of questions — some of them seemed pertinent, you thought; others seemed unrelated and almost ridiculous.

The doctor circled the examining table, thumping you here and squeezing you there. At long last a diagnosis was made: a slipped vertebral disc.

How did the doctor arrive at this conclusion?

The answer is complex and lies in his or her ability to assess symptoms. Assessment is defined as the "systematic evaluation of a person's health status through using the examiner's special senses of sight, hearing, touch, and smell, and special instruments when needed."[1] The answer is also dependent upon the doctor's ability to conduct a meaningful and revealing examination, measure your vital signs properly, and make a diagnosis based on the findings and on your past medical history.

You may eventually be faced with somewhat the same task: examining yourself or a family member or friend—and determining his or her need for medical help. "Home [assessments] physical examinations are the first step in taking responsibility for family health. You are the person who knows your family [or friends] best: good home physicals help you learn what's normal for each family member or friend so you can recognize a problem when it arises."[2] Assessment in the home can also promote a good atmosphere for teaching the entire family and friends good health practices.

Remember, though, you are merely making an **assessment**—not a diagnosis. In certain sections of this book, abnormal signs are listed with an explanation of their probable cause. Again, this is not given so that you will be able to make a diagnosis—it is presented to help you know that a certain sign is abnormal and may need to be checked by a physician. Diagnosis, in most cases, cannot be made by even the best-read lay person. There are many situations in which it is difficult to assess whether signs and symptoms are serious or not. **When in doubt, always ask your doctor.** This book will not qualify you as an ear-nose-throat specialist or a cardiologist, but it can make you aware of preliminary observations and screening measures that can aid you in knowing who **needs** to see a doctor.

CONDUCTING AN ASSESSMENT EXAM

Whenever you examine someone to determine whether he or she should have medical attention, be as thorough and complete as possible. Take concise notes in a readable form that you can give to a doctor in case you decide to call one.

Taking a History

Basic Considerations

The history of the person's complaint is important—sometimes a doctor can make a diagnosis from what is learned in the history-taking alone. You should get as much information as you can from the person regarding his or her current problems and past illnesses.

Before you begin, make sure that the interview environment is pleasant and non-threatening and that there will be no interruption, distraction, or discomfort. Optimum temperature and lighting in the room should be established for the comfort of both the examiner and the person.

You should face the person for maximum observation of person reaction and nonverbal communication.

Good communication and sensitivity on your part may be the most important examination skills for assessment in the long run. Make sure that the person takes an active role in the interview and history-taking by allowing for complete expression of the his or her thoughts and feelings. You should not monopolize the conversation and, most important, you should listen carefully. Let the person know that he or she is in control of the interview.

What to Include in the History

The health history that is obtained through conversing with the person not only records individual problems but gives a whole view of the person in relation to his or her environment. The following information should be included in the health history:

1. **Biographical information:** full name, address, telephone number, birthdate, sex, occupation (usual and present), birthplace, interview date, and usual source of health care.
2. **Chief complaint** (if any). The person should explain any problems and tell you how long the problem has persisted.
3. **Present illness or health status.** This section should include an investigation of the chronic symptoms of any chief complaints as well as a general assessment of the major body systems. The person should be asked if he or she has any of the following problems to report:

    - Head — history of wounds (trauma), severe headaches.
    - Eyes — blurred vision, double vision, pain, yellow color of the white of the eye, pain on looking at light.
    - Ears — loss of hearing, severe dizziness, pain, or drainage.
    - Nose — bleeding, runny, or stuffy.
    - Mouth — sores, pain, trouble swallowing.
    - Neck — stiffness, enlarged glands, tenderness.
    - Respiratory — cough and character of material coughed up, coughing up of blood, chest pain when breathing, shortness of breath.
    - Heart — pain in middle of chest, swelling of both legs, shortness of breath on exercising or when sleeping flat in bed, forceful or rapid heartbeat, history of high blood pressure, heart attack, history of rheumatic fever.
    - Gastrointestinal — poor appetite, indigestion, nausea, vomiting,

diarrhea, constipation, jaundice, pain in stomach, blood in stool or vomited material.
- Genitourinary — pain when urinating, pain in the middle of back, frequent urination, straining to urinate, blood or pus in urine, discharge from penis.
- Neurological — paralysis or severe weakness of a part of the body (an arm or leg), convulsions, or seizure.
- Endocrine disorders — weight change, unusual hunger, unusual thirst, bulging eyes, intolerance to heat or cold.

4. **Past history.** This should include the following items:
   - Past illnesses such as childhood diseases, injuries, hospitalizations, surgeries, obstetric care, and other major illnesses.
   - Allergies such as environmental, food, drug allergies, etc.
   - A record of immunizations.
   - Personal habits that may affect health such as use of alcohol, tobacco, drugs, and coffee or tea.
   - Medications taken regularly (both prescription and/or nonprescription).

5. **Family history.** This should include information relating to the general health of the person's blood relatives, spouse, and children to determine the familial, genetic, or environmental illnesses that may have a bearing on the person's present condition.
6. **Developmental data.** You should look at several aspects when assessing a person's development. Is the person growing normally? Has the person made the proper motor developments for his or her age and maturity? Is his or her body functioning normally for this age? Are the person's mental functions appropriate for this age?

The Physical Examination

General Condition of the Person

Before you start the actual physical examination, note the person's general physical condition and state of health and any outstanding characteristics. Is the person tall and willowy, of an average build, or short and stocky? Is the person's body as a whole symmetrical and balanced? How is his or her posture? How does he or she move — with fluid movements or jerkily? Are the person's hair and hair growth patterns normal? Do you notice any unusual odors of body or breath about the person? How is his or her state of personal hygiene? These and other general questions can help you assess the person's general state of health.

It is much more important to measure the height and weight in children to determine whether or not they are making the proper physical growth and development. It is always necessary to record height and weight and keep the measurements and records in one place. Charts that compare weight and age, height and age, and height and weight are available at most doctors' offices. Often, you can even call a doctor's office and receive the percentile charts without the expense of an office visit.

Measuring Height and Weight

The maximum height for men is reached between eighteen and nineteen years of age, and for women between the fifteenth and sixteenth years of life. Even though height does not change from the time when maximum growth is achieved until old age, height should be measured periodically. In the elderly, stature is decreased because of shrinkage of the discs between the bones of the spine.

Weight should be checked and recorded periodically because weight directly influences the state of health and the capacity to live longer. A person's weight is influenced by genetics, diet, and state of activity. It is known now that being overweight (obese) definitely shortens the life span. If you want to live longer than the average person, it would be helpful to weigh 10 percent less than the average weight for your body build and age. See Tables 3-1 and 3-2 to determine the best weight for your height.

Assessing the Skin

It is important to thoroughly examine the skin — from the heels to the head, under the arms, on the stomach, between the toes, under the breasts, behind the ears, on the folds inside the elbows. Note any abnormality and where you found it.

You should first look at the coloring of the skin. Normal skin color is whitish pink or brown — depending upon the race of the person. Skin color may be a good indicator of personal habits or abnormal conditions. For example:

Brown skin color	over a general area is usually genetic.
	in an exposed area such as the face, ears, back of the neck, and backs of the hands and arms usually indicates exposure to sunlight.

Table 3-1
Weight According to Frame (Indoor Clothing), Women of Ages 25 and Over*

Height†			Small Frame		Medium Frame		Large Frame	
Feet	Inches	cm	Pounds	Kilograms	Pounds	Kilograms	Pounds	Kilograms
4	10	147.3	92-98	41.7-44.5	96-107	43.5-48.5	104-119	47.2-54.0
4	11	149.9	94-101	42.6-45.8	98-110	44.5-49.9	106-122	48.1-55.3
5	0	152.4	96-104	43.5-47.2	101-113	45.8-51.3	109-125	49.4-56.7
5	1	154.9	99-107	44.9-48.5	104-116	47.2-52.6	112-128	50.8-58.1
5	2	157.5	102-110	46.3-50.0	107-119	48.5-54.0	115-131	52.2-59.4
5	3	160.0	105-113	47.6-51.3	110-122	49.9-55.3	118-134	53.5-60.8
5	4	162.6	108-116	49.0-52.6	113-126	51.3-57.2	121-138	54.9-62.6
5	5	165.1	111-119	50.3-54.0	116-130	52.6-59.0	125-142	56.7-64.4
5	6	167.6	114-123	51.7-55.8	120-135	54.4-61.2	129-146	58.5-66.2
5	7	170.2	118-127	53.5-57.6	124-139	56.2-63.0	133-150	60.3-68.0
5	8	172.7	122-131	55.3-59.4	128-143	58.1-64.9	137-154	62.1-69.9
5	9	175.3	126-135	57.2-61.2	132-147	59.9-66.7	141-158	64.0-71.7
5	10	177.8	130-140	69.0-63.5	136-151	61.7-68.5	145-163	65.8-73.9
5	11	180.3	134-144	60.8-65.3	140-155	63.5-70.3	149-168	67.6-76.2
6	0	182.9	138-148	62.6-67.1	144-159	65.3-72.1	153-173	69.4-78.5

For women between 18 and 25, subtract 0.5 kg (1 pound) for each year under 25.
*Courtesy of the Metropolitan Life Insurance Company.
†With shoes on—5.1 cm (2-inch) heels

on the face, nipples, areola of the breast, or vulva may occur during pregnancy.

Reddish-blue skin color	of the lips, mouth, and nails may indicate an excess of red blood cells.
Reddish skin color	of the ears, fingers, nose, and other exposed extremities usually indicates that the body part is cold or sunburned.
	of the face and neck may indicate high blood pressure.
Yellow skin color	of the white of the eye or generalized over the

Table 3-2
Weight According to Frame (Indoor Clothing), Men of Ages 25 and Over*

Height†			Small Frame		Medium Frame		Large Frame	
Feet	Inches	cm	Pounds	Kilograms	Pounds	Kilograms	Pounds	Kilograms
5	2	157.5	112-120	50.8-54.4	118-129	53.5-58.5	126-141	57.2-64.0
5	3	160.0	115-123	52.2-55.8	121-133	54.9-60.3	129-144	58.5-65.3
5	4	162.6	118-126	53.5-57.2	124-136	56.2-61.7	132-148	59.9-67.1
5	5	165.1	121-129	54.9-58.5	127-139	57.6-63.0	135-152	61.2-68.9
5	6	167.6	124-133	56.2-60.3	130-143	59.0-64.9	138-156	62.6-70.8
5	7	170.2	128-137	58.1-62.1	134-147	60.8-66.7	142-161	64.4-73.0
5	8	172.7	132-141	59.9-64.0	138-152	62.6-68.9	147-166	66.7-75.3
5	9	175.3	136-145	61.7-65.8	142-156	64.4-70.8	151-170	68.5-77.1
5	10	177.8	140-150	63.5-68.0	146-160	66.2-72.6	155-174	70.3-78.9
5	11	180.3	144-154	65.3-69.9	150-165	68.0-74.8	159-179	72.1-81.2
6	0	182.9	148-158	67.1-71.7	154-170	69.9-77.1	164-184	74.4-83.4
6	1	185.4	152-162	68.9-73.5	158-175	71.7-79.4	168-189	76.2-85.7
6	2	188.0	156-167	70.8-75.8	162-180	73.5-81.6	173-194	78.5-88.0
6	3	190.5	160-171	72.6-77.6	167-185	75.8-83.9	178-199	80.7-90.3
6	4	193.0	164-175	74.4-79.4	172-190	78.0-86.2	182-204	82.6-92.5

*Courtesy of Metropolitan Life Insurance Company.
†With shoes on—2.5 cm (1-inch) heels.

body may indicate jaundice or some other liver disease.

White skin color (pale) — of the face, mouth, and nails may accompany fainting or fright.

of the face, eye membranes, mouth, and nails may indicate an anemic condition.

of the face may indicate a state of physiological or psychological shock.

Bluish skin color (cyanosis) — of the face, lips, and nail beds may indicate lack of environmental oxygen or heart problems.[3]

For blacks or persons with dark skin, the tissues inside the mouth may have a normal freckling coloration. Gums may have a normal dark blue, blotchy color, evenly distributed. Also, minor yellow pigmentation in the eyes is normal. However, skin color changes and disorders are more difficult to assess in this person, because he or she will not exhibit the marked skin color changes.

The skin should be felt for temperature and moisture. The following chart may help you detect skin abnormalities in the area of temperature and moisture:

Skin Temperature and Moisture	*The Person May Be Experiencing*
Cool and clammy (moist)	trauma, bleeding somewhere in the body, physical shock, nervousness
Cool and dry	exposure to excessive cold
Hot and dry	fever, heatstroke
Excessively dry	dehydration, old age, underactive thyroid, kidney problems, overexposure to the sun
Excessively moist	nervousness, fever, overactive thyroid[4]

In examining the skin, pay special attention to and look for:

- Pimples
- Warts
- Welts
- Spots
- Swelling
- Inflammation
- Rashes
- Boils
- Insect bites
- Wounds
- Patches
- Lumps
- Heat
- Moles
- Sores
- Splinters
- Unusual markings
- Masses
- Pain
- Abnormal coloring
- Scars
- Venous patterns
- Callouses
- Stains

The fingernails and toenails should also be inspected. You should note the color and shape and any lesions that may be connected with the nails. The nails are normally a slightly convex shape, and, for Caucasians, are generally a pinkish color similar to that of healthy skin.

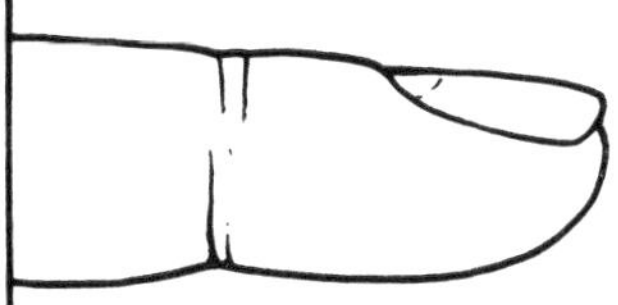

Figure 3-1
Nails are normally a slightly convex shape. When you are inspecting nails, also look for any occurrence of lesions. From: Barbara Bates, *A Guide to Physical Examination* (Philadelphia: J. B. Lippincott Company, 1974), p. 16.

Examining Childrens' Skin

In children, you should thoroughly examine the skin. Note any unusual pigmentation or marking; fungus infections such as ringworm, pimples, sores, warts, swelling, inflammation, rashes, wounds, lumps, moles, sores; insect infestations such as lice; or other skin disorders. Record these.

Next, note the color of the skin. Generally, the skin of an infant has a reddish cast to it because of the thinness of the skin and the presence of increased red blood cells. As the child grows older, the skin becomes a pale pink color. It is not uncommon for a newborn infant to develop jaundice or a yellowish coloration of the skin. This is usually not serious. If a child has a bluish tint to the skin, it may mean that he or she has some malfunction of the lungs, that the blood is not getting the proper oxygen, or that the child has a malformation of the heart. Skin that is paler than normal may mean the presence of anemia or a malformed heart.

While you are checking the color of the skin, also note the color of the fingernail and toenail beds. The nail beds should also be a pale pink similar to the color of the skin. When the nail beds are pressed, they should turn white, but they should return to their normal pink color when the pressure is released. If the pinkish color doesn't return, it may indicate that the blood is not receiving sufficient oxygen.

It is especially important to palpate the skin of children to check for consistency of the tissue, fat deposition under the skin, and amount of moisture in the skin. To do this, a fold of the abdominal skin should be rolled between the thumb and forefinger. This will give you an idea of the consistency of the skin and its fat layer. When the skin fold is released, it should return to its normal position very quickly. If the skin does not quickly return to normal position and coloring, the child may be dehydrated.

Assessing the Hair

Healthy hair that has not been treated by chemicals will be springy, elastic, and slightly oily. Again, the hair is a valuable indicator of general health. Write down what you see. Is the hair dull? Shiny? Covered with chemicals, such as hair spray? Run your fingers through the person's hair. Is it thick or thin? Does it feel dry or excessively oily? What is the texture of the hair?

Examine the roots of the hair and the area immediately around the roots. Look for areas that seem red and moist or dry and scaly.

Assessing the Skull

Note the size and shape of the skull. Is it symmetrical? Feel the skull with your fingertips — cover the entire area of the skull with a firm, gentle motion. Record any incidence of soreness, and make special note of any bumps or unusual bone formations.

In infancy, the head accounts for one-fourth of the body length and one-third of the body weight. In adulthood, the head contributes one-eighth of the body length and one-tenth of the body weight, so you should be aware that the head of an infant or child may be larger in proportion to the rest of the body.

Assessing the Eyes

Checking Their Physical Appearance

If the person is wearing glasses or contact lenses, ask him or her to remove them. Look at the eyelashes and eyelids. The lashes should be evenly distributed along the eyelid, and they should curve outward. The lashes should also be examined for any crustiness or puslike material clinging to them. The lids should be noted for position, color, sores of any kind, infection, and swelling.

The sclera of the eye is normally known as the white of the eye, and as such, its normal color should be white. Often, fatigue and eye strain will make the tiny blood vessels in the sclera swell to make the eyes appear bloodshot. The sclera should be observed for color and any lesions or other abnormalities.

The iris is the colored portion of the eye — either blue, brown, or a variation of these colors. It should be a round shape, and, of course, the color will vary according to each individual, but you should be aware of any abnormal colors such as a red spot or coloration that may indicate the presence of blood.

The pupils are the black portions of the eye inside of the iris. Most often, you think of your pupils in connection with accommodation to light. The pupils should be round and equal in size. If the pupils are unusually dilated or constricted or are unequal in size, a disease condition may be present. Constricted pupils may indicate drug addiction, a central nervous system disease, use of depressant drugs, head injury, or stroke. Dilated pupils, on the other hand, may mean the presence of a relaxed or unconscious state, use of stimulant drugs, shock, or brain damage. Unequal pupils indicate that a person may have head injuries, a stroke, or other type of brain damage.[5]

Check to make sure that the pupils constrict properly. Turn out the lights and have the person face you. Slowly run a flashlight or penlight, starting about a foot above his head, downward across his eyes. As the light strikes the center of the pupil, the pupil will constrict. Both pupils should constrict the same amount and at the same rate of speed. Record any differences between pupils, and record the information if either pupil does not constrict.

Indicators of Vision Problems

The following may be signs of vision problems:

- Tilting the head to one side, frowning, or squinting.
- Difficulty in reading.
- Holding reading material or objects too close to the eyes or head.
- Frequent headaches or nausea.
- Excessive blinking or frequent rubbing of the eyes.
- Not being able to read material that is distant.
- Inflammation of the eyes.
- Excessively watery eyes.
- Crossed eyes.
- Unequal pupil size.
- Flashes of light.
- Blurred vision.
- Double vision.
- Lights surrounded by a halo.
- Loss of peripheral vision.

In a baby, look for the following signs that may indicate vision problems:

- Inability to pick up small objects.

- Missing objects when reaching for them.
- Stumbling over or bumping into things.
- One eye wandering.

Testing Visual Acuity

Other tests can be done to assess eye function. To test visual acuity, a Snellen chart is most often used. The person stands twenty feet from the

Figure 3-2

A simple eye test that you can give to a child. Point to each letter and ask the child to point in the direction that the letter faces — up, down, left, or right. Once the child understands, seat him or her 10 feet away from the chart in a well-lighted room. Have the child cover one eye. Point to each letter on the chart, and have the child point with the left hand in the direction that the letter faces. Note the smallest letter that he or she can see. Now test the other eye. If in repeated tests your child cannot see line 3, or if the child can see better with one eye than with the other, take him or her to a specialist for a complete eye exam. Eye Test from the National Society for the Prevention of Blindness, New York, New York.

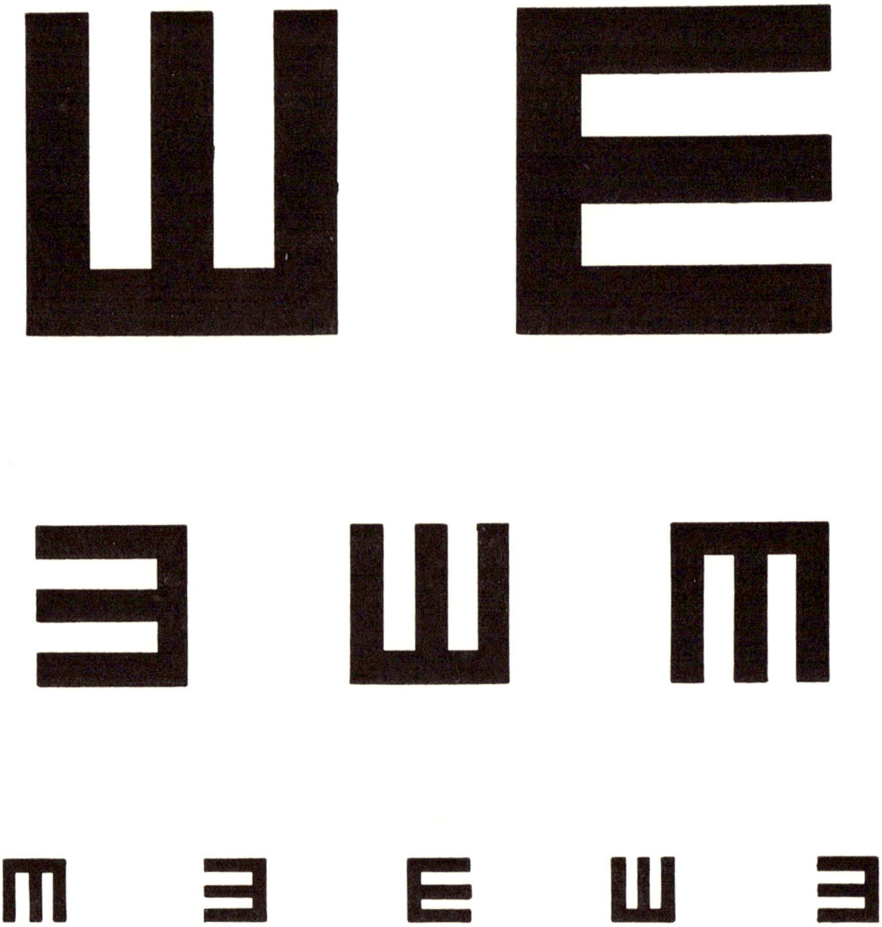

chart and is directed to read each line. The person should progress from the lines of larger print to those of smaller print. The test continues until the person comes to the smallest line in which he or she can identify **half** of the letters. That line is given a number value. Vision is assessed with a two-number figure such as 20/20, 20/30, 20/40, etc. The top figure of any Snellen test result is 20, meaning that the patient is standing twenty feet from the chart. The bottom number indicates the distance from where the person can correctly read the smallest line of print.

Testing the Visual Field

You should also test the visual field. In this test, your field of vision is compared to that of the person. Do not conduct this test if you have an abnormal field of vision. Sit opposite the person about one and one-half to two feet apart with your eyes on the same level as the person. You and the person should cover opposite eyes and stare into each other's eyes. Then move a small object from the sides, above, and below. The person indicates when he or she is able to see the object, and you can compare his or her responses with your own responses. This examination tests peripheral vision.

Testing Eye Muscle Function

You can test eye muscle function by having the person stare at an object or your finger and then moving the object or finger toward the bridge of the person's nose. As the person continues to stare at the object or finger, and as the object or finger gets within five to eight centimeters of the bridge of the nose, the eyes should become temporarily "crossed." Then the eyes become "uncrossed" and look ahead normally.

The person should also follow movements of your hand as you move it up and down and from side to side. Can he or she move both eyes together up, down, and from side to side? Is there any abnormal twitching of the eyes in any position?

Testing Children for Pupil Constriction and Blinking

If you are examining an infant, the two functions that you normally check are pupil constriction and blinking. By shining a penlight in the eyes of the infant, you should be able to note whether the pupils constrict properly. Note whether both pupils constrict at the same time.

You can check pupil function and constriction in an older child by playing peek-a-boo. Have the child cover his or her eyes, and when you say "peek-a-boo," and the child drops his or her hands, immediately observe the pupil reaction. Again note whether the pupils constrict at the same rate, and note whether both pupils constrict to the same size.

To test the blinking response, bring an object toward the infant, close to his or her eyes. The baby should blink when the object gets close to the eyes, and in this way you will know that the child is able to see objects in his or her surroundings.

Testing for Amblyopia (Lazy Eye Syndrome)

In older children, it is wise to check for amblyopia. Amblyopia, or the lazy eye syndrome, means that the muscles of both eyes are not equally strong. As a result, the eye with the weaker muscles does not work as hard, and the other eye takes over most of the visual function. Amblyopia is a problem that characteristically shows up in childhood, so you should be especially aware of the symptoms. Regardless, a child's eyes should be tested professionally when he or she enters school.

Children from ages three to five should be checked for amblyopia in the following manner:

1. Make sure that you are in a well-lighted room but that a light is not shining directly in the child's eyes.
2. Hold your hand up (or make a tracing of your hand) about three feet from the child.

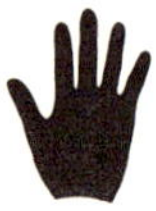

3. Have the fingers of the hand in the picture pointing upward, and ask the child to point his hand in the same manner as the pictured hand.
4. Hold the picture so that the fingers point respectively to the right, left, or downward (this may be done in any order you desire), and again ask the child to mimic the position of the hand in the picture. Repeat any two positions.
5. Cover the child's eye with a sterile gauze pad or with his or her own hand. Remind the child to keep both eyes open regardless of the fact that one eye is being covered. Repeat the test that you previously did.
6. Uncover the eye, and have the child cover the other eye. Repeat the test.
7. Move back to twelve feet and repeat the entire test. A child may have an early case of amblyopia if he or she cannot answer correctly at least four of the six positions at a distance of twelve feet. If you suspect that a child is having such difficulties, see your doctor or an eye specialist as soon as possible.[6]

Assessing the Ears

Examining the Outer Area

Examine the skin of the outer ear. Look for sores, redness, lumps or bumps, moistness, or scaliness on or around the outer ear structure.

Also feel the mastoid area, which is the bony portion just behind the lower ear. Check for swelling, tenderness, and lumps of any kind. The mastoid area is easily infected, especially in children, and these infections can spread.

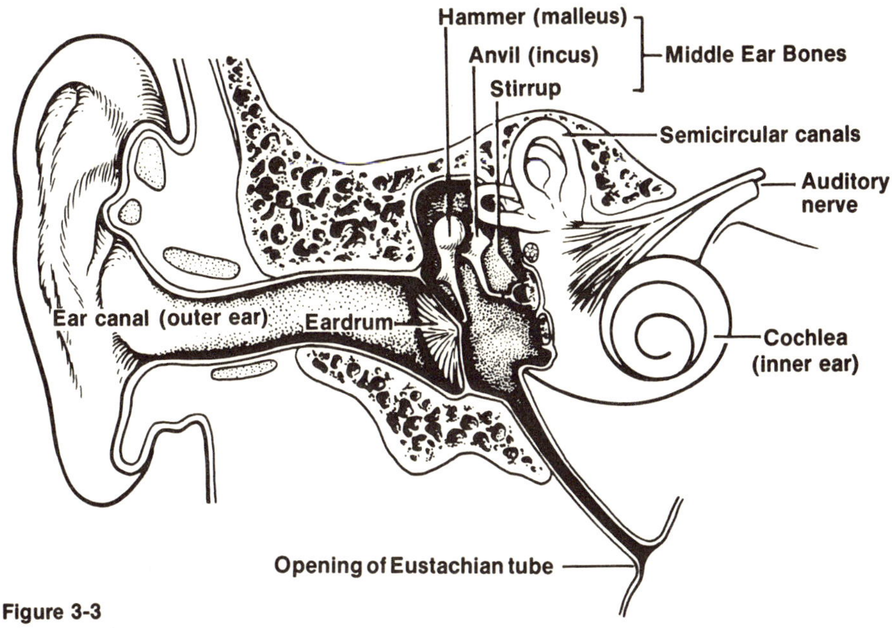

Figure 3-3
Anatomy of the ear.

Examining the Ear Canal and Removing Ear Wax

Pull up and back gently on the ear to straighten out the ear canal. Use your flashlight to look inside: a healthy ear canal will look pink and slightly glossy. You will see a slight accumulation of wax. New ear wax is light yellow or pink in color; the older ear wax becomes, the darker in color it gets. Note that ear wax is darker in darker pigmented people. Record any redness, scaliness, or excess wax buildup. If the person complains of pain when you tug on the ear, look especially for redness or pus inside the ear canal.

There are two accepted methods for removing wax:

1. **Curettement** (or scraping), which is used with soft wax buildup and when a perforation of the eardrum is suspected. This method should only be performed by a doctor or trained nurse.
2. **Irrigation,** which is used for removal of dry, hard wax. Irrigation can be performed at home, but it should never be done if the eardrum has been perforated. To irrigate the ear, use an ear syringe and lukewarm water. Squirt the water from the syringe into the ear canal several times. This should moisten and loosen the wax so that it will be washed out of the canal. If the wax is not easily removed, the person should see a doctor.

Examining the Eardrum

To examine the eardrum, you need an otoscope cup and flashlight or a lighted otoscope. An otoscope may be purchased at some pharmacies and at most medical supply firms. Follow this procedure:

1. With your dominant hand, hold the otoscope upside down so that you can rest your hand against the person's head.
2. Using your other hand, pull the outer ear gently upward and backward so that the ear canal is straightened.

Figure 3-4
When examining a person's ear, hold the otoscope upside down, and pull the edge of the ear up and back with your other hand.

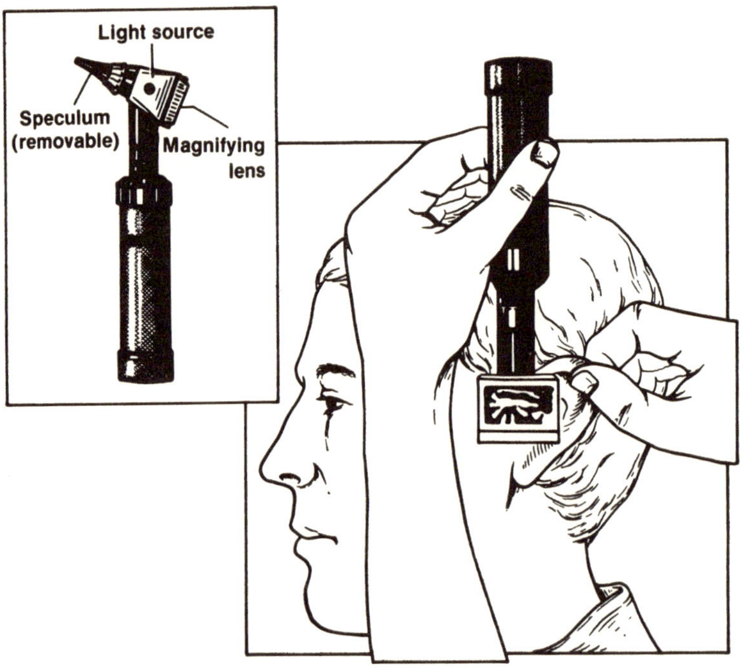

3. Tilt the person's head slightly backward and away from you, and insert the otoscope speculum slowly and cautiously so as not to cause any trauma to the walls of the ear canal. If pain is still caused, use a small otoscope tip (speculum).

The eardrum should be pearly gray or pale pink and shiny, appearing almost metallic or mirrorlike. Behind the eardrum is the malleus handle, which extends downward in the center of the eardrum. The malleus is one of three little bones that conduct the nerve impulse that helps you hear. If the eardrum is properly positioned and healthy, a cone of light will appear

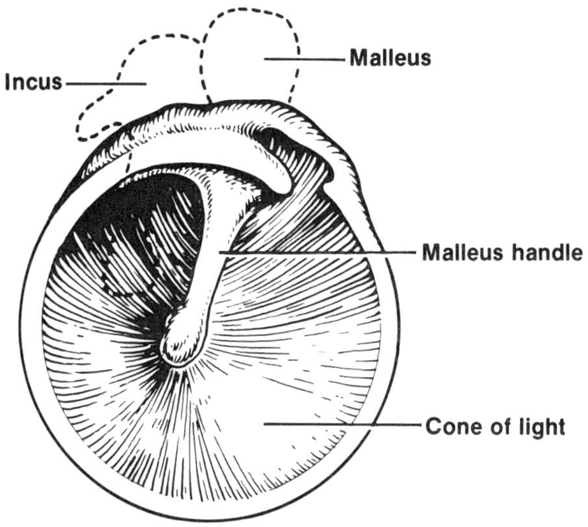

Figure 3-6
The eardrum should be a shiny pearl-gray color. The eardrum may be inflamed if the color is red or a deep pink. You should also see a cone of light at the 5 o'clock position in the right ear, and at the 7 o'clock position in the left ear. If this light is absent or appears in the wrong place, the eardrum may be inflamed or bulging. A white eardrum may mean drainage in the middle ear; a blue eardrum indicates accumulated blood. The malleus handle is located behind the eardrum and extends downward in the center of the eardrum.

Figure 3-5
Examine the person's eardrum by slowly moving the speculum of the otoscope into the ear canal. Some wax may be visible along the walls. Be sure to note any lesions, swelling, or redness.

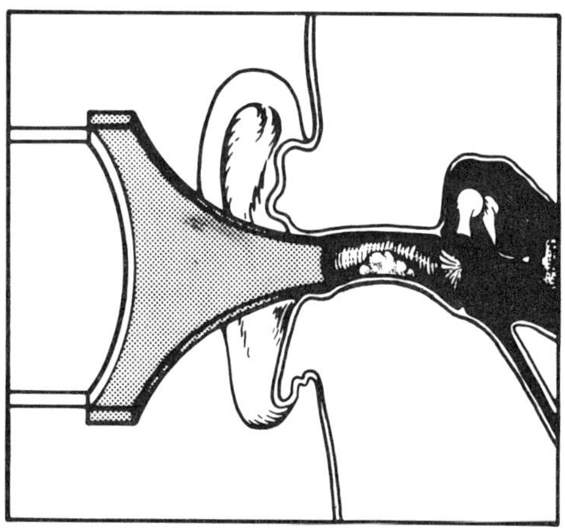

at about the 5:00 position in the right ear and at the 7:00 position in the left ear. If the cone of light is absent, the eardrum may be bulging, pulled back, or inflamed.

Note whether the eardrum is red or dull-looking or if it fails to reflect light. The eardrum may be pink when it is inflamed and white if pus has formed in the middle ear. The eardrum may also bulge from pus formation in the middle ear. If the eardrum retracts (or is drawn back), it may mean that there is an obstruction of the eustachian tube, which leads from the ear to the nasal area.

If an inflammation (red) is in the ear's outer canal, the canal appears swollen and pink or red in the light of the otoscope. The eardrum is usually unaffected and retains its normal pearly color. The sign of an infected middle ear is a reddened eardrum, bulging with fluids. An adults ear generally resists infection because the eustachian tube runs downward, aiding drainage.

Children may be apprehensive about your looking into their ears. You may need assistance in holding a child to examine the internal structure of the ear.

Checking the Person's Hearing

After you have checked the structures of the ear, you need to assess the person's hearing. One test that can be performed without the individual's awareness is to see how well the person hears words that you speak as you are conversing. Do you have to talk in an abnormally loud voice? Does the person ask you to repeat things several times? Does the person turn his or her head to one side to listen to you?

Conduct a simple hearing test by holding your hand about three inches away from the person's ear and rubbing your thumb and forefinger together lightly (you are aiming for a rustling sound, not a rough, rubbing sound). Ask the person if he or she can hear it. Check the other ear, and record any differences in hearing ability.

Next, try a voice test. Move to a position where your lips are about one to two feet from the person's ear. Instruct the person not to try to read your lips, as this will give false results in the test. Have the person plug the ear on the side of the head away from your lips. Then softly whisper numbers and have the person repeat them. Repeat this exercise using a medium whisper, a loud whisper, a soft tone of voice, a medium tone of voice, and a loud tone of voice. Then move to the other side of the person, have him plug the opposite ear, and repeat the entire examination. If the room is quiet, a person with normal hearing will be able to correctly interpret a quiet whisper at a distance of two feet.

Another test can be performed with a watch, but make sure that it is a ticking watch and not one that runs on batteries and so produces no sound. Have the person close his or her eyes and plug one ear. Move the watch away from the person's unplugged ear until the watch tick can no longer be heard. Note the distance on your record form. Then perform the same examination with the other ear.

In an infant, you can test hearing function by making a sharp and sudden sound. If the child hears the sound, he or she will blink his or her eyes. In older children, you can use other tests to note hearing acuity. The whisper test is especially useful for this purpose. You should have the child's ears subjected to an audiometer test right before he or she enters school to have the hearing acuity assessed professionally.

NOSE AND SINUSES

Watch the person breathe for a few minutes prior to beginning the exam, and record whether the person breathes through the nose or the mouth. Observe the size and color of the external nose. Also check the nostrils for discharge and flaring.

Ask the person to tip his or her head back slightly so that you can focus light into the nasal passage. If the nostril is small, you may want to lift the outside edge of it slightly to allow better vision. Note the appearance of the septum, which is the structure that divides the nostrils. The septum may deviate slightly to the left or right in most individuals, but you should look for only very pronounced deviations.

The lining (mucosa) of the nose should be soft, moist, and slightly pink. Note any tissue that is swollen, red, or bluish or that is bleeding. Nasal mucosa that is red and swollen indicates the presence of a viral infection. When the mucosa is paler than normal, the patient may have an allergic condition.

To test whether the nose is functioning properly, cover or plug one of the nostrils, and have the person breathe through the opposite nostril. Repeat the procedure with the other nostril plugged. The person should be able to breathe equally well through either nostril.

Have the person close both eyes and plug one nostril. Then put objects with a familiar smell several inches from the nostril. Use items such as coffee, a burning cigarette, an orange, etc. that are easily identifiable by odor. Bottles of food flavorings such as vanilla, almond, cherry, and peppermint extract are also good. The person should be able to quickly and correctly identify each smell. Repeat this test with the other nostril plugged. The person should be able to identify smells correctly with either nostril.

It is interesting to note that small babies breathe through their noses — they learn mouth breathing later in life. To check whether the nostrils of an infant or child are plugged, close the child's mouth and one nostril at the same time. Make sure that the infant or child is breathing easily and correctly through that nostril, then examine the function of the other nostril. Record any breathing difficulties, swelling, or unusual discharge.

MOUTH

Dentures should be removed before you begin an examination of the mouth. But remember to check the fit of the dentures before they are removed. Be aware of sores in the mouth of a denture wearer that may indicate ill-fitting dentures.

Checking the Lips

Examine the lips first. Check them for symmetry, color, swelling, moisture, lumps, ulcers, and cracking. Feeling the lips will test for any surface abnormalities such as lumps and bumps.

Checking the Gums

Next examine the gums. Healthy ones should be pink or coral (occasionally with a slightly gray cast to them). Variations in color are correlated to complexion and the degree of pigmentation of the person, or to disease conditions. For example, an anemic person will have exceptionally pale gums. A patient with jaundice will have a yellowish cast to the gums, and a child with measles will have Koplik's spots on the gums (these appear as blue-white spots surrounded by a red border). The gums should be firm, strong, and tightly sealed around each tooth. Record any tenderness, puffiness, bleeding, and pulling away of the gums from the teeth. Incidentally, it is normal for the gums to pull away from the teeth slightly as a person ages.

Checking the Tongue

Examine the tongue. Disorders in other parts of the body may reveal themselves in the tongue. It can be stained almost any color as a result of food and drink and can vary in texture from smooth to hairy. The tongue should be moist, smooth, and beefy red, and it should fit the mouth. Record any parts of the tongue that are bright red or that have curd-white patches. A reddish (brighter red than normal) or purplish tongue may indicate certain nutritional diseases. When a person has jaundice, the tongue may be a yellowish color. A black tongue may be present with tobacco use or penicillin treatment.

Grasp the tip of the tongue with gauze-wrapped fingers, and swing it to the left and to the right. Examine the mucosa and the border of the tongue. Have the person touch the palate with the tip of the tongue. Inspect the floor of the mouth for any irregularities, and note the appearance of the underside of the tongue. Ask the person to move his or her tongue from side to side, up and down, in and out of the mouth, and around the inside of the mouth. Record any difficulties in movement.

Checking the Inside Lining of the Mouth

Note the inside lining of the mouth. Examine between the lower lip and the gums, between the upper lip and the gums, and along each cheek. Again, record any spots that are bright red or curd-white.

Checking the Teeth

Check the teeth for cavities, loose or absent teeth, shape, location (crooked teeth), and color. An adult should have thirty-two teeth.

Checking the Pharynx

Ask the person to open his or her mouth wide and say "aah" so that you can examine the pharynx (the fleshy area that you can see farthest back in the throat). You will need a flashlight; if the person has a difficult time keeping his or her tongue flat in the mouth, you will also need a tongue depressor (the flat end of a butter knife works, too). When you use the tongue depressor, note the response of the soft palate. Normally, the soft palate should rise upon depression of the tongue.

When looking at the pharynx and inside of the mouth, check the pillars at the back of the mouth, the uvula (or punching bag), and the tonsils. They should be moist and pink. You should also check for symmetry, unusual swelling, ulcers or other sores, tonsil enlargement, and any discharge (other than saliva). Mucous drainage may leave a whitish or yellowish coating on the tongue or pharynx. Record any variation in the throat, the pharynx, or the tonsils, especially areas that are red, swollen, white, or yellowish, or that are covered with mucus.

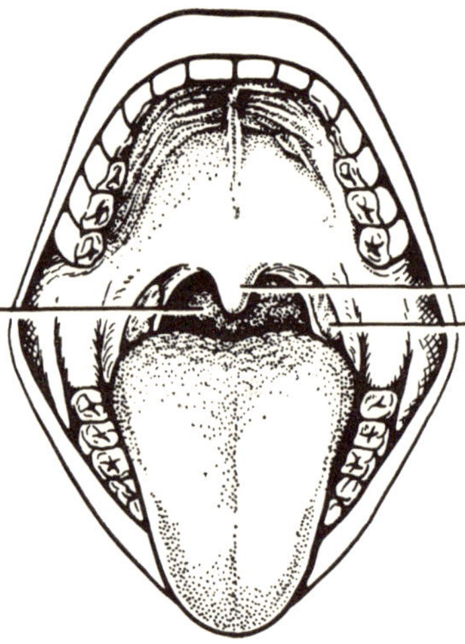

Figure 3-7
Examining the back of the throat and inside of the mouth. From Tom Ferguson, "Teaching Medicine to Kids," *Medical Self-Care: Access to Medical Tools,* Spring 1977 (No. 2), p. 11.

Checking for Breath Odor

Note the breath odor while examining the inside of the mouth. Bad breath may indicate that an infection is present or that the person does not observe proper hygiene. Breath that smells like ammonia may indicate that the person has uremia (a condition in which substances that are normally eliminated in the urine accumulate in the blood). Uncontrolled diabetes mellitus produces a breath that may smell sweet, flowery, or like acetone (a smell similar to fingernail polish remover).

Checking for Oral Cancer

Oral cancer is a disease that often goes undetected. But there are some simple guidelines to follow so that early detection can be accomplished:

1. **Check face symmetry.** Are there any new lumps, bumps, or changes in facial color? Is there a change in a mole or other pigmented spot? Is the face proportioned as usual?
2. **Examine the lips.** Is there a lump when the lips are pressed together? Are there ulcers or other sores present that haven't healed during the last two weeks? Does the lip have a normal borderline?
3. **Note the health of the gums.** Are there any new lumps, bumps, or swellings? Are ulcers or other sores present? Are there white areas on the gums? Is there unusual bleeding?
4. **Examine the cheeks.** With the thumb on the inside of the cheek and the index finger on the outside of the cheek, press and squeeze the tissue between the fingers. Repeat the process on both cheeks. Are there rough areas, lumps, bumps, or swellings inside the cheeks? Do the inside of the cheeks have a white coating? Are there white, red, or dark patches on the insides of the cheeks?
5. **Check the tongue on all sides, underneath, and on the upper surface.** Are ulcers or other sores present that have hard borders?
6. **Examine the floor of the mouth.** Are there color changes or sores? Are ulcers or sore spots present?
7. **Examine the roof of the mouth.** Are there unusual lumps, bumps, sores, or swelling? Are there changes of color such as white, red, or dark patches? Does any area of the mouth feel painful or have a loss of feeling?
8. **Observe the side of the neck.** Are there lumps that do not go away?
9. **Look at the center of the neck.** Watch the Adam's apple. Are there any lumps or bumps? Has the person experienced continued hoarseness?[7]

Checking for Joint Mobility

Finally, have the person open and close the mouth so that you can check for mobility. You should palpate the joint where the jaw joins the skull while the mouth is wide open and when it is closed. Have the person move his or her jaw from side to side also.

Examining a Child's Mouth

Infants in the first three months of life do not produce much saliva, so the lack of saliva should not alarm you. Children do not usually like to have their mouths examined, and you may have to gently restrain the child with the assistance of another person.

A child has twenty teeth in his or her mouth (whereas the adult has thirty-two). These teeth are called deciduous teeth because a child loses them and they are replaced by permanent teeth. Note the presence of crooked teeth and misalignment of teeth in the child. With the improvements and convenience of orthodontic work, the malocclusion and misalignment of teeth may be remedied before adulthood.

Children often experience problems with swollen or inflamed tonsils and adenoids. Check the back of the mouth and the throat carefully, especially noting the size and color of the tonsils. The adenoids cannot be seen unless they are swollen. In the case of persistent swelling and inflammation, both the tonsils and adenoids may have to be removed.

Exercise much care in examining the throat for unusual color or markings, such as white or yellow patches. These may indicate the presence of strep throat, which should immediately be referred to the care of a doctor. Strep throat can lead to rheumatic fever in children, which, in turn, may cause damage to the valves of the heart. Thus, it is especially important that any extremely sore throat be checked by a doctor so that antibiotic therapy can be given to remedy the condition and prevent further complications.

NECK

First, check to make sure that the neck is in a centered position. Ask the person to tilt his or her head backward as far as possible without straining; now have the person swing his or her head forward, to the right, and to the left. Record any discomfort, pain, or difficulty in movement.

Next examine the neck for swollen glands or lymph nodes. Normally, lymph nodes are so small that they cannot be felt by a manual examination; a slight infection will make them firm and may make them swell to the size of a lima bean. Severe infections may make them as large as walnuts. To examine the lymph nodes, use the tips of the fingers in a to-and-fro motion. The person should relax the neck muscles as much as possible, and the neck should be bent slightly forward.

BACK

Examine the back with the person undressed. Note the person's posture. Correct posture should show the body extended with the head held upright and thrown slightly backward. The chest should protrude somewhat, and the abdomen should curve slightly inward in relation to the chest. Inspect the spinal profile, noting the normal cervical (neck), thoracic (chest), and lumbar (lower back) curves.

Many people suffer unnecessary back pain from incorrect posture while standing, sitting, unloading luggage from a car trunk, scrubbing a floor, and carrying or chopping. See the accompanying illustrations that show correct and incorrect postures for various activities.

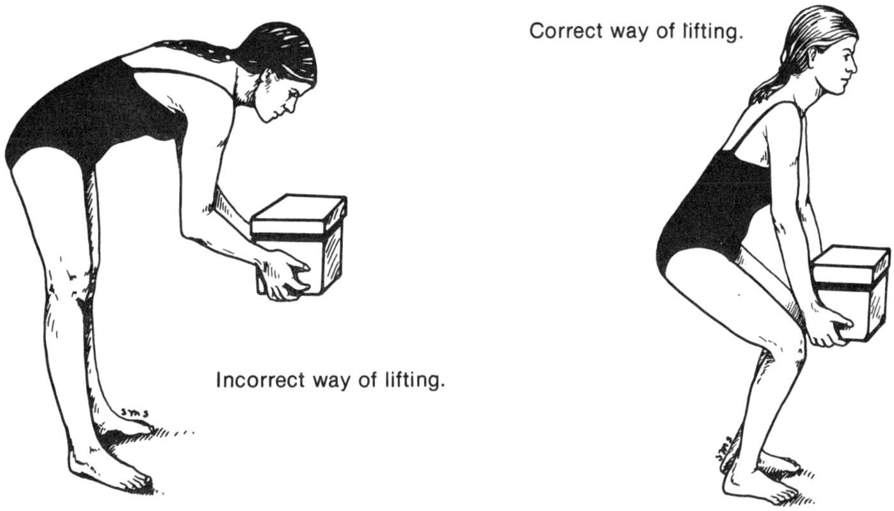

Figure 3-8
To avoid back strain, squat down to lift objects, and keep your back straight. Do not bend from the waist.

Figure 3-9
Place your knees on some sort of pad, and keep your back straight.

Incorrect way to wash the floor.

Correct way to wash the floor.

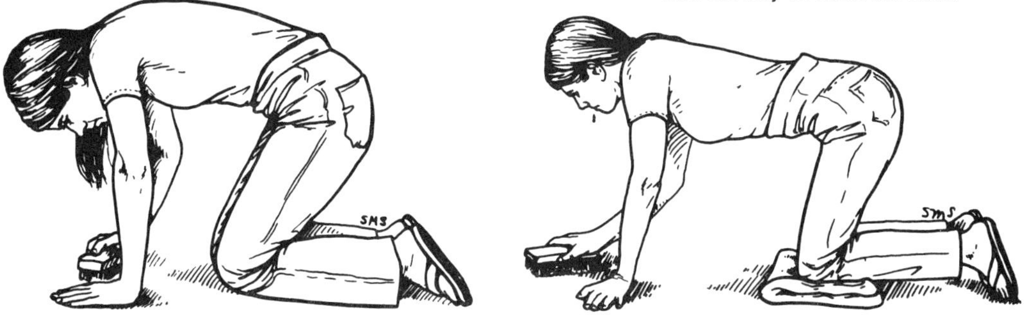

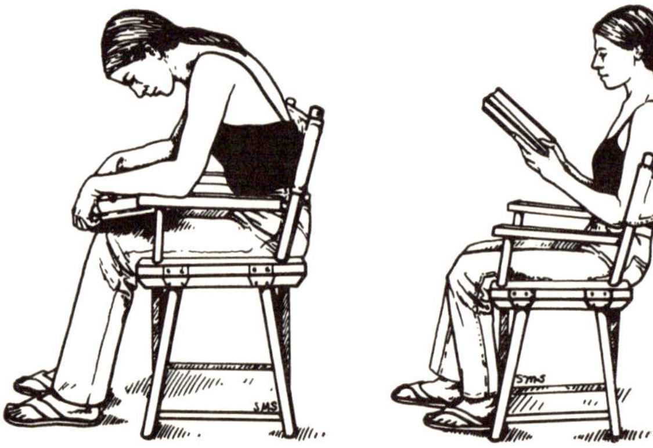

Figure 3-10
When you sit in a chair, keep your back straight against the chair. If you are reading, do not lean over the book. Instead, bring the book up toward you.

Figure 3-11
When you are going to carry a heavy object in one hand, bend your knees to reach down and pick it up, and lean forward slightly. Again, try to keep your back straight. Use your other arm to balance the load.

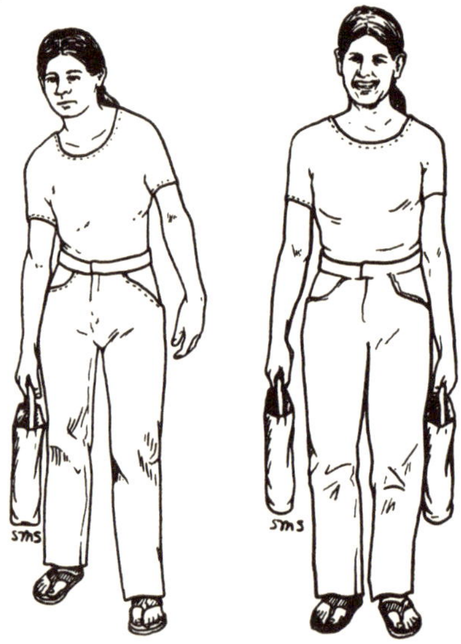

Incorrect way to stand at a sink.

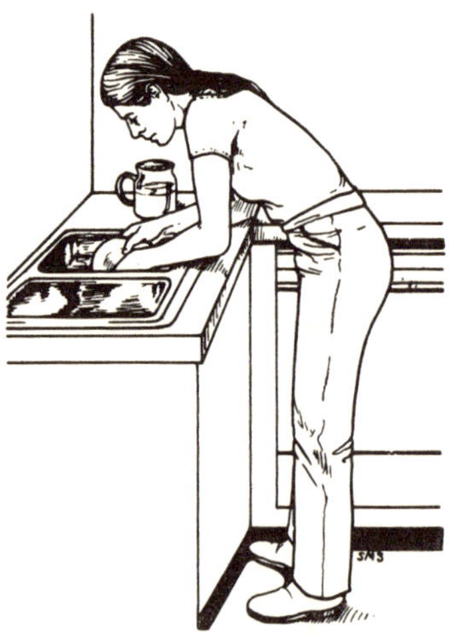

Correct way to stand at a sink.

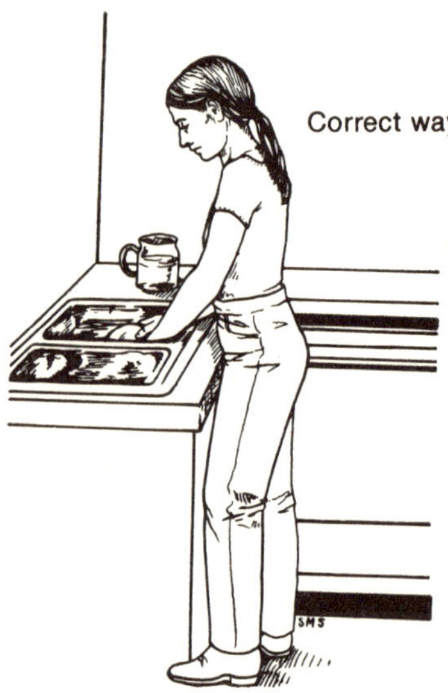

Figure 3-12
When working at the sink, be sure that your back is kept straight. It also helps to bend one knee slightly.

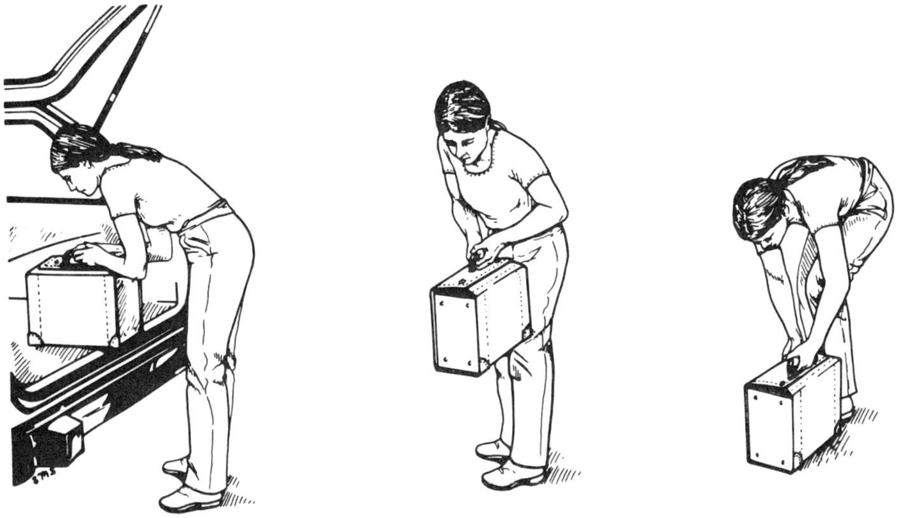

Incorrect way to take luggage from a car trunk.

Figure 3-13
Taking luggage out of a car trunk can be dangerous to your back if you do it the wrong way. Most people stoop down to pick up the luggage, turn, and then bend at the waist to drop it. This strains the back muscles and twists the spine.

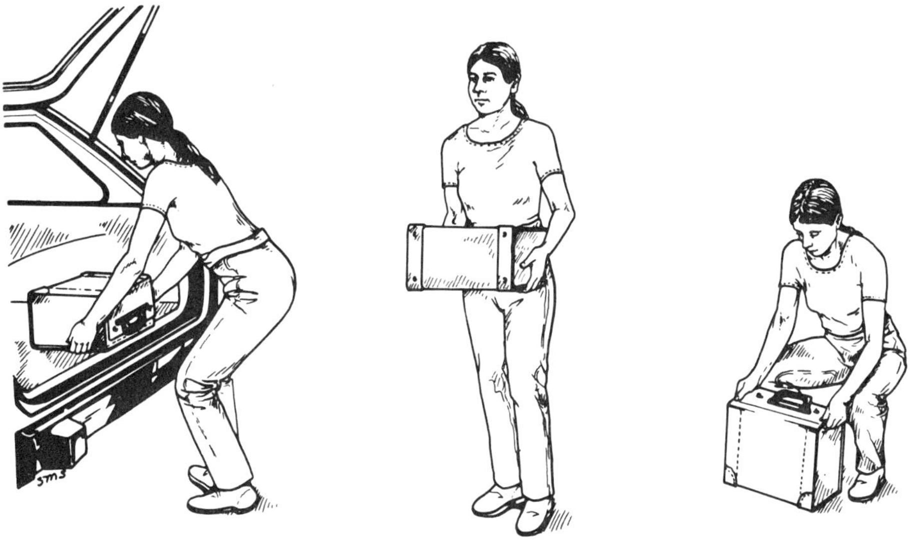

Correct way to take luggage from a car trunk.

Note any abnormal curvature of the spine as you observe the patient from the side. Illustrations have been provided so that you may see some of the more common **abnormal** spinal curvatures.

Note any curvature of the spine from side to side as you stand behind the person. It is important to conduct an additional test for **scoliosis.** Although it is usually quite easy to see the side-to-side curvature of the spine when you look at the person from the back, a slight curvature may not be so apparent. In any case, you should have the person bend over at the waist with the hands clasped. If the person has scoliosis in any degree, it will show by one side of the back being raised and prominent and the other side of the back being flattened.

When checking a child for scoliosis, observe him or her from the back and ask yourself the following questions:

1. Does the head line up over the crease of the buttocks, or does it lean to one side?
2. Is one shoulder higher than the other, or is there a fullness on one side of the neck?
3. Is the "wing" of one shoulder blade higher or more prominent than the other?
4. Is the waistline the same on both sides, or is there a greater distance between the arm and flank on one side?
5. Does there appear to be a curve when you run your fingers down the spine?
6. Are the hips level and symmetrical, or is one side high or more prominent?
7. The child should then bend forward with the back parallel to the floor and the hands clasped. Again, are both sides of the back symmetrical, or is there a prominence or bulge on one side of the back or flank?

If the answer to any one of these questions is "yes," the child has scoliosis to some degree and should be seen by a doctor. If scoliosis is diagnosed before the child has reached his or her full growth, it may be partially or completely corrected so that major deformity is avoided. The child may have to do special exercises, wear a back brace, or have surgery, but any one or a combination of the treatments is surely preferable to the deformity that accompanies scoliosis.

BREASTS

Observing the Person

Ask the person to sit facing you with her arms hanging loosely at her sides. Study her breasts carefully — note whether they are symmetrical in shape and size. (Most women have one breast that is larger than the other, but both should be about the same general shape and contour.) Note the color of the breasts. They are normally a pinkish color, but during pregnancy and as a woman gets older, they may darken. Note the surface characteristics of each breast. Check for any dimples or bulges that occur in one breast but not the other. Examine the breasts for unusual pigmentation patterns, moles, ulcers or other sores, an abnormal amount and distribution of hair, swelling, and venous patterns that may be abnormal.

Examine the areola of each breast. This is the more darkly pigmented area around the nipple. Note its size, symmetry, shape, color, and surface characteristics. Also observe any bulging or sores. Record any abnormalities.

While the woman is sitting, look closely at her nipples. Nipples vary greatly from one person to the next in size, coloration, and shape. Check to see if the nipples are pointing the same way. Make sure that the nipples do not adhere to any underlying mass of tissue. The nipples may change during or be affected by menstrual periods or pregnancy. Note any tenderness, redness, discharge, rashes, wrinkled appearance, or sores.

Before a manual breast examination is begun, observe the appearance of the breasts in several positions. Again, you are looking for any unusual lumps, bulges, or dimples in the breast tissue. You have already observed the person sitting with her arms hanging loosely at her sides. Now have the person raise her arms over her head. Observe the breasts and record any unusual findings.

Next, have the woman lean over so that the breasts are allowed to hang freely. Make your observations and notations. Then have the person seated with her hands pushing on her hips. When the woman is in these different positions, the breasts should move upward and outward freely.

If you suspect a mass in one breast or the other, gently move or compress the breast and watch for dimpling.

Manual Breast Examination

To perform a manual breast examination, have the person lie down and put a small pillow under the shoulder on the side that you will examine first. This spreads the breast tissue more evenly over the chest. In your mind, divide the breast into quadrants. Each quadrant should be palpated by the person with the tips of the fingers moving gently in a circular, massagelike motion. The palpation should begin at the outside of the breast and move in toward the areola and nipple. The quadrants should be examined in a clockwise direction. Note any lumps, irregularities, and masses. If you find an irregularity in one breast but not the other, it is probably abnormal; a lump in the same general place in both breasts is probably normal for that woman. Describe any lumps that you find, noting firmness, tenderness, location, shape, and size.

Breast tissue should normally be soft and homogenous in a young adult, but there are certain normal variations in breast tissue. In a very young woman, the breast tissue may feel firm and elastic. In a post-menopause woman, breast tissue may feel nodular and stringy. Right before the menstrual period, breast tissue may become engorged and feel

Figure 3-14
Self-examination of breasts (looking).

Stand in front of a mirror with the upper body unclothed. Look for changes in the shape and size of the breast and for dimpling of the skin or "pulling in" of the nipples. Any changes in the breast may be made more noticeable by a change in position of the body and arms.

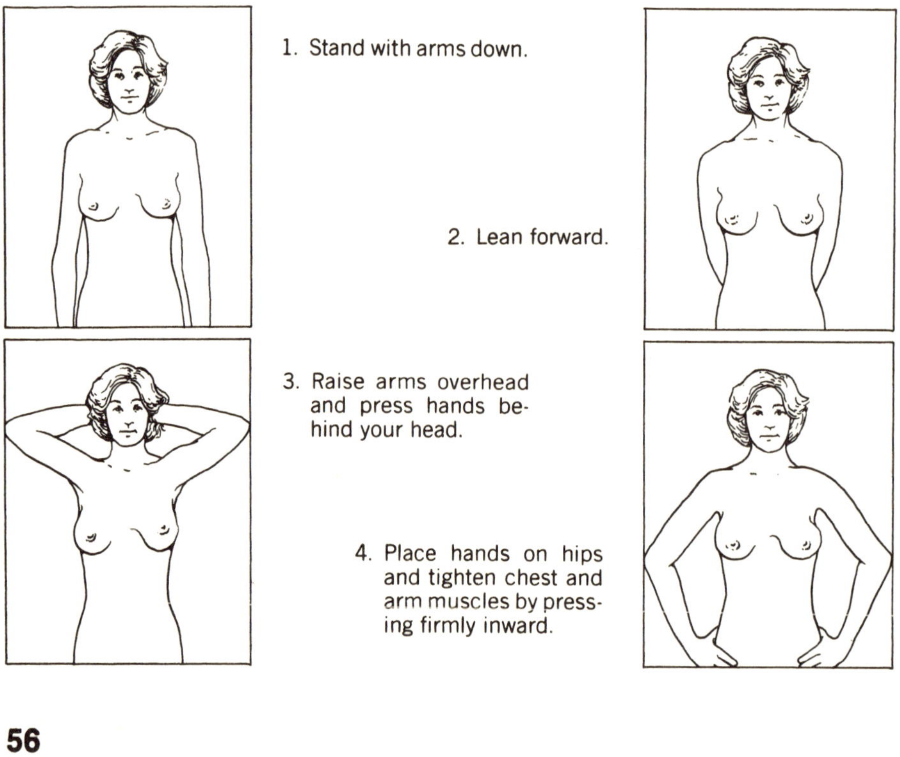

Figure 3-15
Self-examination of breasts (feeling).

Lie flat on your back with a pillow or folded towel under your shoulders and feel each breast with the opposite hand in sequence. With the hand slightly cupped, feel with flattened finger tips for lumps or any change in the texture of the breast or skin; also, note any discharge from nipples or scaling of the skin of the nipples. Feel gently, firmly, carefully and thoroughly. Do not pinch your breast between thumb and fingers. This may give the impression of a lump that is not actually there.

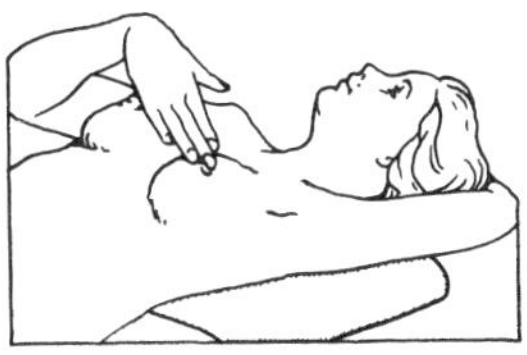

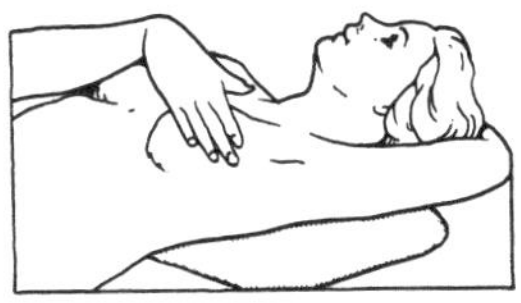

1. Place a pillow or folded towel under your left shoulder. This raises the breast and makes examination easier. Place your left arm over your head. With your right hand, feel the inner half of your left breast from top to bottom and from nipple to breastbone.
2. Feel the outer half from bottom to top and from the nipple to the side of the chest. Begin at outermost top of your right breast for 12 o'clock, then move to 1 o'clock, and so on around the circle back to 12. A ridge of firm tissue in the lower curve of each breast is normal. Then move in an inch, toward the nipple, keep circling to examine *every part of your breast,* including nipple. This requires at least three more circles. Now slowly repeat procedure on your left breast with a pillow under your left shoulder and left hand behind head. Notice how your breast structure feels.

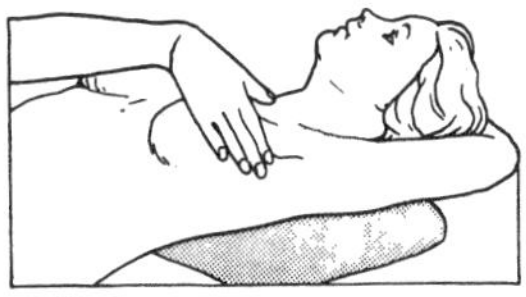

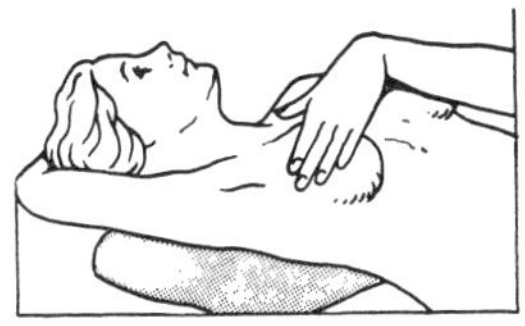

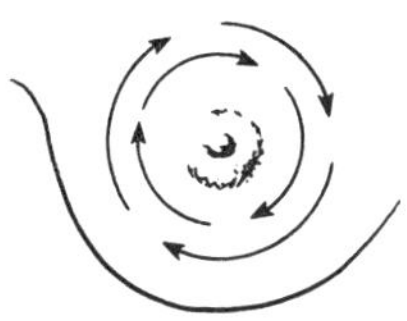

Pay special attention to the area between the breast and armpit itself.

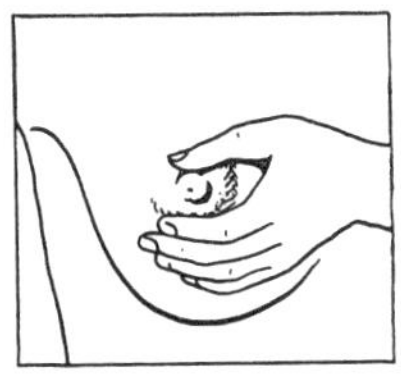

Finally, squeeze the nipple of each breast gently between thumb and index finger. Any discharge, clear or bloody, should be reported to your doctor immediately.

Now, place the pillow or folded towel under your right shoulder. Repeat this same process for your right breast using the fingers of your left hand to feel.

tender with accentuated lobes and glands. For purposes of examination, the best time is usually one week after the menstrual period.

Finally, squeeze the nipple of each breast gently between the thumb and index finger. Any discharge, clear or bloody, should be reported to a doctor immediately.

Ninety-five percent of all lumps are discovered by the woman herself, and not all lumps are malignant.[8] A woman should establish a regular time each month for a self-examination of the breasts. As was mentioned previously, the best time is a few days after the menstrual period, and for women who are in the menopause, the first day of each month is preferable. By performing the examination at the same time each month, the woman will know what is normal for her breasts.

Examination of the breasts can also be done in the shower or bath. When the hands are warm and soapy, glide the hands gently over every part of the breasts. The left hand should be used for examination of the right breast, and the right hand should be used to examine the left breast.

Next, examine the breasts before a mirror. Look for dimpling, puckering, and any other changes that may occur in breast shape and contour. Lift the arms over the head and inspect the breasts again. Put the heels of the hands together and press. Again look for dimpling, puckering, and any other skin changes.

Facts about Breast Cancer

A word about breast cancer will emphasize the importance of regular breast self-examination and frequent examinations by your physician. One out of fifteen women will develop breast cancer in her lifetime. Breast cancer is the leading cause of cancer deaths among women, and it is the leading cause of death for females of ages forty to forty-four. Certain factors may precede, predispose a woman to breast cancer, or be related to breast cancer in some way. These are: age, family history of breast cancer (especially mothers and aunts), whether or not a woman has borne children (particularly whether a woman has borne her first child before age thirty), previous cancer in one breast, precancerous fibrocystic disease, prolonged total menstrual activity, cancer in other body organs, high dietary fat intake, chronic stress, high radiation exposure, deficiency in the immune system, virus, trauma, or taking certain drugs.[9]

CHEST

Observe and inspect the person's thorax (chest area). Especially note its symmetry, paying attention to deviations in size and shape. These deviations may help you detect other problems.

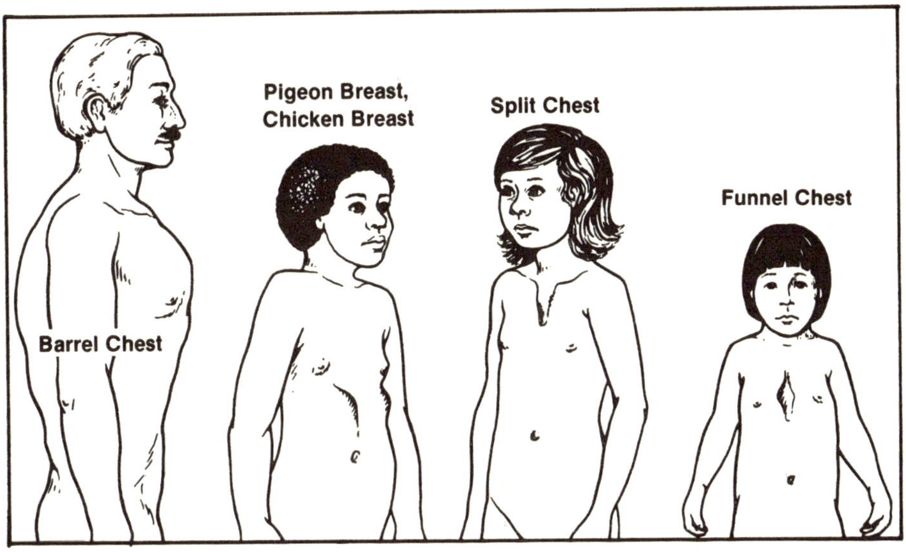

Figure 3-16
Barrel Chest: enlarged back and chest dimensions; ribs appear more horizontal than sloped.
Pigeon Breast: projection of breastbone.
Split Chest: complete or partial separation of breastbone.
Funnel Chest: sinking depression of lower breastbone.

HEART

The first step in assessing the function of the heart is to observe the chest. You should find that the heart beats at a normal rate and rhythm. (For further information on the normal heart rate and rhythm, refer to the chapter on vital signs.) Any abnormal pulsations, dimpling, heaves, lifts, vibrations, skipped beats, or thrills (abnormal tremors) should be noted and described.

Next, listen to the heart with either a stethoscope or your ear placed against the chest. You will normally hear two heart sounds and in rare instances a third. The first sound characteristically is referred to as a "lub" sound, which is louder and lower than the second heart sound. The second heart sound is shorter and higher than the first and is described as a "dub."

Heart murmurs occur from either excessively turbulent blood flow through the heart or vibrations of the heart and large blood vessels that come into or go out of the heart. Murmurs may produce a variety of sounds, but some of the more common are a rushing, a rumbling, a blowing, a hissing, or a whizzing sound. The presence of any abnormality such as a murmur should be recorded and referred to a physician.

Certain characteristic signs appear when a child has some form of heart disease, and you should be aware of some of these physical indicators. Poor weight gain, delayed development, respiration that is faster than normal, excessively rapid heartbeat, cyanosis (or bluish tinge to the skin, lips, or nail beds), clubbed fingers, and chest abnormalities and deformities may indicate the presence of some type of heart disease. Be sure to note any of these irregularities in the child's record and refer them to a doctor.

LUNGS

Watch the person breathe. Breathing should be quiet, relaxed, rhythmic, and smooth: both sides of the chest should expand at the same rate during the breathing process.

Remember that there is a difference between the way men, women, and children breathe. Women breathe using the chest muscles while men and children breathe with the diaphragm. Therefore, you will notice more chest movement with women and more stomach movement with men and children.

After watching the person breathe while standing in front of him or her, examine the person as you stand behind him or her. Have the person fold his or her arms over the chest so that you can get a more accurate picture. It is also helpful to place one of your hands flat on different parts of the person's chest to check for abnormal vibrations or tenderness.

A stethoscope should be used to listen to all areas in the front and back of the chest area. Normally, when a person breathes, the air can be heard moving in and out of the lungs, sounding like wind blowing through trees. Listen for wheezes, bubbling, or other sounds that seem abnormal.

ABDOMEN

Suggestions for Examination

To examine the abdomen, have the person lie on his or her back with the hands resting loosely on the chest or to the side. The person should be unclothed (at least from the chest to the topline of the pubic hair) and should be relaxed. A small pillow under the knees or head may help to relax the person, as well as breathing deeply through the mouth.

Make sure that the person has emptied his or her bladder before the examination. You can help the person by making sure that your hands are warm. When you listen to the bowel sound with a stethoscope, warm the bell of the stethoscope with your hands or under warm water before you place it on the abdomen. It is often helpful to distract the person with conversation and questions at the beginning of the exam. Later, after the exam has begun, this will probably be unnecessary. If the person is frightened or ticklish, use his or her own hand under yours at the beginning of the manual examination.[10]

The Abdominal Quadrants

In order to record accurately any findings, divide the abdomen into four quarters with an imaginary line across the abdomen through the navel, and another line from top to bottom, again through the navel. See the accompanying illustration for more detail regarding the placement of the organs in the abdominal cavity.

Figure 3-17
The abdominal quadrants.

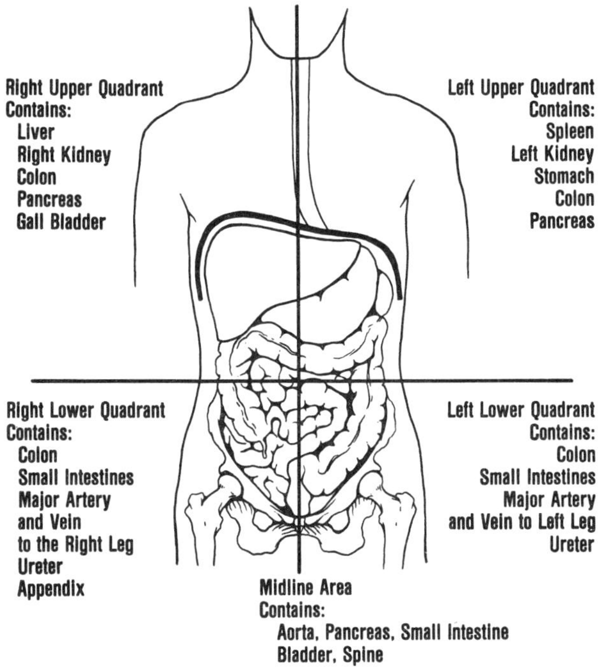

Examining the Abdomen

1. First, step to either side of the person and bring your eyes on a level with the top of the abdomen so that you are looking across the area. Note any abnormal swellings, distention, inflammation, or sores.
2. Note the navel area. Observe its contour and location (whether it is in the middle of the abdomen). Record any inflammation, sores, or hernias.
3. Observe the respiratory movement of the abdomen in males (remember that women breathe using primarily the chest muscles).
4. Note any digestive movements that may be taking place. These movements are generally not seen unless the patient is very lean. You will want to listen for bowel sounds with your stethoscope or your ear. (If you use your ear, place it snugly against the abdomen, but not so snugly that the pressure creates pain for the person.) This procedure should precede palpation (feeling) so that bowel sounds will be more regular. Normal bowel sounds occur every five to fifteen seconds but may be more irregular. To get an adequate assessment of bowel sounds, listen to the sounds for at least five minutes in each quadrant. Listen for the normal sounds of digestion: quiet, slow, and gurgling. Record any sounds that are constantly gurgling or that are extremely loud. Also note an instance where you can hear no sounds at all for one minute.
5. Palpation (feeling) is especially helpful in assessing the health of the abdomen. Use your fingertips and press very lightly initially to determine tenderness, the presence of large masses, and lumps. When using a light palpation, maintain pressure on the area that you are examining during both inhalation and exhalation. If you feel the person tense up as you press an area, ask if there is any pain (a tensing-up generally means that the person is "guarding" a tender area). A healthy abdomen will feel soft, and you will not be able to feel any organs or masses.

If the person has complained of pain in the abdomen before you even start the examination, begin palpation at the point furthest from the painful area and work your way gradually toward it—If you start with the area of pain, the person will probably not relax enough to permit a thorough examination.

The appendix cannot normally be felt, but in cases where the appendix is inflamed and swollen, you can feel this part of the intestine by palpating (feeling) halfway between the navel and the crest of the right hipbone. If the appendix is inflamed or infected, you should not only be able to feel its structure, but when you press on the area, the person should feel some tenderness or pain. Make a note of any swelling, tenderness, or pain.

—Special Considerations for the Infant and Child—

In infancy, the abdomen normally protrudes because of the poorly developed musculature, so do not be alarmed at the protrusion.

It is especially important to check the navel and its surrounding area in the infant. Note whether the navel has healed properly after the umbilical cord has fallen off. It is not uncommon for infants or children to have umbilical hernias. These characteristically do not show up unless the infant is crying or straining in the abdominal area. Have the child strain against the abdominal area and check to see if there are any bulges around the navel. Also note the presence of any inflammation in that area, and make a record of any other irregularities.

Remember that infants and young children breathe with the diaphragm, so there may be more movement in the abdominal area concurrent with respiration. This is perfectly normal.

MALE GENITALIA

Look closely at the penis shaft: note any pimples, sores, lumps, swelling, or red spots. Look at the top of the penis and examine the urethral opening. Record any redness of the mucosa, discharge, sores, or swelling. (If you are a man and are uncircumcised, pull back the foreskin; check the urethral opening and note any sores, pimples, or red spots under the foreskin. A waxy substance along the inside of the foreskin is a normal lubricant for the folds of flesh.)

Palpate (feel) the penis shaft for the presence of any lumps or unusual swelling. Record any abnormal findings.

Look closely at the scrotum (the sac of flesh holding the testicles). Observe the size, superficial appearance, and symmetry of the scrotum. Usually the left testicle will be slightly lower than the right one, so this is not a cause for alarm. Note any red spots, sores, or pimples. Check the insides of both thighs and the underside of the scrotum for red areas, sores, or pimples.

A testicular self-examination is especially important for men ages fifteen to thirty-four because of the increased incidence of cancer of the testes. In fact, cancer of the testes is one of the most common forms of cancer in men under the age thirty-four.[11] Eighty percent of those who develop cancer of the testes are under forty years of age.[12]

The self-examination should take place after the bath or shower when the scrotum is the most relaxed. Using the index and middle fingers on the underside of the testicles and the thumb on top, roll the testicle between the thumb and fingers. They should normally feel firm, smooth, and freely movable in the scrotum. Feel for the epididymus, which is on and behind the testicle. Normally, it should feel spongier than the testicle tissue.

FEMALE GENITALIA

Look closely at the genital area. Examine the area covered by hair, and note any red areas, sores, or pimples. It is best to examine yourself while not menstruating; menstrual discharge tends to mask sores, abnormalities, or abnormal discharge.

A woman can lie on her back using a mirror, draw her knees up, and spread them apart, letting them fall to the table. Examine the flesh of the labia, around the vaginal opening. The labia should be round, full, and a pinkish color. In a woman who has had multiple childbirths, the large labia are thinner and do not quite meet at the midline. As a result, the smaller labia underneath are visible. Record any sores, redness, or discharge (other than menstrual).

ANUS AND RECTUM

An examination of the anus and rectum should be done by a physician, as should a complete examination of the internal female reproductive system.

EXTREMITIES

When you examine the extremities, you are generally looking at the physical characteristics of the limb.

Have the person stand before you with the arms at the sides. Note the symmetry, shape, and physical characteristics of the arms. Are both arms the same size? Is one arm longer than the other? Are there sores, unusual markings, unusual areas of pigmentation, or other skin problems?

Look at the hands. Do the hands tremble? Are the hands enlarged? Are the fingers unusually slender and long? Also note the fingernails.

Next, examine the legs. Note the color and texture of the skin of the legs and feet. Check the legs for venous (vein) patterns and enlargement that may indicate varicose veins. Note the temperature of the legs and feet with the back of the hand. These extremities should not feel excessively cold or warm to the touch. Examine the toenails.

You can tell if a person has flat feet by immersing the feet in water and then having the person stand on a dry newspaper. The outline that the wet feet have left on the paper will depict whether the feet are normal or flat.

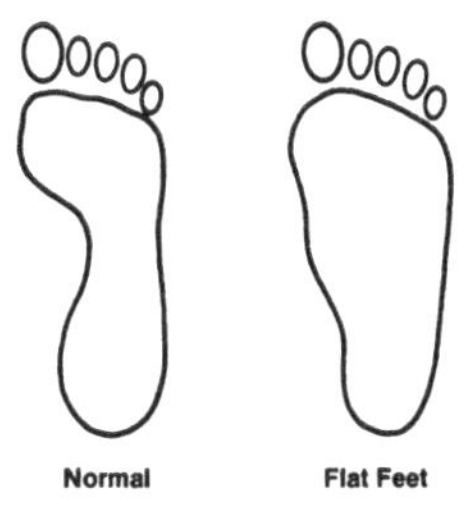

Figure 3-18
Outline comparing flat and normal feet.

TESTING THE REFLEXES

There are many reflexes in the body that can be tested, but only the two most common ones are listed here.

1. **Patella.** The person should be sitting on a table or chair so that the legs are hanging freely. Strike the area directly below the kneecap on the midline. This reflex response should produce an extension of the leg. Repeat the test on the other leg.

2. **Plantar.** Using a key, the dull end of a pin, a tongue blade, an applicator stick, or the handle of the reflex hammer, stroke the bottom of the foot, beginning at the heel and moving upward toward the ball of the foot. The person's toes should flex (curl).

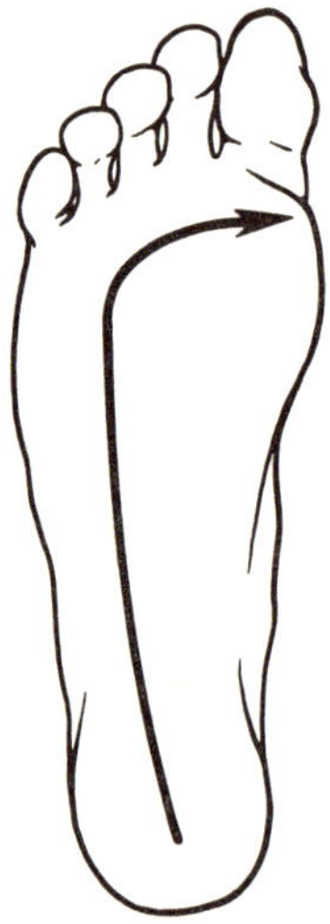

Figure 3-19
When testing the plantar reflex, stroke the bottom of the foot, beginning at the heel and moving toward the ball of the foot.

It is rather difficult to test the responses of an infant to the sensory stimuli. But a gentle stroking of various parts of the body will usually elicit various movements and responses. Infants have certain reflexes that adults do not. These reflexes disappear within a matter of months, but you can check a few of them while the infant is still young:

- **Blinking (dazzle reflex).** The eyelids close in response to a bright light. This reflex disappears after about the first year of life.
- **Acoustic blink.** Both eyes blink in response to a loud noise. There is no set time for disappearance of this reflex.
- **Rooting.** When you touch the infant's cheek, his or her mouth opens, and the infant turns his or her head to the side that was stimulated. This reflex disappears at about three to four months.
- **Startle (Moro) reflex.** Hold the baby in a suspended and prone position. Then, suddenly lower the entire body about two feet and stop abruptly. The baby's arms abduct (draw away) and extend with the hands open and the fingers extended. The legs flex slightly, the hips abduct, and the arms return in a clasping motion.[13]

In older children, you should have the child draw some pictures and write. Observe the pictures and handwriting and note any gross irregularities or abnormalities. Also, observe the child as he or she walks, rises from the floor from a supine position, and sits and stands. Note any jerky motions, inability to accomplish any of the before-mentioned, and weakness. Record these abnormalities.

Any abnormalities or unexplained concerns found during your assessment should be referred to a physician.

NOTES

1. Ruth Murray, et al., *Nursing Assessment and Health Promotion Through the Life Span* (Englewood Cliffs, New Jersey: Prentice-Hall, Inc., 1975), p. 4.
2. Toni M. Roberts, Kathleen McIntosh Tinker, and Donald W. Kemper, *Healthwise Handbook* (Garden City, New York: Doubleday & Co., Inc., 1979), p. 13.
3. Barbara Bates, *A Guide to Physical Examination* (Philadelphia: J. B. Lippincott Company, 1974), pp. 11-12.
4. Brent Q. Hafen and Keith J. Karren, *First Aid and Emergency Care Workbook*, Second Edition (Denver: Morton Publishing Company, 1980), pp. 24, 26-27.
5. Ibid., pp. 19, 27.
6. Shirley Linde, "Medical Tests and Checkups You Can Do Yourself at Home," *Family Circle*, November 20, 1979, p. 119.
7. Nguyen Thanh Nguyen with Patty de Roulf, *Your Mouth: Oral Care for All Ages* (Radnor, Pennsylvania Chilton Book Co., 1979), pp. 96-97.
8. Roberts, p. 16.
9. Henry P. Leis, Jr., "Risk Factors in Breast Cancer," *AORN Journal*, November 1975, pp. 724-725.
10. Bates, p. 161.
11. Michael Castleman, "A Field Guide to Men's Reproductive Health," *Medical Self-Care: Access to Medical Tools*, No. 5, 1978, p. 27.
12. Margaret Conklin, et al. "Should Health Teaching Include Self-Examination of the Testes?" *American Journal of Nursing*, December 1978, p. 2073.
13. Bates, pp. 357-360.

CHAPTER 4

SELF-CARE LAB TESTS

INTRODUCTION

There are several laboratory tests that you can do at home to assess your health. A simple urinalysis can be done using inexpensive materials and taking very little of your time. This test identifies the presence of eight ingredients in urine that may be a key to a state of health or disease. Early pregnancy test kits have also been put on the market. The advantages and disadvantages of these kits will be discussed. The guaiac test for blood in the stool can identify the presence of colon or rectum cancer long before symptoms become apparent to you.

Self-care lab tests are not diagnostic tools. They merely serve to assess the health of the systems that they test. If you find an abnormality, see your doctor immediately — he will perform a diagnosis that will identify the cause of the problem.

URINALYSIS AT HOME

You can do a nearly complete, laboratory quality urinalysis at home inexpensively. And the procedure will probably take no more than three to four minutes. The home urinalysis will give you basic information concerning various body systems, and it will tell you when you need to go to a doctor for prevention of a serious condition or remedy of a disease.

How To Obtain Reagent Strips

To conduct the home urinalysis, you need to obtain reagent strips at your local pharmacy or a hospital supply house, or from two companies that manufacture the reagent strips. Of course, the local pharmacy or hospital supply house will provide the strips more quickly, but they are likely to be more highly priced than the strips ordered from the manufacturing companies.

The following information is needed for making requests to the manufacturers:

Name:	N-MULTISTIX™
Order number:	#2829
Description:	"One bottle of 100 Dip-and-Read Test Reagent Strips for in-vitro diagnostic urinalysis of pH, protein, glucose, ketones, bilirubin, blood, nitrite and urobilinogen."
Company:	AMES COMPANY Division of Miles Laboratories, Inc. Elkhart, Indiana 46514

Name:	CHEMSTRIP-8™
Order number:	#10208
Description:	"One container of 50 Dip-and-Read Reagent Strips for in-vitro diagnostic urinalysis of nitrite, pH, protein, glucose, ketones, urobilinogen, bilirubin, and blood."
Company:	BIO-DYNAMICS/bmc Subsidiary of Mannheim/Boeringer 9115 Hague Road Indianapolis, Indiana 46250

The shelf life of each of these products is about one year, so each container has enough strips to test yourself once a week for a year. If you want to test other family members, you will have to order more than one container per year. If you notice that the color test zones on the strips have turned brown, the strips are no longer potent and are not usable for testing urine.

Urine contains waste products of metabolism and several other key ingredients, and these reagent strips measure the presence and/or overabundance of eight important elements that may indicate a state of health or disease. The strips show the presence of the elements by color changes in the test zone areas.

—How To Conduct the Reagent Strip Urinalysis—

To conduct the urinalysis, moisten the strip in urine by either one of two means: (1) dipping the strip in a urine specimen that has been caught in a special container or (2) passing the strip through a urine stream while urinating. To correctly obtain a reading from dipping the strip into urine, make sure that the container is large enough to allow you to fully submerge the strip. The urine should be caught halfway through the process of urination in a clean container that is free of dust, dirt, detergents, or other foreign matter. To obtain a reading from passing the strip through a urine stream, wait until you are about half finished urinating. Then pass the strip through the stream so that the strip is fully moistened for about one second. Excess urine should be tapped off the strip, and the force of the urine stream should not be excessive, because this may give an incorrect reading.

To check the results of the test, you should have a watch with a second hand or a stopwatch to time various color zones on the strip. After the time has elapsed for each color test zone, compare the test zone with the color chart on the bottle. Be sure to read the color test zone in a well-lighted area.

Testing for Other Factors

Before you begin your test with the reagent strips, you can test for three other factors. First, you can test for urine volume. A normal adult passes between one pint and one quart of urine per day. With older adults, the volume may be slightly more or less — from one-half pint to one and one-half quarts per day.

Urine volume may be decreased when you drink less fluids, when perspiration is increased, or when you are subject to prolonged vomiting and/or diarrhea. Cardiovascular shock or a collection of fluid in the tissues known as edema (swelling) can also cause a decreased urine output.

Urine volume will increase if you increase your consumption of fluids, if you are nervous, or if you take diuretics such as caffeine, alcohol, or drugs. Diseases such as diabetes mellitus (sugar diabetes) may also cause you to have an increase in urine volume.

To test for normal urine volume, merely collect urine for a twenty-four-hour period in a container that holds from one to two quarts of liquid. In this way, you will know if your urine volume is normal, too high, or too low.

Urine color can also give you a clue to certain abnormalities in the body. Normally, urine varies from a pale straw to an amber or yellow amber color. Urine color will vary with the amount of liquid taken in during the day — the more liquid taken in, the paler yellow will be the color of the urine; the less liquid taken in, the more amber will be the urine.

Urine colors that you may want to discuss with your physician include: cloudy, smoky, very yellow, yellow-brown or green-brown, red or red-brown, orange or orange-brown, dark brown or black, fluffy or bulky surface deposits.

You can also test the urine by noting its smell. Urine normally has an aromatic or nutty smell. Urine with an unpleasant odor may be produced from eating asparagus or garlic or from a bacterial infection. The urine of a diabetic may smell like acetone — slightly fruity or resembling the smell of fingernail polish remover. Bacterial infections may make the urine smell like ammonia.

PREGNANCY TESTING AT HOME

Women are now offered an over-the-counter, do-it-yourself pregnancy test kit for use at home. The United States Food and Drug Administration, after reviewing data from several makers of the kits, finds the various pregnancy test kits to be reasonably accurate for preliminary personal checkups if special care is used in testing and a number of variables are taken into account.

The first at-home pregnancy test kit was E.P.T., manufactured by Warner-Chilcott. Since then, other products have been introduced, such as "Answer" by Diagnostic Testing, "Pregna-B" and "R-U" by North American Biologicals, "Predictor" by Organon, and "Acu-Test" by J. B. Williams.

How Does the Pregnancy Test Work?

All of these tests use the same method of diagnosing pregnancy. A pregnant woman's urine contains the hormone HCG (human chorionic gonadotropic hormone). When a few drops of urine are exposed to rabbit anti-HCG serum, the HCG in the urine will combine with the antiserum and form a bond. Sheep cells coated with HCG (antigen) are then added to the urine and rabbit antiserum. If the HCG in the urine has bonded with the antiserum, the sheep cells (antigen) can find no free cells with which to form a bond, so the cells settle in the solution and form a ring on the bottom of the test container. So, a ring on the bottom of the container indicates that the woman is pregnant.

If the woman is not pregnant, there will be no HCG in the urine. Therefore, the rabbit anti-HCG serum can find no HCG with which to bond. When the sheep cells (antigen) are added, they form clumps in the solution, creating a smooth, milky fluid with no ring in the bottom of the container. Thus, the test indicates that the woman is not pregnant.

Factors That Affect the Accuracy of the Test

There are several factors that home pregnancy test kit users should keep in mind:

1. Even though the test kits stress that diagnosis of pregnancy can be accomplished early by use of the kits, product accuracy claims are actually based on tests run fifteen or so days after the missed menstrual period.
2. Results of the test can be easily and inadvertently misinterpreted or botched. Any dirt in the test container may give a faulty reading, as can unusual vibrations in the room, exposure to sunlight, and reading the test results too soon or too late.
3. A woman should check her urine before beginning the test. Normal urine should be clear, straw-colored, and free of particles.
4. Women who have had a recent difficult pregnancy may receive a "false positive" reading on the test.
5. A "false negative" reading may occur with an ectopic (outside the uterus) pregnancy, because the HCG level is generally very low in the early weeks of an ectopic pregnancy, and the test may not detect this low HCG level.

While an at-home pregnancy test can give an accurate diagnosis, consultation with a doctor is essential to assure proper medical care. The at-home pregnancy test kit is only a method of making a preliminary diagnosis.

THE GUAIAC HOME TEST FOR COLON CANCER

The guaiac test is used to detect trace blood (or blood that cannot readily be seen by the human eye) in the stool. Specifically, the test detects the possible presence of colon cancer, which is on the rise and constitutes a major cancer problem. Frequently, the test finds colon tumors while they are small enough to be surgically removed, thus providing a cure.

The guaiac test is sold by SmithKline, Inc. and is marketed under the name *Hemoccult.* It can be purchased at most pharmacies. The retail price of the test is approximately one dollar, but a lab fee is charged for test analysis. The test itself comes in a cardboard kit that looks like a matchbook. Inside is a special filter paper.

How To Conduct the Guaiac Test

To conduct the test, you must follow a special diet that is prescribed within the instructions. First, you catch three successive stool samples, smearing the thinnest amount on the windows of the kit. You will be taking two samples from each stool for the smears.

Then the test kit is taken to a laboratory (one that is located near you or that you normally patronize). At the lab, a technician adds one drop of water and two drops of a special solution to each window of the test kit. If one window turns blue, the test is positive — indicating the presence of blood in the stool. You should then consult with your physician. He will probably give you a thorough rectal and internal colon examination to locate the source of the problem.

A new guaiac test has been developed recently called *Hemoccult II.* In this test, you take two samples from three consecutive bowel movements. Each of the samples is then smeared on *Hemoccult II* filter papers, and a few drops of developing solution are added to the specimens within four days of the bowel movement. A bluish discoloration of any of the specimens is considered a positive result (meaning that blood is present in the specimen), and you should seek further evaluation by a professional. The test is accurate and useful, but the developing solution is expensive. Most people use the previously mentioned method of sending specimens to a laboratory.

HOME THROAT CULTURES

Throat cultures can be partially performed at home. This can be a very effective means of preventing complications that can occur with streptococcic bacteria, which can cause rheumatic fever and kidney disease. Physicians take throat cultures to prevent the development of such complications and to avoid unnecessary antibiotic use.

In Maryland, some parents have been taught by the Columbia Health Plan to perform throat cultures. Parents who learned the procedures determined accurate and reliable results, and their participation in this program reduced pediatric office visits by 15 to 20 percent. Taking home throat cultures caused greater parental participation in child care, better understanding of early treatment, decreased contagion by other family members, and efficient screening for family members other than the sick child.

Although the procedures for taking home throat cultures will not be discussed here, you can ask your doctor to teach you the procedure, and you can ask him or her to help you make arrangements for culture growth and analysis by a local laboratory. Note that you will not grow the culture at home, nor will you analyze the results, but you can take the culture itself and deliver it to the lab where the proper procedures can be followed for diagnosis.

HOME GONORRHEA TEST

Gonorrhea is on the increase and is the number one reportable communicable disease in the United States. An FDA scientific advisory panel has now recommended approval of an over-the-counter, do-it-yourself specimen-collection kit for gonorrhea. The kit, designed and manufactured by Bio-Medical Innovations of Glenview, Illinois, is intended for men only. The user is able to collect his own specimen and mail it to a designated laboratory for staining and microscopic study.

The "Gonorrhea Screen Kit for Males" is similar in concept to the home pregnancy test kits now on the market. In practice, a man would collect and prepare a smear of discharge from the penis, following a set of illustrated instructions. Each kit has a coded identification number that permits the user to get his results anonymously by phone within three days. Positive responders would be advised to see a doctor or health clinic for the required treatment. The specimen collection procedure is simple enough for most men to follow without difficulty.

HOME BREAST CANCER TEST

By 1984, women may be able to buy (on prescription) flexible foil designed to detect heat buildups in breast tissue and, in some cases, help detect breast abnormalities, including cancer.

The woman will mold a twenty-four-by-eight-inch strip of the sheeting on her breasts, tucking it under and around and covering all surfaces. Then she will look in the mirror for patterns of heat.

If any parts of the picture of the sheeting covering the breasts show asymmetrical, bright blue patterns — signs of heat buildup — the woman would go to the doctor, who would check further for the possibility of breast cancer.

The pattern of heat also will be apparent to the naked eye, but the doctor would take special pictures to make a permanent record.

The Food and Drug Administration has just approved the heat-sensitive sheeting as an aid for doctors in breast disease detection. Clinical studies show that it works, because cancer tissue is hotter than normal tissue surrounding it. For example, if a tumor is present — even one that is too small to be felt in an examination — it will turn the plastic sheeting bright blue over the cancer.

The special sheeting contains liquid crystals — heat-sensitive microparticles made from processed sheep wool grease and encased in a gelatin film. The very thin layer of heat sensitive capsules then is sandwiched between flexible mylar foil.

It is estimated that a piece of foil that will work for five years will cost around fifty dollars. The trade name for the product is *Thermascan.* The sheeting is made by Eurand America Inc. in Dayton and will be marketed by BCD Products Inc. in New York.

The government may soon approve another version of thermographic devices that employs two heat-sensitive pads worn inside the bra to record "hot" spots that can mean tumors or other breast disease.

The device consists of two foil-wrapped pads bearing eighteen rows of blue dots divided into three sections. To do the test, a woman simply puts the pads in the refrigerator to activate the chemicals, then inserts the pads in her bra. In fifteen minutes, the blue dots change to different shades of pink, each shade corresponding to a certain temperature. She matches each section of dots with the shades of pink on a chart provided with the BCSI kit. She then compares the dots from the left pad with the dots in the same section on the right pad, noting any significant color difference between them.

The BCSI is expected to sell for about ten dollars a box and will be available at first through physicians only.

CHAPTER 5

EMERGENCIES AND COMMON COMPLAINTS

The most serious problem for the injured occurs when those on the scene are plagued with indecision as to what kind of self-care or emergency care to offer; in many injuries, delay of even a few minutes can spell the difference between life and death or between full recovery and permanent disability.

Every person should know how to obtain medical assistance rapidly and what to do until professionals arrive on the scene. Remember, too, that most first aid is rendered to people who will never seek professional medical attention due to the nature of their injuries (a child who falls off a bicycle and suffers abrasions, for example, will probably not be treated further than initial first aid treatment offers). As a general rule, self-care should be performed until professional medical help arrives at the scene, while a victim is being transported to a medical facility, or if a victim has a minor injury that does not require professional medical attention.

GENERAL RULES FOR EMERGENCIES

Self-care in emergencies is that treatment offered before professional medical help arrives at the scene. In cases of severe injury, self-care is performed to prevent death by:

- Preventing further injury
- Counteracting shock
- Restoring breathing
- Controlling bleeding
- Removing poisons

While each emergency case will be different, the following general rules apply to situations where emergency self-care is required:

HOW TO GET QUICK EMERGENCY HELP

In order to receive the best emergency medical help fast, you should keep a list of the phone numbers for the people listed below near your telephone. If you have no such list, clip this section from the book and write the appropriate phone numbers on the lines.

In many communities, all that is required to receive emergency assistance of every kind is dialing the numbers 911. Check to see if this is true of your community.

1. The Rescue Squad ______________________
Often part of the local fire department, these specially-trained paramedics are likely to respond swiftly and competently.

2. The Police ______________________
They may or may not be able to respond with medically trained personnel. However, they can get someone to the hospital quickly.

3. Ambulance Service ______________________
Some services have trained paramedics, others don't. Contact the local medical society for the name of the best service in your area.

4. Your Doctor ______________________
Your own doctor may not be available, but he or she should be alerted if an emergency has occurred.

5. Poison-Control Center ______________________
In some communities, this service will give information to doctors only. Call before an emergency occurs to find out.

Give the following information over the phone:

1. **The victim's location.** Give city or town, street name, and street number. If calling at night, describe the building.
2. **What has happened?** Tell the nature of the emergency—woman is bleeding badly, child has fallen and is unconscious, man has had a heart attack, and so on.
3. **Identify yourself.** Give your name. If it is different from the name of the homeowner or the apartment dweller, give that person's name as well.
4. **Give your phone number.**
5. **Tell them if they will need extra help.** If the victim is overweight, if there are several flights of stairs and no elevator, and so on.
6. **Ask for questions and advice.** Let the person on the other end of the line ask you questions and tell you what to do until help arrives.

1. Recognize your limitations. Don't attempt a procedure that is complicated if you are unfamiliar with it or if, for some reason, you can't properly perform it. Instead, wait for medical help to arrive, and do what you *can* while you are waiting.
2. Evaluate the victim rapidly before you begin any kind of first aid work. Check him or her over thoroughly; if you pay attention only to the broken arm that is obvious, for example, you might miss a third-degree burn on the back of the leg.
3. Keep the victim lying down (an essential in shock control) *unless* he or she is vomiting, bleeding from the mouth, experiencing breathing difficulties, or in severe shock. A victim of severe shock should be kept on the back with the head lower than the body (unless there are head and/or chest injuries), while a victim of an injury should be left with the head level with the body until the extent of injuries is determined.
4. Don't move a victim unless it is necessary. There are some cases where the victim is in further danger if he or she is not moved — you must take someone out of a burning building, for instance, and you must move someone far enough way from a burning building so that falling debris will not hit him or her. If no danger is present, don't move the victim.
5. Remove only clothing that you absolutely have to — otherwise you may aggravate the injuries. In some cases, you will **have** to remove some clothing to examine the victim; if so, remove enough to get a clear idea of the extent of the injuries. If you do remove clothing, tear it along the seams and then make sure that the victim stays warm (if possible, keep the victim covered).
6. If the victim is conscious, reassure him or her. If you can, keep the victim from seeing his or her own injury. Make sure that the victim understands that you know about his or her injuries, that you are doing everything you can to help, and that medical professionals are on the way.
7. Do whatever you can to prevent infection. Never touch an open wound or a burn with your fingers or with other objects that have not been sterilized. It is preferable to use sterile bandages or comresses. There is one important exception to this rule: **if a person is bleeding to death and no sterile bandage is available, use whatever you can to stop the bleeding (including your hand, a piece of your clothing, or a piece of the victim's clothing).**
8. Never try to feed an unconscious person any solid or liquid food —this may cause choking.
9. If you must move a victim due to environmental dangers, carefully

assess the possibility of a broken bone (including back injury). Make sure that the affected part is completely immobilized before you move the victim.

10. If you move a victim on a litter or stretcher, always move him or her feet first. This allows the carrier by the head to keep a constant watch for development of breathing problems.

Figure 5-1

EMERGENCY MOVES

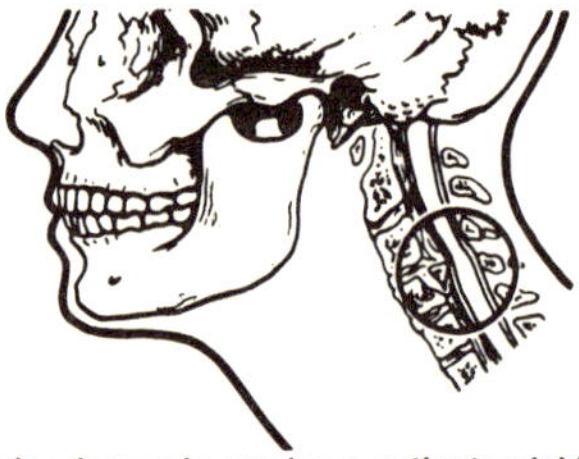

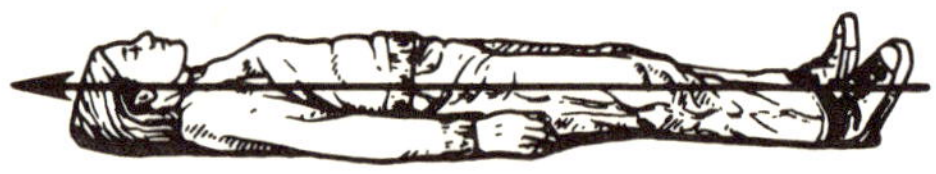

1. The major danger in moving a patient quickly is the possibility of spine injury.
2. In an emergency, every effort should be made to pull the patient in the direction of the long axis of the body to provide as much protection to the spine as possible.
3. It is impossible to remove a patient from a vehicle quickly and, at the same time, provide protection for his spine.

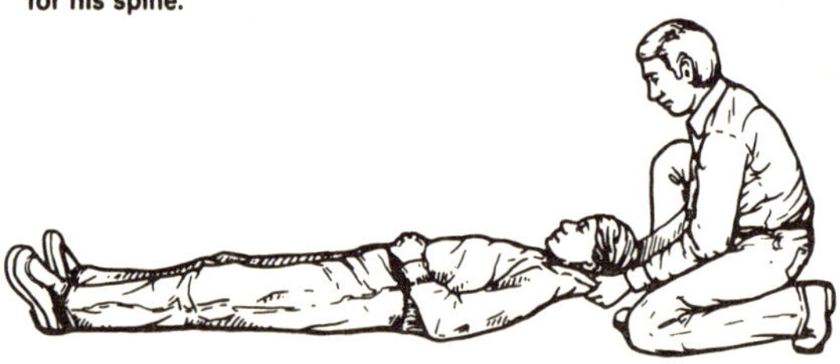

4. If the patient is on the floor or ground, he can be dragged away from the scene by tugging on his clothing in the neck and shoulder area.

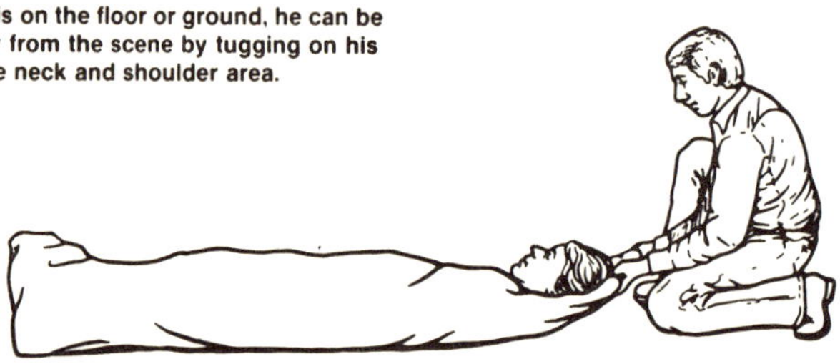

5. It may be easier to pull the patient onto a blanket and then drag the blanket away from the scene.
6. Such moves are emergency moves only. They do not really protect the spine from further injury.

7. Where possible, all injuries should be immobilized as much as possible prior to movement.
8. All injuries should be protected as much as possible during movement.

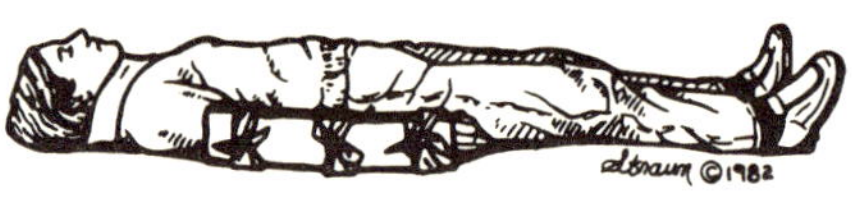

11. Don't try to do too much. Keep the victim safe and comfortable (as much as possible), and take measures to reverse life-threatening situations (such as bleeding), but don't try to be heroic when you don't need to be. It *is* possible to do too much for a victim; use the self-control necessary to do what is needed and then wait for help.
12. Keep bystanders away from the victim. You may need to enlist the help of others to accomplish this, but it's a critical part of first aid.

SELF-CARE EMERGENCY EXAMINATION OF THE SICK AND INJURED

Throughout any examination of the sick or injured you should briefly and in a general way explain what you are doing, why you are doing it, and what should be done about it. This will help alleviate the concern of the victim and involved bystanders. It will help you and others know what should be done and in what order. If the victim is conscious, ask questions about what he or she feels as you proceed. Table 5-1 lists those factors that you should check and gives you guidelines regarding signs and symptoms and their possible causes.

CHOKING

Choking is the inability to breathe caused by blockage of the throat; infection can cause choking, as can foreign bodies (usually food) lodged in the throat. Children often get objects such as marbles, coins, hard candy, and small pebbles lodged in their throats; in most cases, these objects do not completely obstruct breathing and can be dislodged easily. Any victim of choking aggravates the situation because of fear, panic, and anxiety.

Self-Care for Choking

An initial attempt at dislodging a blockage should be made by

TABLE 5-1

Assessing the Sick and Injured

CHECK	OBSERVE	SIGNS	POSSIBLE PROBLEMS/ CAUSES
BREATHING	Watch and feel for chest to rise and fall; listen for breathing; check skin color	No respiration; cyanotic; ashen-gray color or general death-like appearance	Respiratory arrest
		Rapid, shallow breathing	Airway obstruction; heart failure; shock
		Deep, gasping, labored, choking breathing	Hypertension, pain, hyperventilation
		Frothy blood at nose and mouth; coughing	Lung damage; fractured ribs; foreign bodies (bullets); pulmonary edema; severe lung contusions
PULSE	Feel carotid artery	Absent	Cardiac arrest; death
		Rapid, strong	Fright; heat stroke; hypertension; apprehension
		Rapid, weak	Shock; heat exhaustion; bleeding (hemorrhage); diabetic coma
		Slow, strong	Stroke; concussion
BLEEDING	Look for wounds Check body openings Feel clothing Feel body	Serious	Hemorrhage; shock
		Minor	Wound
		Internal	Closed wound
POISONING	Look in mouth Look for container Look at surroundings Listen to victim Ask observers Smell odors	Burns on mouth	Caustic poisoning
		Nausea	Drug overdose; ingested poison; poison inhaled in gas form; poison or drug injected; plant poisoning
LEVEL OF CONSCIOUSNESS	General observation	Brief periods of unconsciousness	Simple fainting; concussion
	Ask victim questions	Confusion, disorientation	Slight blow to head; psychiatric disorder; concussion; hysteria; alcohol or drug overdose; cerebral oxygen insufficiency; emotional disturbance
		Stupor	Cerebral oxygen deficiency; alcohol intoxication
		Deep coma	Concussion; brain damage; skull fracture; severe blow to head; diabetic shock; hysteria; poisoning
		Convulsions	Insulin shock; epilepsy

Table 5-1 (continued)

ABILITY TO MOVE	Ask victim to move extremities; use hand pressure test	Limited use of any or all extremities	Injury to spinal cord in neck
		Paralysis on one side	Injury to spinal cord in lower back
		Inability to move arms and hands	Pressure on spinal cord or in brain
		Inability to move legs and feet	Stroke; head injury with brain damage or hemorrhage
SKIN COLOR	Check extremities and fingernails; check inside of lips on dark-skinned victim	Red skin	High blood pressure; carbon monoxide poisoning; heart attack; skin burn
		White skin	Fright; shock; heart attack
		Blue skin (cyanosis)	Asphyxia; anoxia; heart attack; electrocution; poisoning
PUPIL REACTION	Lift victim's eyelids and check pupil response to light	Dilated	Shock; unconsciousness; cardiac arrest; brain damage; drug use or overuse; disorder of the central nervous system
		Constricted	Head injury; stroke
		Unequal	Head injury
		No response to light, eyes rolled back in head	Death; coma; false eye; cataracts
SKIN TEMPERATURE	Take temperature with thermometer, orally or rectally; feel with back of hand	Cool, clammy skin	Trauma; hemorrhage; shock; heat exhaustion; nervous stimulation; bleeding
		Cool, dry skin	Exposure to excessive cold
		Hot, dry skin	Fever (in illness); exposure to excessive heat (heat stroke)
REACTION TO PAIN	Touch victim in various spots	Numbness or tingling in extremities	Injury to spinal cord
		Severe pain and no pulse extremity	Occlusion of main artery to that extremity
		No feeling of pain or sensation with obvious injury	Hysteria; violent shock; excessive alcohol or drug usage; spinal cord injury
		General pain with injury	Body injury; probably no spinal damage
		Local pain in extremity	Fracture

slapping the victim sharply on the back between the shoulder blades. You can perform this technique whether the victim is standing up, sitting down, or lying on the floor. Blows to the back should be forceful, quick, and applied in rapid succession.

If your attempts at back-slapping are unsuccessful and if you are unable to see the object that is lodged (or if your attempts to dislodge the object with your fingers have forced the object further down into the throat where you can no longer reach it), use manual thrusts.

— Manual Thrusts — The Heimlich Maneuver —

Manual thrusting — also called the Heimlich Maneuver — can be performed on a victim who is either conscious or unconscious and who is standing, sitting, or lying down. The Heimlich Maneuver can be successfully used on any victim ranging in age from infants to adults. You can even perform it on yourself if you are choking and no one is present (or if those who are present do not know how to help you).

Heimlich Maneuver for Victims Who Are Standing or Sitting

If the victim is standing or sitting (even if the victim is unconscious), use the following technique:

1. Stand behind the victim.
2. Wrap your arms around the victim's waist.
3. Grasp your hands together in front of the victim.
4. With one hand, form a fist; place the thumb side of your fist against the victim's abdomen. The fist should be positioned slightly below the tip of the breastbone and slightly above the navel.
5. With your hands grasped, press your fist into the victim's abdomen with a quick, upward thrust.

If the object is lodged tightly, it may be necessary to repeat the thrusting motion several times. Watch for the object — it will come flying out of the victim's mouth with some force. Repeat the thrusting motions until you see the object (the victim may reach into his mouth and remove the object if it is forced into his mouth).

Heimlich Maneuver for Victims Who Are Lying Down

If the victim is lying down (whether the victim is conscious or unconscious), use the following technique:

1. Place the victim on his or her back.
2. Position yourself either by kneeling close to the victim's side or by straddling his or her hips or one of his or her thighs; assume the position that is most comfortable for you and that allows you the most strength in the thrusting. The size of the victim will probably determine which position you assume.
3. Place one of your hands on top of the other; the heel of your bottom hand should rest in the middle of the victim's abdomen, slightly below the rib cage and slightly above the navel.
4. Move forward so that your shoulders are directly over the victim's abdomen.
5. Press your hands quickly and forcefully toward the victim's diaphragm. The thrust should be rapid and upward.

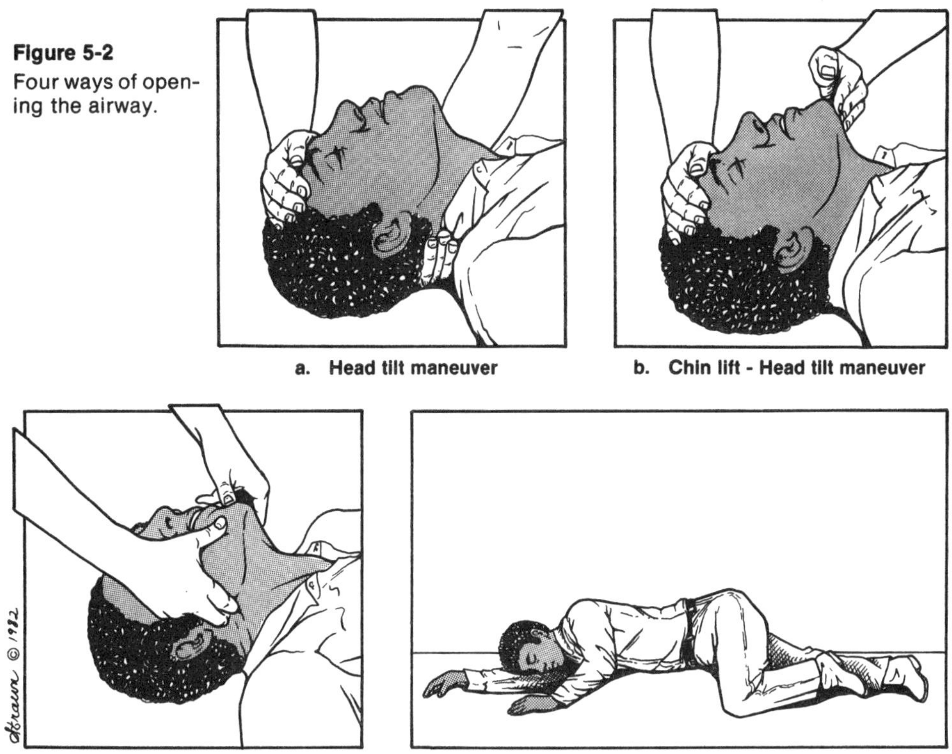

Figure 5-2
Four ways of opening the airway.

a. **Head tilt maneuver**

b. **Chin lift - Head tilt maneuver**

c. **Jaw thrust maneuver**

d. **Face down maneuver**

6. In the case of a small child or infant, rest the child on your forearm or thigh and use two or three fingers to accomplish the maneuver.
7. The above procedures are best learned under the direction of a qualified instructor. Such sessions are available through the American Red Cross.

Figure 5-3

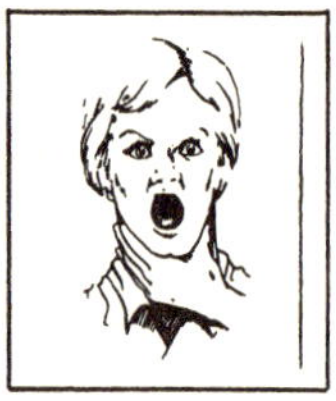

SUMMARY OF FIRST AID FOR CHOKING

1. If victim can cough, speak, breathe ▶ Do not interfere
2. If victim *cannot* cough, speak, breathe . . .
   a. Have someone call for help. Telephone ____________ (number)
   b. TAKE ACTION

FOR CONSCIOUS VICTIM

1

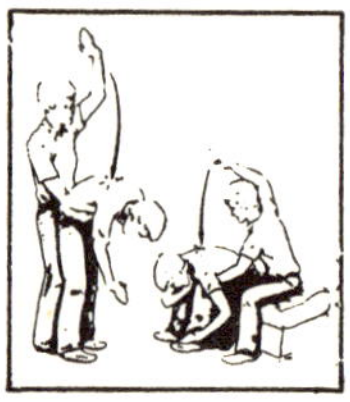

4 QUICK BACK BLOWS

2.

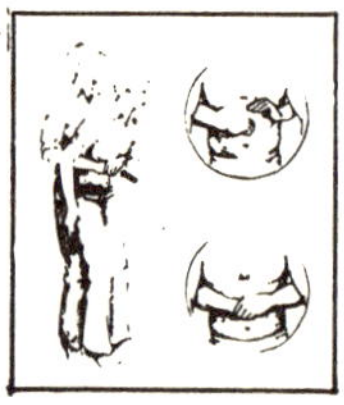

4 MANUAL THRUSTS

Repeat steps until effective or until victim becomes unconscious.

FOR UNCONSCIOUS VICTIM

1.

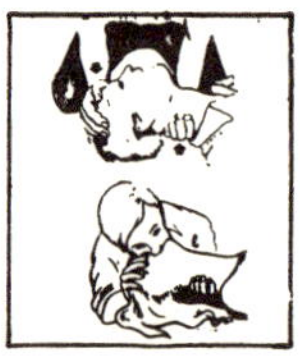

OPEN AIRWAY — TRY TO VENTILATE

2

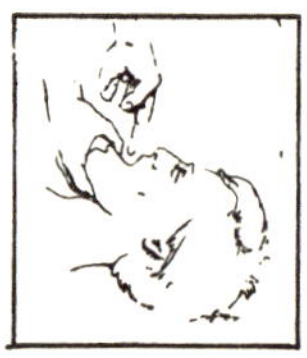

FINGER PROBE

3.

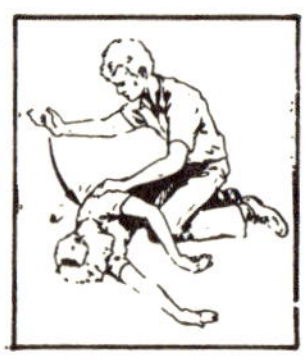

4 BACK BLOWS

4.

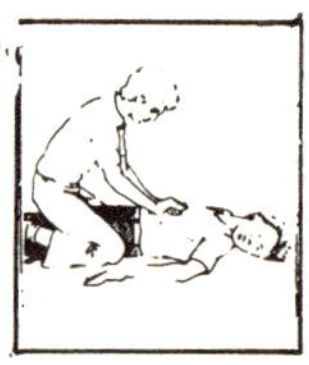

4 MANUAL THRUSTS

Repeat steps until effective.

Continue artificial ventilation or CPR, as indicated.

Source: Adapted from American Red Cross.

STOPPAGE OF BREATHING AND CIRCULATION

The respiratory (pulmonary) and the circulatory systems are vital body systems. If either fails for more than a short time, death will follow quickly. In terms of self-care, respiratory and circulatory emergencies must be treated at once in order to preserve life and prevent irreparable body damage.

Self-Care for Stoppage of Breathing

The instructions in **Figure 5-5** from the American Red Cross provide the necessary procedures for caring for a victim who has stopped breathing. Always call for emergency aid and have the victim transported to a hospital.

Self-Care for Stoppage of Breathing and Heart Beat

Cardiopulmonary resuscitation (CPR) is an emergency self-care procedure that combines artificial respiration with artificial circulation. It is

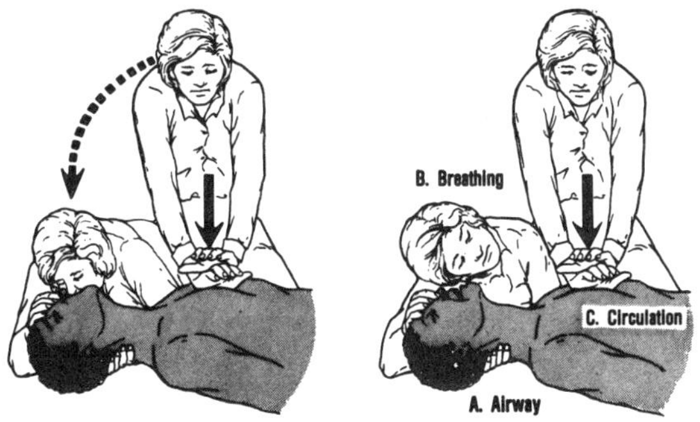

One-rescuer cardiopulmonary resuscitation (CPR)
15 chest compressions
— At rate of 80 per minute
2 quick lung inflations

Two-rescuer cardiopulmonary resuscitation (CPR)
5 chest compressions
— At rate of 60 per minute
— No pause for ventilation

1 lung inflation
— After each 5 compressions
— Interposed between compressions

Figure 5-4
One-rescuer and two-rescuer CPR.

used in self-care emergencies in which both circulation and breathing have stopped.

The administration of successful CPR requires special training. CPR must be learned through classroom instruction and practice under the direction of qualified personnel. It is strongly recommended that you avail

Figure 5-5

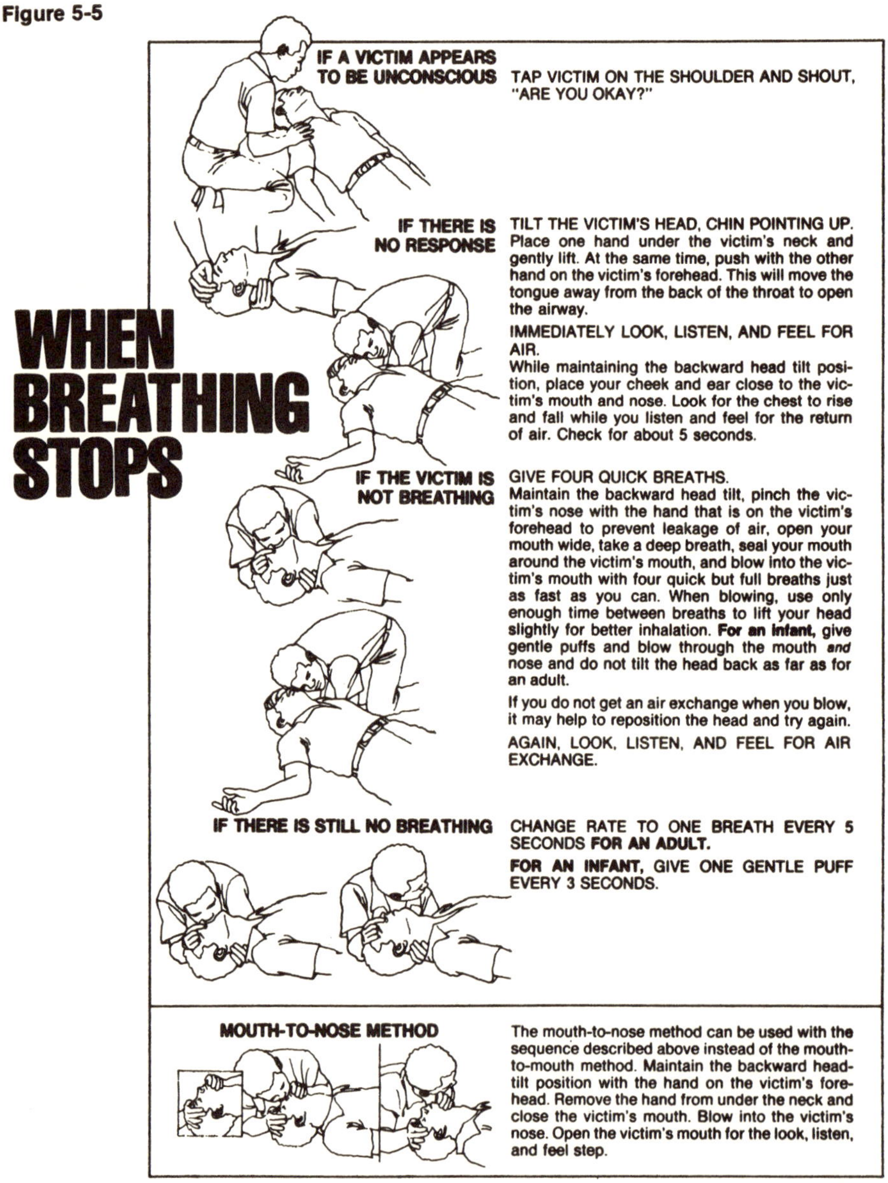

Source: American Red Cross

yourself of such training through either the American Red Cross or the American Heart Association in your community.

BLEEDING

The control of bleeding is secondary only to maintenance of air passages and restoration of breathing. A person's survival can be threatened by loss of a quart or more of blood.

Self-Care for Bleeding

The simplest and most preferred method to control severe bleeding is to place a dressing over the wound and apply pressure directly to the bleeding site with the palm of the hand. Although a sterile dressing should be applied, one may not be available at the time of the emergency, so the cleanest cloth on hand may have to be used. In the absence of a dressing or cloth, the bare hand may be used until a dressing is available. If the dressing becomes soaked with blood, another dressing should be applied over the first one with firmer hand pressure. The initial dressing should **never** be removed, because removal will disturb the blood clotting process.

Always see a physician for anything other than minor bleeding. And even with minor wounds, particularly puncture wounds, check with your physician to see if you need a tetanus shot.

POISONING

Over a million times each year in the United States alone, someone is poisoned. That poisoning may be the result of ingestion (such as the child who drinks his mother's kitchen cleaner), of contact with poisonous chemicals (resulting in dermatitus), of insect stings or bites, of snakebite, or of contact with poisonous plants.

Oral Poisoning

Basic Instructions

It is a medical emergency when anyone swallows a poison. Every nonfood substance should be considered a potential poison. Follow these procedures in poisoning emergencies:

1. Try to determine the probable poison and the amount swallowed. Carefully assess the person's condition.
2. If the poison container is available, read the label for ingredients of the poison.
3. Call the Poison Control Center and/or a local hospital emergency room.
4. While waiting for medical help, provide the following treatment.

Treatment for Oral Poisoning

1. Keep the person warm.
2. Make the person vomit, but remember that there are conditions in which the person should **not** be made to vomit:
   - When the person is unconscious or convulsing
   - When the poison swallowed is a strong corrosive, such as acid or lye
   - When the swallowed poison contains kerosene, gasoline, lighter fluid, furniture polish, or other petroleum distillates, unless instructed to do so by Poison Control Center. (Exception: If these are mixed with dangerous insecticides, then the poison must be removed.)

   To make the person vomit, give two tablespoonfuls (30 ml) syrup of ipecac. (Children under twelve—one tablespoon; infants—two teaspoons.) Follow this with one to two cups of water. If no vomiting occurs after twenty minutes, this dose may be repeated one time only. To stimulate vomiting, gently tickle the back of the throat with a spoon or similar blunt object.
3. Administer activated charcoal (two to four tablespoonfuls in a glass of water) after vomiting has occurred or if ipecac has failed to cause vomiting within an hour. Do not give activated charcoal before ipecac has had an opportunity to cause vomiting. Both ipecac and activated charcoal are available in most drugstroes and should be kept in your home, particularly where there are little children.
4. All poison victims should be seen by a physician.

Poison Ivy, Oak, and Sumac Poisoning

Signs and Symptoms

The signs and symptoms of poison ivy, oak, and sumac poisoning commonly include initial redness of the affected area followed by development of bumps and blisters; oozing lesions appear and crust over; severe itching accompanies symptoms; symptoms appear anywhere from four to seventy-two hours after exposure and are usually self-limiting.

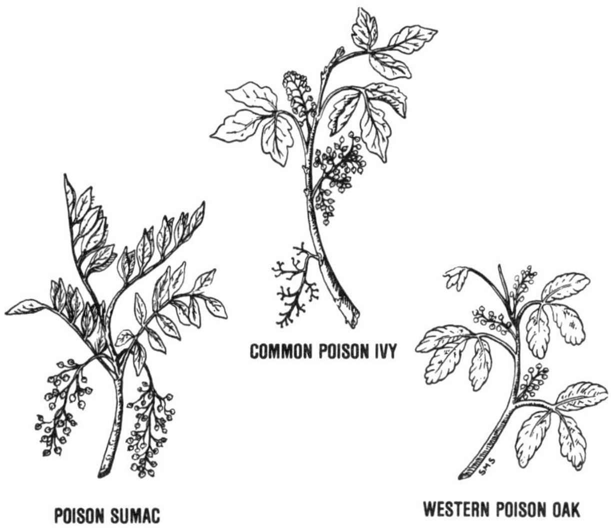

Figure 5-6
Common poisonous plants.

Self-Care

Self-care includes:

- Washing skin and clothing with soap and water, making sure that all soap is removed
- Wipe skin with solution of 70 percent alcohol
- Use wet compresses of cold water, boric acid, or liquid aluminum acetate to relieve inflammation while lesions are oozing
- Use calamine lotion to relieve itching
- Obtain allergy shots if you are in constant contact with plants or if symptoms are severe

Snakebite

Symptoms

Mild to moderate symptoms include mild swelling or discoloration and mild to moderate pain at the wound site with tingling sensations, rapid pulse, weakness, dimness of vision, nausea, vomiting, and shortness of breath. Severe symptoms include rapid swelling and numbness, followed by severe pain at the wound site. Other effects include pinpoint pupils, twitching, slurred speech, shock, convulsions, paralysis, unconsciousness, and no breathing or pulse.

Self-Care for Snakebite.*

Poisonous or nonpoisonous, a snakebite should have medical attention. A snakebite victim should be taken to a hospital as quickly as possible, even in cases when snakebite is only suspected. Meanwhile, take the following self-care measures:

- Keep the victim from moving around
- Keep the victim as calm as possible, preferably lying down
- Immobilize the bitten extremity and keep it at or below heart level
- If a hospital can be reached within four to five hours and no symptoms develop, this is all that is necessary

If mild to moderate symptoms develop, apply a constricting band two to four inches above the bite but **not** around a joint (i.e., elbow, knee, wrist, or ankle) and **not** around the head, neck, or trunk. The band should be three-fourths to one and one-half inches wide, **not** thin like a rubber band. The band should be snug but loose enough to slip one finger underneath. Be alert to swelling; loosen the band if it becomes too tight, but do not remove it. To ensure that blood flow has not been stopped, periodically check the pulse in the extremity beyond the bite.

If severe symptoms develop, incisions and suction should be performed immediately. Apply a constricting band, if not already done, and make a cut in the skin with a sharp sterilized blade through the fang mark(s). Cuts should be no deeper than just through the skin and should be one-half inch long, extending over the suspected venom deposit point (because a snake strikes downward, the deposit point is usually lower than

*American Red Cross leaflet

the fang mark). Cuts should be made along the long axis of the limb. **Do not** make cross-cut incisions; **do not** make cuts on the head, neck, or trunk. Suction should be applied with a suction cup for thirty minutes. If a suction cup is not available, use the mouth. There is little risk to the rescuer who uses his or her mouth, but it is recommended that the venom not be swallowed and that the mouth be rinsed.

If the hospital is not close (cannot be reached within four to five hours):

- Continue to try to obtain professional care by transportation of the victim or by communication with a rescue service
- If no symptoms develop, continue trying to reach the hospital and give the general self-care described above
- If **any** symptoms develop, apply a constricting band and perform incisions and suction immediately, as described above

BURNS

Over two million burn accidents occur each year in the United States. Of those who are burned (in fires, by chemicals, by the sun, in automobile accidents, or in other kinds of accidents), more than 70,000 require hospitalization; almost 10,000 of them die as a result of their burns. Of those that don't die, 1.9 million require medical treatment that may range from long-term rehabilitative surgery to simple self-care.

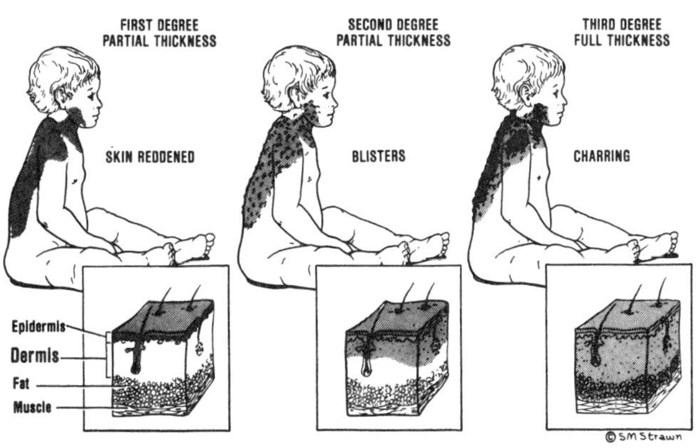

Figure 5-7
Classification of burns by degree of injury.

	Burn	Treatment	Consequence
1	First degree is red, sore, not blistered.	Cool the burn with tap water or cool compresses.	Heals without scarring in about six days.
2	Second degree is blistered and painful. It may ooze fluid.	Apply cool water. Remove clothing that is not stuck to the wound; remove jewelry. Lay victim flat. Use cool compresses on the way to the hospital. Don't cool a large portion of the body — shock may occur. If the burn area is large, cover the person loosely with a clean sheet. If he has chills, cover him with a blanket too. Second and third degree burns require emergency care, maybe hospitalization.	Heals in two weeks with slight scarring.
3	Third degree is white, brown, or charred; it may be painless at first.		Can take months, even years to treat. Grafting operations reduce scarring and deformity, but scars are inevitable.

Self-Care for Burns

1. If clothing is on fire, immediately extinguish flames. Use the means that will be the quicker — either water or whatever other nonflammable liquid is at hand — or smother the fire with a heavy wrap (coat, blanket, or rug) followed by rapid cooling with water. Never allow the victim to run.
2. For scald burns, cool immediately by immersing the extremity or holding it under running, cool water. If the trunk is involved, pour cool water on the affected area.
3. Lie the victim flat. Rapidly remove any overlying clothing and constrictive articles such as rings, bracelets, or boots, before swelling occurs. Compress the injured area with cool, moist dressings. If an extremity is injured, soak it in cool water.
4. For a serious injury, arrange rapid transportation to a hospital, maintaining cool compresses to injured areas during transport.
5. Don't cool a large portion of the body — shock may occur. If the burn area is large, cover the person loosely with a clean sheet. If he or she has chills, cover the victim with a blanket, too.
6. Remove clothing that is not stuck to the wound; remove jewelry. Lie the victim flat. Do not attempt to remove clothing stuck to a burn.
7. Don't break blisters, and do not put any grease, ointment, petroleum jelly, or medication on severe burns.
8. Anything other than a mild burn should be seen by a physician.

FROSTBITE

Exposure to abnormally cold temperature can cause extensive tissue damage.One of the most common and dangerous cold injuries involves frostbite—the actual freezing of body cells.

Symptoms of Frostbite

The body part that has become frostbitten will have gone from being very painful to being absolutely numb, whether it is your hands, feet, ears, or nose. (That is the order in which parts of the body are most apt to become frostbitten.)

When you look at the frostbitten part, it will be pale and cold to touch and may feel like a chunk of marble or a stick of wood.

All frostbite, regardless of how mild or severe it is, looks and feels this way at first.

Self-Care of Frostbite

Rapidly rewarm the frozen part unless the body tissues have already been thawed and refrozen.

1. The best method of rapid rewarming is to immerse the frozen part in a large container, preferably a bathtub or whirlpool bath if available. Use water between body temperature 102° F. and 108° F. It will take twenty to forty-five minutes to thaw the frozen part in water at this temperature. Avoid water hotter than 108° F. Continually monitor the water temperature. As the water cools, hot water should be added, but do not pour it directly on the injured part.
2. If a tub is not available, the next best method is to use a hot, moist towel. Constantly change the towel to maintain the recommended temperature level. Place the towel gently on the frozen area without rubbing.
3. If the frostbite is superficial and wet heat is not available, hands can be rewarmed by placing them under the armpit, against the abdomen, or between the legs. Feet can be warmed by placing them in the armpit or against the abdomen of a friend.

4. When the part is warm, encourage the victim to move it gently to aid in the restoration of circulation. But if the affected parts are feet or legs, do not allow the victim to walk.
5. Get the victim to a physician. All frostbite, no matter how mild, should be seen by a doctor.

HYPOTHERMIA

Hypothermia — literally meaning a low amount of heat inside the body — results when the body's inner core lowers in temperature.

Symptoms of Hypothermia

If a person's temperature starts to drop from a normal of 98.6° F. and is not reversed, the consequences can be fatal.

The first response to cold in the body's attempt to conserve heat is a constriction of the blood vessels close to the surface of the skin, then of the tissues under the skin. This causes the skin to grow pale and allows more blood flow to the brain and internal organs in an attempt to maintain heat.

As the body continues to lose heat, it attempts to produce more by shivering (involuntary action of muscles to generate heat). The shivering eventually becomes intense and uncontrollable.

As heat loss continues, the more severe effects of hypothermia set in. Basically, the body slows down. The blood is sluggish. The brain is starved for oxygen. Efforts to produce heat have exhausted the victim. He or she also suffers from a lack of sugar in the blood, which causes dizziness, a lightheaded feeling, and even nausea. The victim becomes disoriented and starts to stumble. Shivering begins to subside, and muscles become more rigid, causing incoordination and stumbling. The exposed skin may become blue and puffy. Speech becomes thick and thinking disoriented, and amnesia may develop.

Self-Care of Hypothermia

A hypothermia victim may deny that he or she is in trouble. Believe

STAGES OF HYPOTHERMIA
(General Body Cooling)

1) Shivering - an attempt by the body to generate heat.
2) Apathy.
3) Unconsciousness with a glassy stare, slow pulse and slow respiration rate.
4) Freezing of the extremities.
5) Death.

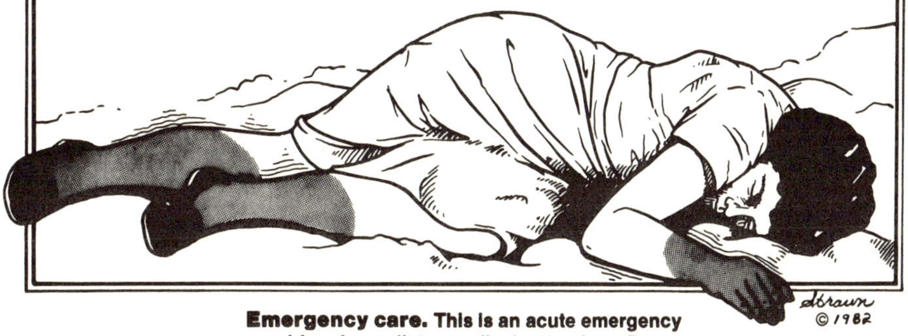

Emergency care. This is an acute emergency requiring immediate medical attention. Emergency care includes:

Keep the patient dry - replace wet clothing.
Apply external heat to both sides of the patient using whatever heat sources are available including the body heat of rescuers.
If the patient is conscious and in a warm place have him breathe warm moist air or oxygen if available.
Monitor respirations and pulse and provide pulmonary and cardiopulmonary resuscitation as required.
Do not give hot liquids by mouth.
Do not allow patient to exercise.
Handle the patient gently.

Figure 5-8

the **symptoms** — not the victim. Even mild symptoms demand immediate, drastic treatment, especially in camping or hiking situations when shelter, heat, and help are not readily available. The following steps should be followed for a hypothermia victim:

1. Get the victim out of the wind and rain.
2. Strip off all wet clothes.
3. If the victim is only mildly impaired:
   - Give warm drinks
   - Get him or her into dry clothes and a warm sleeping bag
   - Well-wrapped, warm (not hot) rocks or canteens placed close to victim's body will hasten recovery

4. If the victim is semiconscious:
   - Try to keep the victim awake. Give warm drinks if the victim is alert enough
   - Leave the victim stripped. Put him or her in a sleeping bag with another person (also stripped). If you have a double bag, put the victim between two warm donors. Skin to skin contact is the most effective treatment
5. Build a fire to warm the camp.
6. **If available,** have the victim breathe warm, moist air or oxygen.
7. Get to a hospital as soon as possible.

HEAT EMERGENCIES

Excessive exposure to extreme heat may result in heat exhaustion or heat stroke. Although the external cause of heat injuries is the same, there are important differences between heat injuries that must be clearly

Figure 5-9

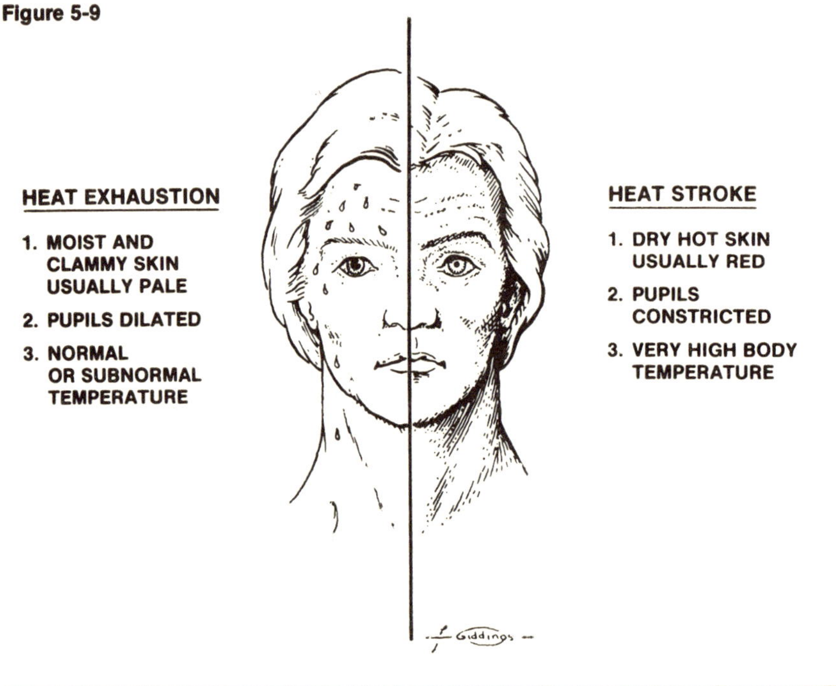

understood. Each condition represents a different bodily reaction to excessive heat, and for this reason, the signs, symptoms, and self-care are also different.

Symptoms of Heat Emergencies

The symptoms of **heat exhaustion** are pale, moist, clammy skin with dilated pupils and normal or subnormal temperature, while symptoms of **heat stroke** — a life-threatening condition — are dry, red, hot skin with constricted pupils and a very high body temperature.

Self-Care of Heat Emergencies

Self-care of heat exhaustion involves moving the victim to a cool spot and trying to get him or her to drink salty liquid. Also, remove the victim's clothing and cool the victim off by bathing him or her with cloths soaked in cool water or alcohol. Usually the person feels better promptly. If not, the person should be seen by a physician.

If the person is obviously feverish, the injury is probably heatstroke, and minutes count. You **must** get the victim's temperature started down immediately. Call for an ambulance, then strip off the victim's clothes and start cooling with whatever means you can find. A bath in a tub of cold water and ice is ideal, but a massage with ice cubes or ice packs is more likely to be practicable. Rub the victim's arms and legs with handfuls of ice cubes. Get others to help if possible.

The patient should be rushed to the hospital emergency room as soon as possible to allow professionals to take over.

SPRAINS

A sprain is an injury to the ligaments around a joint or to the joint covering itself, producing undue stretching or tearing of these tissues.

Symptoms of Sprains

Symptoms include pain around the joint, inability to use the joint, rapid and marked swelling, and discoloration of the area around the joint.

Self-Care for Sprains

1. Place the joint at rest in an elevated position.
2. Pack the sprained area in ice to reduce swelling, control internal bleeding, and reduce pain. Do not apply heat.
3. Wrap the joint firmly with a bandage.
4. Keep the injury elevated for at least twenty-four hours, and continue ice treatment periodically. Do not cause frostbite.
5. If pain and swelling continue or if a fracture is suspected, get medical attention.
6. After twenty-four to forty-eight hours, moist heat can be applied.

STRAINS

A strain is an overstretching of muscles and/or tendons, causing muscle bundles and tendons to stretch and possibly rupture.

Strains usually occur in the back area due to lifting improperly or lifting something that is too heavy.

Symptoms of Strain

Symptoms include stiffness when moving back and leg muscles and muscle spasm in the low back region with terrible pain that may radiate down the leg.

Self-Care for Strains

1. Rest the affected area and apply warm, moist heat.
2. Use of a board under the mattress or lying on a firm surface like the floor is recommended for a strained back.
3. Severe strains should be seen by a physician.

Figure 5-10

WHEN TO APPLY HEAT, WHEN COLD

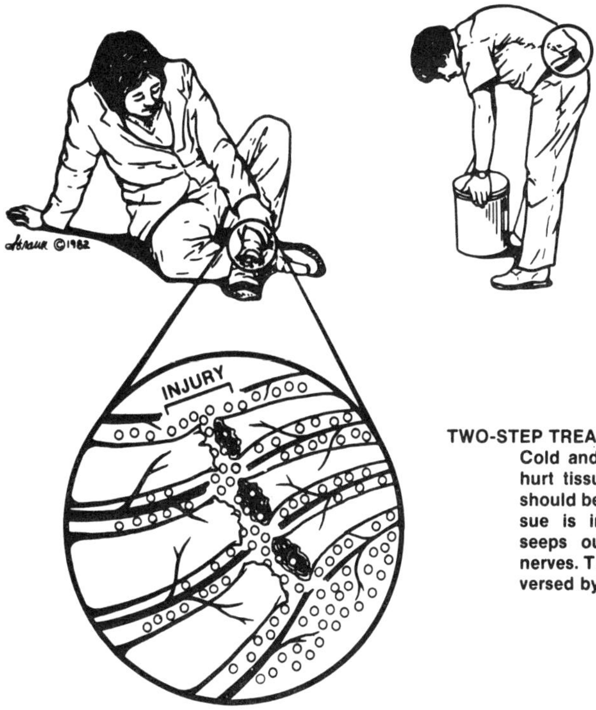

TWO-STEP TREATMENT FOR A STRAIN OR SPRAIN
Cold and heat are common prescriptions for hurt tissues of a sprain or strain, but which should be used? The answer is both. When tissue is injured, inflammatory fluid (circles) seeps out around torn blood vessels and nerves. The damage is slowed by cold, then reversed by heat.

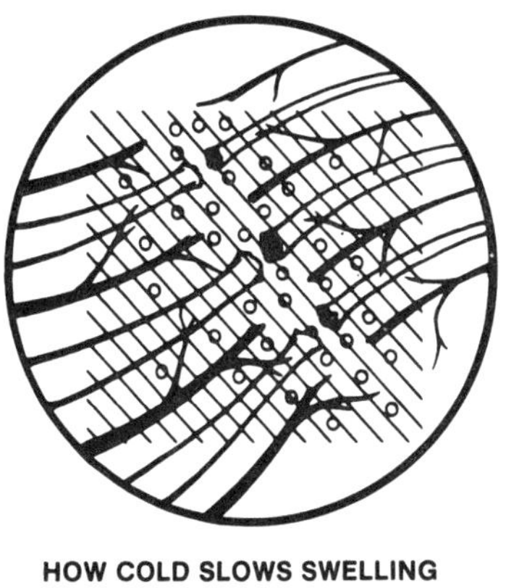

HOW COLD SLOWS SWELLING
Cold packs should be applied immediately after injury and used off and on for the first 24 to 72 hours, to reduce inflammation and start recovery. The cold (line pattern) constricts swollen blood vessels, restricting bleeding and fluid seepage. Cold also relieves pain by reducing muscle spasms and slowing nerve impulses.

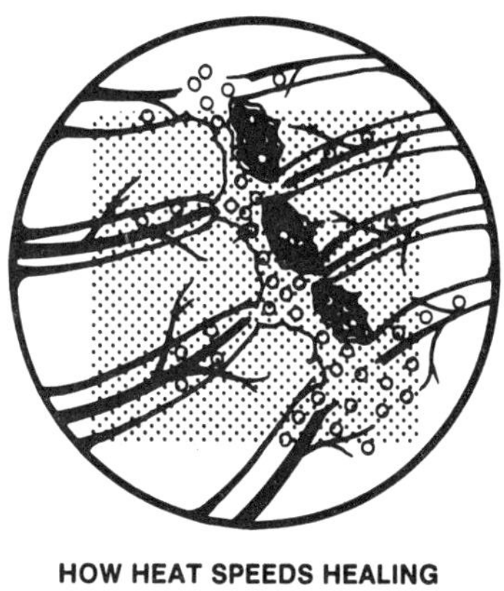

HOW HEAT SPEEDS HEALING
After cold reduces inflammation, heat (dot pattern) dilates blood vessels to increase blood flow, bringing in nutrients and repair agents such as scar-tissue cells and white blood cells that carry debris away. Heat also accelerates chemical processes, speeding the growth of cells to repair breaks in tissue.

FRACTURES AND DISLOCATIONS

A fracture is a broken or cracked bone that may either be open or closed. In an open fracture, the bone is broken and a wound is present. In a closed fracture, the bone is broken but no open wound is present.

A dislocation is when one or more of the bones forming a joint slips out of a normal position.

Signs and Symptoms

- Pain or tenderness in the region of the fracture
- Deformity or irregularity of the affected areas
- Loss of function (disability) of the affected area
- Moderate or severe swelling
- Discoloration
- Victim's information, if conscious (the victim may have felt the bone snap or break.)

Self-Care for Fractures and Dislocations

Splints are used to support, immoblize, and protect parts with injuries such as known or suspected fractures, dislocations, or severe sprains. When in doubt, treat the injury as a fracture and splint it. Splints prevent movement at the area of the injury and at the nearest joints. Splints should immobilize and support the joints or bones above and below the break.

Certain guidelines should be followed when splinting:

- Gently remove all clothing from any suspected fracture or dislocation.
- Do not attempt to push bones back through an open wound.
- Do not attempt to straighten any fracture.
- Cover open wounds with a sterile dressing before splinting.
- Pad splints with soft material to prevent excessive pressure on the affected area and to aid in supporting the injured part.
- Pad under all natural arches of the body such as the knee and wrist.
- Support the injured part while the splint is being applied.
- Splint firmly, but not so tightly as to interfere with circulation or cause undue pain.

- Tie all knots on or near the splint.
- Do not transport the victim until the fracture or dislocation has been supported.
- Elevate the injured part and apply ice packs when possible.

Examples of various splinting procedures are shown in the accompanying illustrations.

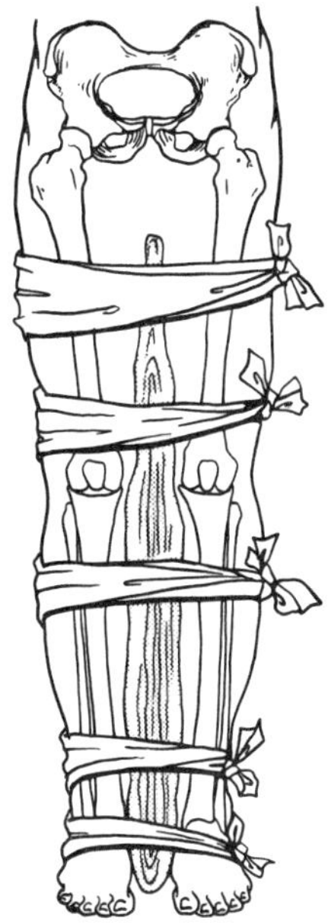

Figure 5-11
Improvised self-splint. Improvised splints may be made from pieces of wood, broom handles, heavy cardboard, newspapers, magazines, or other firm materials.

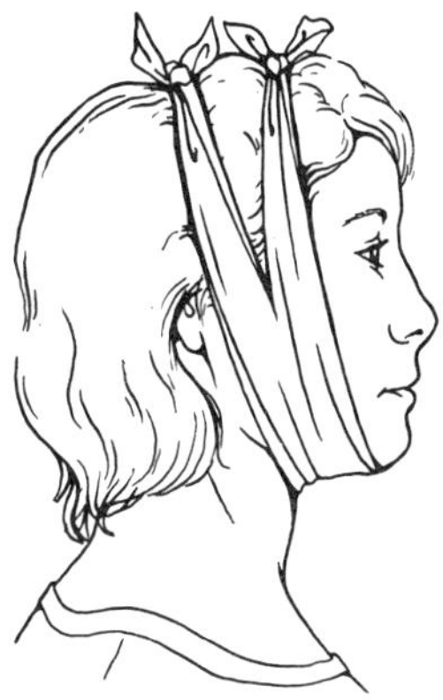

Figure 5-12
Immobilizing a fractured jaw with a four-tailed bandage.

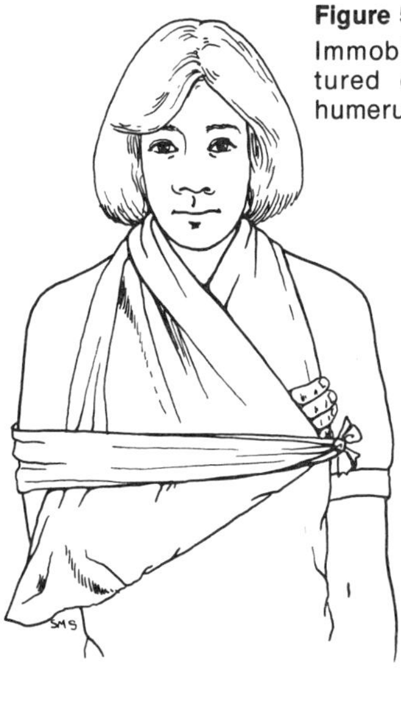

Figure 5-13
Immobilizing a fractured collarbone or humerus.

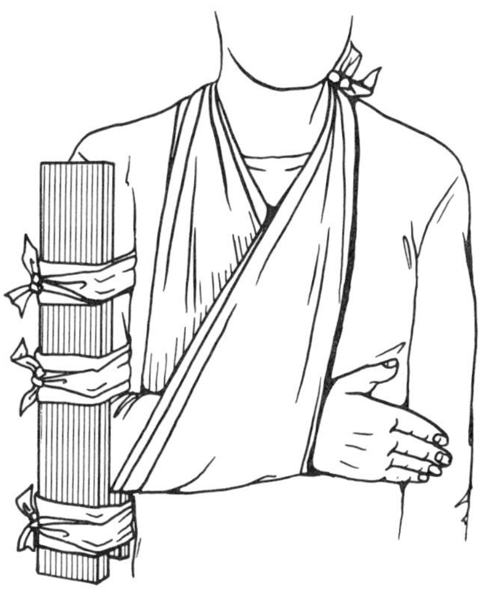

Figure 5-14
Immobilizing a fractured upper arm.

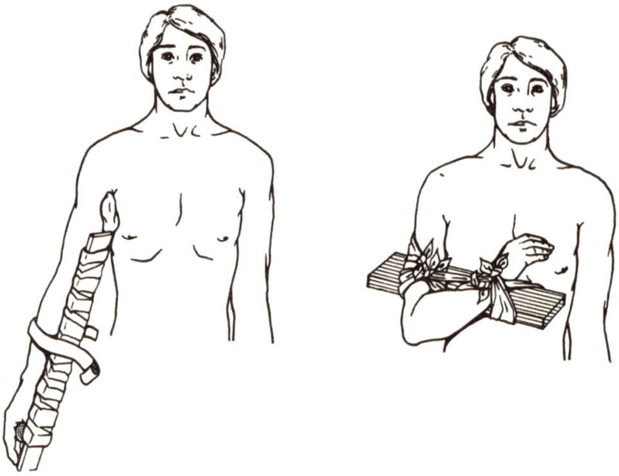

Figure 5-15
Immobilizing a fractured elbow. Do not bend or straighten the arm. Splint the elbow in the position in which it is found.

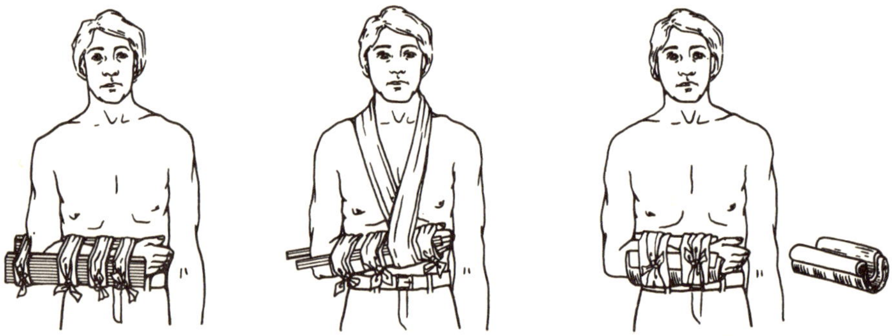

Figure 5-16
Immobilizing fractures of the forearm, wrist, and hand.

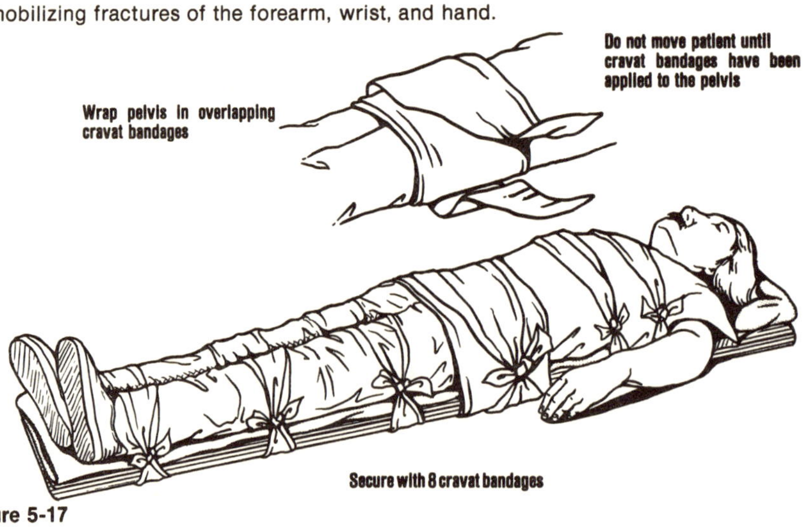

Figure 5-17
Immobilizing a fractured pelvis. Do not move the person until cravat bandages have been applied to the pelvis. A cravat bandage is a triangular bandage that is folded.

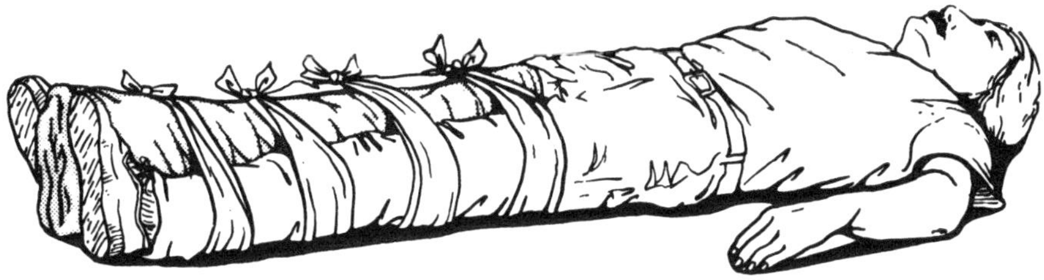

Figure 5-18
Improvised splint of the thigh and knee.

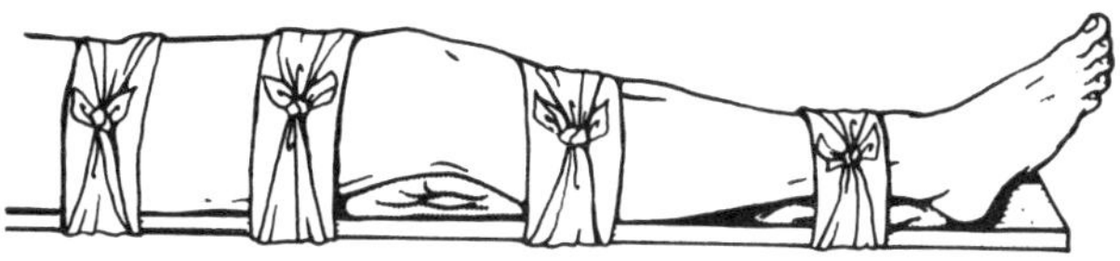

Figure 5-19
Immobilizing a fractured kneecap.

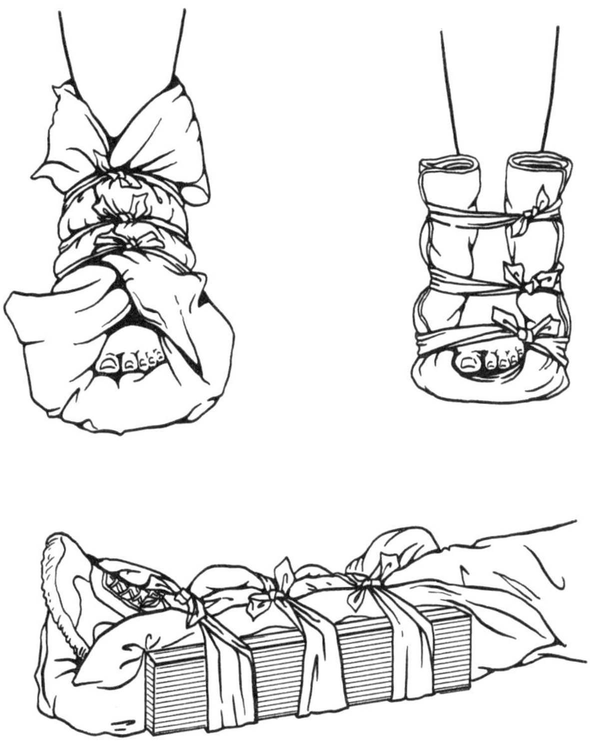

Figure 5-20
Immobilizing a fracture of the ankle and foot.

CONVULSIONS

What Causes Convulsions?

A convulsion is an attack of total or partial unconsciousness accompanied by rigidity and spasm of the muscles. Convulsions are often symptomatic of an underlying condition, although they do not always indicate disease. Possible causes include low blood calcium, congenital defects, lack of oxygen, severe gastrointestinal illness, or the onset of acute infectious diseases. Low salt intake, acute or chronic kidney disease, stroke, chronic alcoholism, poisoning from strychnine and lead, injury (especially fracture of the skull), malaria, neurotic disease, tetanus, congenital injury, meningitis, sinusitis, infection in the middle ear, encephalitis, brain tumors, heat stroke, hysteria, and low blood sugar may also cause convulsions. In children, any general infection, gastroenteritis, ear infections, pneumonia, urinary infections, and a high fever (over 105° F.) can bring on convulsions. Convulsions in children between six months of age and four years of age **usually** do not indicate any serious ailment; however, convulsions that develop during later stages of measles, mumps, and other childhood diseases are serious and may indicate central nervous system complications. Convulsions sometimes occur when a woman develops a condition called toxemia during pregnancy. This attack of convulsions is called eclampsia.

Signs and Symptoms

Convulsions usually have a violent onset and last from a few minutes to half an hour. The muscles go rigid, followed by jerky spasms with bluish facial and lip discoloration and foaming or drooling at the mouth. The victim may stop breathing, bite the tongue severely, or lose bladder and bowel control.

In some nonepileptic seizures, the victim staggers but doesn't fall, makes purposeless movements, utters unintelligible sounds, and is confused.

As the convulsion subsides, the victim may be irritable, drowsy, or disoriented. Quiet stupor or deep sleep may follow. Convulsions seldom cause death. If the victim dies, it is usually from an injury or disease, not from the convulsion itself.

Self-Care Treatment

1. If the victim starts to fall, lower him or her gently to the ground. Do not forcefully restrain the victim, but protect the victim from hurting him or herself.
2. Turn the victim's face to the side to prevent choking on saliva. If necessary, help the victim onto his or her stomach — the victim is better off on the stomach than on the back because of the danger of choking. Do not shake or scream at the victim.
3. Do not place anything in the victim's mouth. Jamming objects in the mouth can do more harm than good.
4. If the attack is long and breathing stops, give mouth-to-mouth resuscitation.
5. Give the victim nothing to eat or drink.
6. Loosen any constricting clothing, and allow the victim to pass naturally through the attack.
7. When the victim recovers, do not question or disturb him or her. Protect the victim from embarrassment and from curious onlookers both during and after the attack.
8. Call a physician, particularly if repeated convulsions occur.

EPILEPTIC SEIZURES

What Is Epilepsy?

Epilepsy is a chronic physical disease often accompanied by seizures. The most common types of seizures are grand mal, petit mal, and psychomotor. Little is known about the cause of epilepsy except that it is not hereditary and is not associated with mental illness or insanity. Most epilepsy can be controlled with proper medication and medical care. Seizures rarely result in serious injury.

Signs and Symptoms of Seizures

A grand mal seizure is characterized by sudden loss of consciousness. If the victim is standing, he or she falls with boardlike rigidity; this soon changes to rapid, generalized, jerking muscle movements. Gradually the spasms disappear; the victim may pass into a deep sleep that lasts for several hours. When the victim awakens, he or she may be confused or ill-tempered. The victim probably will have no recollection of the seizure. He or she may also manifest abnormal behavior, such as incoherent speech, extreme restlessness, and confusion.

Petit mal seizures last only from five to twenty-five seconds. The victim pales and seems to stare vacantly into space. The eyes may roll back into the head, and the head, eyes, or upper extremities may jerk slightly. The victim is usually alert and able to continue normal functioning when the spell has passed.

Psychomotor seizure is characterized by automatic, stereotyped movements or a variety of abnormal behavior associated with clouding of consciousness and partial amnesia. The victim may become belligerent or antagonistic, roam from place to place, have a temper tantrum, or even become destructive.

Regardless of the type of seizure, the epileptic may experience an "aura" — a warning that the attack is about to occur. Almost any strange feeling, such as an unusual feeling of depression, excitement, pain in the limbs or abdomen, trembling, or a strange odor, may warn of the imminent onset of a seizure.

Self-Care Treatment of Seizures

1. Keep calm. You can't stop a seizure once it has started; you shouldn't try to restrain or revive the victim.
2. Don't forcefully restrain the victim, but do what you can to prevent him or her from falling.
3. Loosen any tight clothing, especially around the neck.
4. Put a pillow or a rolled-up coat under the victim's head. Clear any sharp objects or hard objects away from the victim to prevent injury.
5. Place the victim on his or her side so that mucus will drain from the mouth.
6. Don't be concerned if the victim stops breathing.
7. Give mouth-to-mouth resuscitation if the victim does stop breathing. The victim will usually start breathing again quickly.
8. Consciousness will return naturally following the seizure. Allow the victim to rest if he or she is drowsy or disturbed following the seizure; if the victim seems alert and normal, allow him or her to resume normal activities.

When to Seek Medical Help

Call a doctor immediately if the victim passes from one seizure to another without regaining consciousness or if the victim does not regain consciousness quickly following a seizure.

INSULIN SHOCK

When the level of insulin in the body is greater than the body needs or uses, insulin shock occurs. The conditions that foster insulin shock — too much insulin and too little blood sugar — result when a diabetic has not eaten enough, when the diabetic has exercised more than usual and has burned up more carbohydrates, when a diabetic injects too much insulin, or when a diabetic has diarrhea or vomiting.

Signs and Symptoms

The signs and symptoms of insulin shock include dizziness, weakness, nervousness, irritability, rapid pulse, belligerence, hostility, confusion, disorientation, and profuse sweating. Insulin shock mimicks drunkenness: the victim staggers, has poor coordination, and may become stuporous or lose consciousness. The skin is usually pale, moist, cool, and clammy; there is slow, shallow breathing.

Self-Care Treatment

1. If the victim is conscious, ascertain that he or she is diabetic.
2. If the victim is conscious, give him or her orange juice, soft drinks, sugar cubes, or candy to help increase the blood sugar level. Do not give a diabetic in insulin shock a diet soft drink. Some diabetics carry candy or special quick-sugar commercial preparations in plastic, soft-tipped containers that can be squeezed into the mouth.
3. If the victim is unconscious, look for a diabetes identification bracelet or necklace. Rub a sugar cube on the victim's tongue, or place a small amount under the tongue, but give only as much as can be absorbed. Do not give the victim anything to eat or drink.

SYMPTOMS OF LOW BLOOD SUGAR

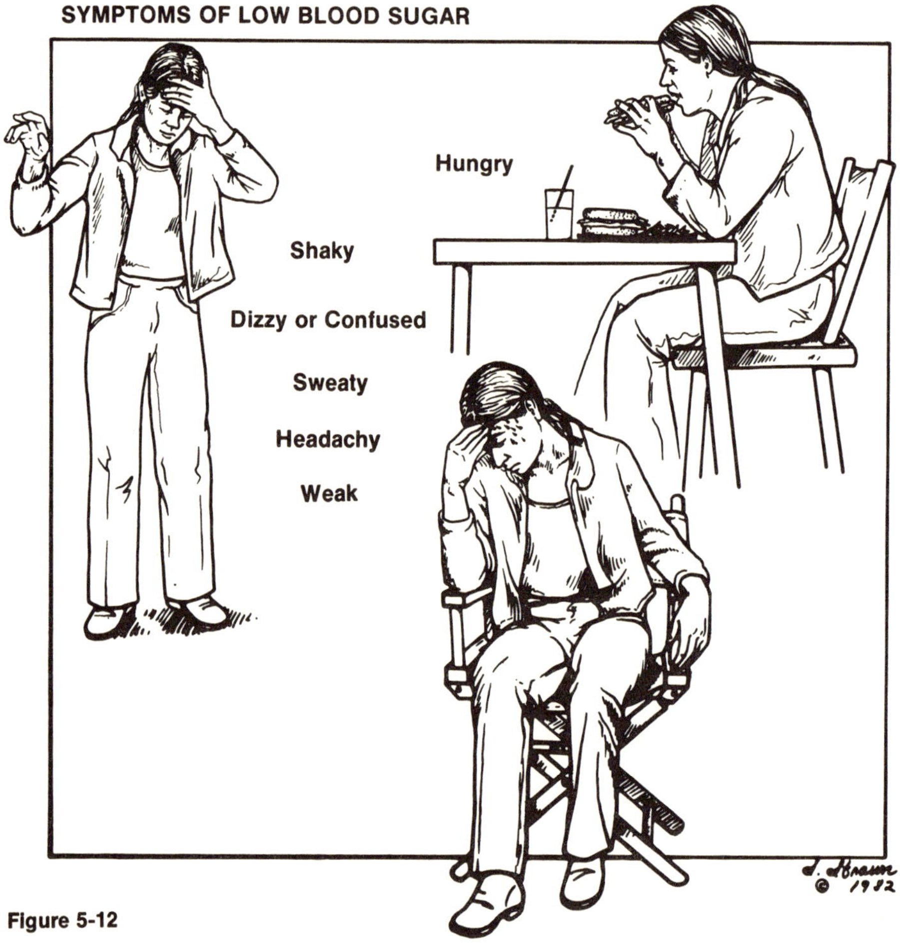

Figure 5-12

When to Call the Doctor

Call a doctor or transport the victim to a hospital immediately if he or she regains consciousness but does not seem to recover, or if the victim does not regain consciousness within ten to fifteen minutes after you have started treatment.

DIABETIC COMA

When carbohydrates are not metabolized quickly enough and gather in a diabetic's bloodstream, the blood sugar level rises above the insulin level and results in diabetic coma. Common situations that lead to diabetic coma are undiagnosed diabetes, a diabetic who forgets to inject insulin at the prescribed time, a diabetic who undergoes stress or illness, a diabetic who does not inject insulin in the prescribed dosage, or a diabetic who eats or drinks too much.

Signs and Symptoms

Diabetic coma comes on gradually, usually over a period of days. Signs and symptoms include thirst, frequent urination, confusion, dis-

Figure 5-22

SYMPTOMS OF HIGH BLOOD SUGAR

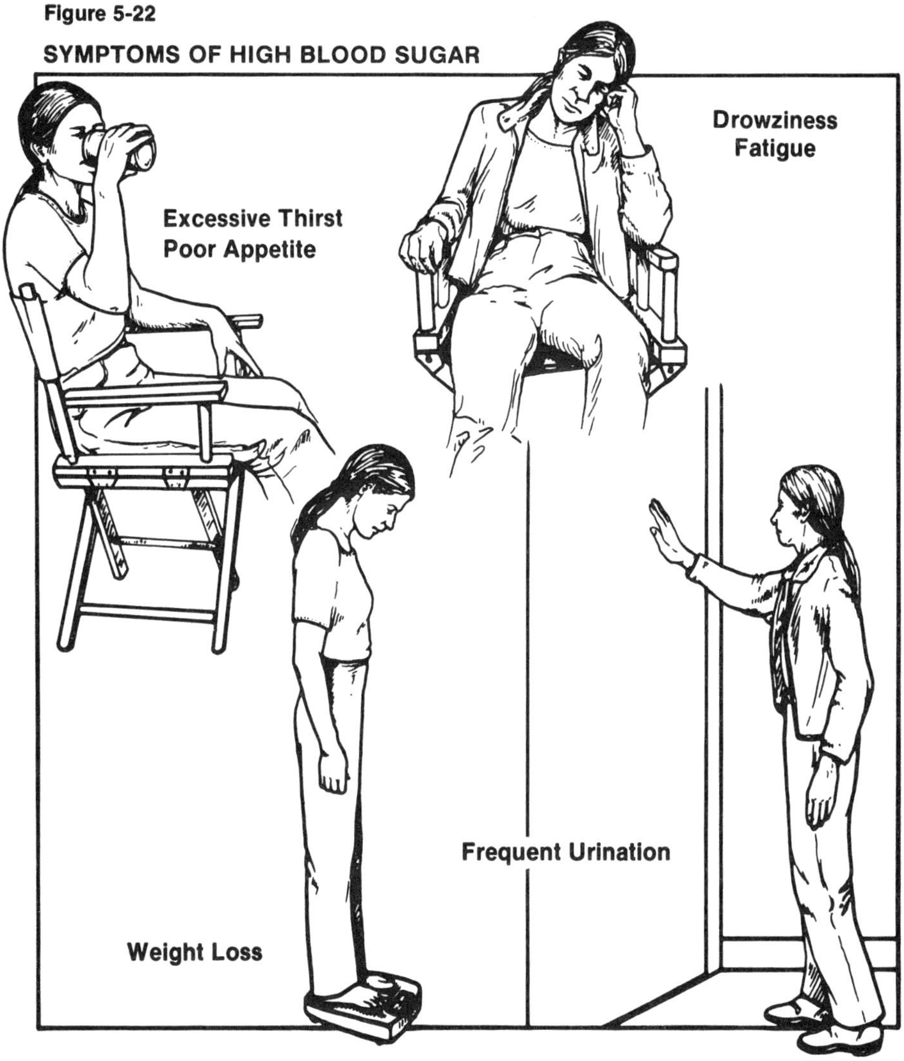

orientation, stupor, a sweet, winelike odor on the breath, an acetone odor on the breath, dry flushed skin, deep red lips, fever, intense hunger and thirst, frequent vomiting, weak rapid breathing, absent pulse, and coma. If the condition is not corrected, the coma leads to eventual death.

Self-Care Treatment

Any victim of diabetic coma should be transported to a doctor or hospital immediately. If you are trained to administer insulin and if the victim is conscious, you should help him or her administer insulin to correct the condition before transportation to a doctor.

If you cannot administer insulin and if there is no doctor or hospital available, follow these treatment guidelines:

1. Keep the victim lying down flat or with head and shoulders raised slightly.
2. Keep the victim warm.
3. If the victim is conscious, give the victim fluids that do not contain sugar or starches. A baking soda/salt water solution is good to use.

FEVER

A fever does not always mean the presence of disease — food, excitement, anxiety, exercise, or wearing too much clothing can all elevate the body temperature. Exercise can result in a fever of as much as 103° F. In most cases, however, fever does signal the onset of disease — generally viral pneumonia, bacterial infection, colds, sore throat, earache, mumps, measles, chicken pox, appendicitis, heat stroke, polio, or tonsillitis.

A fever usually peaks during the late afternoon or early evening. Once a fever has "broken," the skin will feel cool and clammy.

A common symptom of fever is chilling — the body responding to fever as it would to a drop in the outside temperature.

Self-Care Treatment

1. Stay in bed and rest. Sleep if you can.

2. Increase your fluid intake. Aim for at least twelve eight-ounce glasses of clear liquid each day that the fever persists.
3. Take aspirin to relieve muscle aches and control fever.
4. Sponge your skin with tepid (lukewarm) water — the evaporation provides a cooling effect.
5. Take a tepid bath. Even though cold water would increase conduction of heat away from the body, water temperature of about 70° F. is considered tolerable.

Fever in Children

A child can generally withstand a higher fever than an adult can; in cases of extremely high fever, the child may experience convulsions, known as **febrile** convulsions. If the child's fever is above 105° F. orally (106° F. rectally), follow these self-care guidelines:

1. Put the child in a cool bath for up to thirty minutes.
2. Rub the child's skin from head to toe with a solution of equal parts of rubbing alcohol and cool water.
3. Wrap the child in a wet sheet that has been soaked in a quart of water and half a pint of rubbing alcohol. If you don't have a sheet, use wet cloths; keep the cloths wet by changing them frequently.
4. Administer a cool water enema of one teaspoon of salt dissolved in a pint of cool water.

If the child experiences a febrile convulsion, turn the child on his or her stomach and turn the face to the side to prevent choking. Don't put your finger between the child's teeth, and don't shake the child or shout at him or her. If the child begins to turn blue or bites his or her tongue, wrap a cloth around a spoon handle or a stick and put it between the teeth — don't try to force it if the teeth are clenched. Take measures described above to cool the child while someone calls the doctor.

Caution: There has been some recent concern about giving infants and children aspirin for fevers caused by chicken pox and other viruses because it may induce Reye's syndrome—the symptoms of which range from severe vomiting to brain damage and possible death. Consult your physician concerning aspirin use in these cases.

WHAT TO DO WHEN YOUR CHILD IS FEVERISH

Here's what pediatricians recommend.

1. **Keep your child cool.** Dress him lightly. Just a shirt and diaper or underpants is fine.
2. **Use no blankets,** or just a sheet, in bed.
3. **Keep room temperature cool** (65 to 70 degrees).
4. **Give plenty of cool, clear liquids** to replace fluid lost by sweating. Sometimes milk upsets a feverish child's stomach. Give ice water, juice, or fruit drinks instead. Offer them frequently in small amounts. For bottle-fed infants, your pediatrician may suggest temporarily replacing formula with a commercially prepared pediatric solution, like Pedialyte or lytren, containing water, dextrose, sodium, potassium, and other minerals the body needs.
5. **For temperature of 104 degrees F. or over, sponge the child in the bathtub with lukewarm water** for twenty minutes to bring down the fever. Use long, firm, soothing strokes to bring blood, and the heat it carries, to the skin's surface, where the water will help cool it by evaporation. Don't use ice-cold water; this will cause shivering, a body reaction to cold designed to conserve heat and raise body temperature.
6. **Don't give fever-reducing drugs** like baby aspirin or acetaminophen to infants unless the doctor suggests it. If he does use the following dose schedule.
7. **Know about convulsions,** a possible complication of sudden, high fevers. Convulsions can occur with such common conditions as ear infections, colds, or tonsillitis when the fever rises rapidly to the 105 range or higher. Keep calm. Have someone call the doctor. Lay the child down. Place a rolled piece of paper or cloth between his teeth at one side of the mouth to keep him from biting his tongue. Take off his clothes. Sponge him off with cool water until his temperature comes down. Though alarming to parents, convulsions usually are over in a few minutes and seldom are dangerous. Do notify a doctor, however.

Adopted from: Parents Magazine, June 1980 p. 70

When to Call the Doctor

Call the doctor if:

- You have a fever of 101° to 102° F. for two days without explanation (no obvious illness)
- You have a low-grade unexplained fever for five days
- Your neck is stiff (you can't touch your chin to your chest)
- A feverish child looks ill, even though his or her fever is low
- A feverish infant is under four months of age
- A feverish child loses his or her appetite and won't eat or drink
- Fever in a child goes above 106° F. orally or 107° F. rectally

For a description of procedures for taking temperature, see the section on temperature in Self-Determination of Vital Signs (Chapter 2).

SWOLLEN GLANDS

Two types of glands are generally most susceptible to swelling: lymph and salivary. The lymph glands are part of the body's defense mechanism against disease; they appear in the neck, the groin, and the axillary (armpit) regions. They act as filters to trap bacteria so that infection can't spread rapidly throughout the body. When the glands are swollen, it generally means that they are doing their part to contain infection, although glands may swell without the presence of infection.

When the glands in the neck swell, it usually indicates the presence of a sore throat or an ear infection. When the glands in the groin area swell, there is probably an infection in the feet, legs, or genitals. A scalp infection may make the glands behind the ears swell. Swelling in the lymph glands in the front or the side of the neck is seldom serious; most serious is swelling in glands above the collarbone, in the back of the neck, or in both armpits.

If glands become red and tender in addition to swelling, there may be an infection in the gland itself.

Soreness in a gland usually disappears rapidly, but the gland may remain swollen for a longer period of time while the body struggles to fight the infection.

Bacterial infections or the mumps may cause the salivary glands, located in front of and below the ears, to swell.

Self-Care Treatment

No special treatment for swollen glands is required. You should observe them over the period of swelling to see if they enlarge or if others begin to swell. Take aspirin to relieve pain.

When to Call the Doctor

Call the doctor if:

- A gland that is swollen is red and tender
- The salivary glands swell
- Swollen glands persist for more than three weeks
- Glands behind the ears swell

- Swollen glands are present for more than five days when accompanied by a fever

CONCUSSION

Concussion is a brain injury usually caused by a blow to the head. All head injuries are potentially serious. Although the brain is completely surrounded by a protective cerebrospinal fluid and membranes and is completely encased by bone, it can still be injured by a sharp blow. Brain injuries swell, causing pressure within the skull. There is also danger of bleeding inside the skull; continued pressure from bleeding can compress the brain, and eventual brain damage or death is possible due to brain compression or impaired circulation to the brain.

Signs and Symptoms

Symptoms include signs of a bump, blow, or laceration on the head, mild or severe headache, loss of orientation, inability to answer simple questions, unequally dilated pupils, semiconsciousness or unconsciousness, possible leg or arm paralysis, slow pulse, weak and rapid heartbeat, irrationality, persistent nausea or vomiting, leakage of blood or fluid from the ears, nose, or mouth, and black eyes.

If the concussion is severe, the victim cannot be easily awakened after falling asleep. Any loss of consciousness after apparent recovery is a dangerous and serious sign of continued bleeding inside the skull with consequent compression of the brain. Such a condition may produce personality changes months after the injury, amnesia, and increasing lethargy. Vomiting in adults is rare and is indicative of severe injury. The headache associated with concussion should disappear overnight.

Self-Care Treatment

All cases of concussion should receive medical aid. Until you are able to get a doctor to the scene, follow these treatment guidelines:

1. Keep the victim lying down and quiet.

2. If the victim's face is red, elevate the head and shoulders slightly. If the face is white or ashen, do not elevate the head. Remember: "Face is red, raise the head; face is pale, raise the tail."
3. Never give the victim any kind of stimulant.
4. Keep the victim in a darkened room.
5. Keep the victim warm.

A victim who vomits more than twice, who shows marked sleepiness, who has an unsteady gait, who has unequal pupils, who has peculiar eye movements, or who suffers from disorientation or amnesia is more seriously hurt and is in more immediate need of medical care.

UNCONSCIOUSNESS

Unconsciousness refers to complete unawareness of surroundings and inability to make purposeful movement. Sleep is the only normal state of unconsciousness.

Fainting is brief unconsciousness; coma is prolonged, deep unconsciousness; stupor is partial, transient unconsciousness.

The most common cause of unconsciousness is intoxication from alcohol or sleeping pills; the second most frequent cause is head injury. Other leading causes include strokes, diabetic coma, insulin reactions, overdoses of prescription drugs, and poisons (such as carbon monoxide, industrial gases, heroin, and other chemicals found in the environment). Shock and bleeding may bring on unconsciousness, and some psychiatric conditions cause a comalike condition.

Self-Care Treatment

If the cause of unconsciousness is not apparent, and until specific treatment can be given, do the following:

1. Make the victim as comfortable as you can; loosen any tight clothing.
2. Check to see if the airway is obstructed; start mouth-to-mouth resuscitation if the victim is not breathing.
3. Examine the victim carefully. Look for signs of head injury, bleeding,

spinal injury, poisoning, and so on. In the presence of a witness, examine the victim's personal belongings for an identification bracelet or wallet card that indicates that the victim has diabetes, hypertension, or epilepsy.

4. Place the victim on his or her side; turn the victim's face down with the jaw jutting out so that saliva and mucus drain freely from the mouth.
5. Don't move the victim unless you have to to prevent him or her from sustaining further injury (to remove the victim from a burning building, out of a puddle or corrosive chemical spillage, and so forth).
6. Do not flex, extend, or twist the neck if you suspect that the victim might have sustained cervical spine injury.
7. Never give an unconscious person anything by mouth.
8. Do not attempt to stop drainage from the ears or nose; just lightly cover with a dressing.
9. Get medical help as soon as you can.

HEADACHE

Headache is the most common symptom of mankind. Ranging from mild to severe, headache can cause pain that is general or regional, concentrated or intermittent, penetrating or throbbing, radiating or pressured, or bursting. Headache can stem from any of a number of causes —most of them organic (brain tumor, high blood pressure, neck injury, head injury, low blood sugar, allergy, infection, or dental problems) or environmental (sun glare, loud music, freezing temperatures) in nature. There are three general types of headaches: migraine, sinus, and tension.

Migraine Headache

Two-thirds of those who suffer migraines inherit the trait, and 80 percent of all migraine sufferers are women. A **prodrome** — a generalized warning similar to the epileptic's aura — may appear hours or days before the headache, but the headache's onset is generally sudden and harsh. The migraine headache is caused by the vessels in the brain first constricting, then dilating.

A number of factors cause migraine headache — depending on the weaknesses of the individual. Common causes include faulty sleeping patterns, faulty rest, overwork, sudden relaxation following a period of intense strain, certain foods (common among them cheese, yeast, chocolate, wine, and citrus fruits), and certain odors (among them hair spray,

Over the Counter Pain Killers (Analgesics)

Aspirin. By far the most common pain-killer is aspirin, listed as either aspirin or acetylsalicylic acid on labels. It seems to be almost a cure-all, relieving pain, cooling fevers, reducing swelling, and relieving the ever-elusive headache.

Unfortunately aspirin can have some side effects in some people. It can cause an asthma-like attack, chronic hives, ringing in the ears, and bleeding in the lining of the stomach in some people, particularly those taking large doses.

Salicylamide. Salicylamide can be considered a "first cousin once removed" to aspirin. Salicylamide essentially does the same job as aspirin. It relieves pain, cools fevers, and reduces inflammation. And, because it has a slightly sedative effect, it is used in some sleeping pills. Salicylamide does not have many of aspirin's undesirable side effects: Specifically, it is safe for people who are allergic to aspirin, and it does not cause gastric distress or gastric bleeding, as aspirin does.

Unfortunately, there aren't many products on the market that contain only salicylamide—*Sal-Eze* and *Zarumin* are two. It is, for some reason, most commonly combined with aspirin in pain relievers such as *Excedrin, Excedrin P.M.,* and *B.C.*

Phenacetin. Phenacetin, unrelated to either aspirin or salicylamide, reduces fever and relieves pain, but it is not effective in reducing inflammation. It doesn't have many of aspirin's side effects.

But taken in large doses for a prolonged period, it can result in serious kidney impairment and can cause or worsen kidney disease.

It's listed on the labels of the pain-killers that contain it. Some of the more common include *Empirin, A.P.C., Bromo-Seltzer,* and *Duradyne.*

Acetaminophen. Acetaminophen is chemically related to phenacetin, but it is considered the safest of the four pain-killing over-the-counter medications. It reduces fever and kills pain, but it is not effective in treating inflammation. Safe for those who are allergic to aspirin, it produces none of the undesirable side effects that aspirin causes. It is the pain-killer and fever-reducer most often used in children's medications.

Again, you can identify products containing acetaminophen by checking labels. Some of the most common products that contain acetaminophen include *Datril, Liquiprin, Percogesic, Tylenol, Tylenol Extra-Strength,* and *Bayer Non-Aspirin.* Acetaminophen is included as an ingredient and is mixed with other analgesics (including aspirin) in products like *Vanquish, Bromo-Seltzer, Excedrin,* and *Excedrin P.M.*

Caffeine. Although it is not an analgesic, caffeine is used in many pain medications because of its effect on headaches. It constricts the blood vessels, providing relief for some forms of migraine headache.

Caffeine is always listed on the label; it is an ingredient in *Anacin, Cope, A.P.C., Empirin Compound, Vanquish, Excedrin,* and *Excedrin P.M.*

nail polish, perfume, powder, rubbing alcohol, shaving cream, soap, flowers, shoe polish, chalk, copying machines, ink, dry-cleaned or ironed clothing, newspapers, and auto emissions).

Signs and Symptoms

The pressure of swelling blood vessels causes intense, throbbing pain to suddenly appear and worsen, usually on only one side of the head and usually in the same location each time. Other symptoms include nausea and vomiting, irritability, blurred vision, sensitivity to light and sound, constipation or diarrhea, redness and swelling of the eyes and nasal lining, elevated blood pressure, temporary blindness, blind spots, chills, tremor, dizziness, and excessive urination.

The headache generally lasts from two to forty-eight hours.

Self-Care Treatment

Try to sleep or rest in a dark room. Do not bend your head forward or move or stop suddenly. An ice pack on your head can sometimes afford some relief; take aspirin to help relieve pain.

Check with your doctor to see if he or she recommends direct pressure on the blood vessel that runs directly under your jaw angle on the same side as the headache (never apply such pressure to both sides of the neck at the same time, or you will cut off blood supply to the brain). Avoid eating foods that may trigger or worsen your headache — including, besides those listed above, bologna, salami, bacon, t.v. dinners, packaged nuts, potato chips, canned soups, seasoning mixes, and Oriental foods that contain monosodium glutamate.

Recent emphasis has been placed on the benefits of relaxation — such as exercise, yoga, chiropractic manipulation, transcendental meditation, hypnosis, and biofeedback — in migraine therapy. Massage of the head and neck may also be helpful in reducing pain.

Sinus Headache

Congestion, nasal blockage, inflammation, allergy, nasal polyps, the common cold, upper respiratory infections, tooth abscesses or infection, fatigue, poor diet, alcohol, and smoking all cause the sinuses to inflame, resulting in sinus headache. Sinus headache tends to be worse in damp weather and during times of heavy pollution.

Signs and Symptoms

Pain, usually moderate, dull, and aching, occurs over the sinuses, usually between the eyes. The pain is most severe in the morning and lessens throughout the day. Accompanying symptoms include difficulty in breathing, low-grade fever, irritability, sore muscles, or a stiff neck.

Self-Care Treatment

Stand erect with your head steady, or sit in an upright position in bed. Apply hot or cold compresses to the area that is causing pain. Get as much rest as you can, and don't drink alcohol. Do not smoke. Reduce the dust in the atmosphere as much as you can; a humidifier will reduce dust and will increase the moisture content of the air.

Avoid using over-the-counter nasal sprays or decongestants without your doctor's approval.

Tension Headache

One-third to one-half of all headaches are tension headaches — headaches that are brought on by worry, anxiety, strain, muscle tension, or depression.

Signs and Symptoms

Prior warning in the form of nausea, weakness, fatigue, or visual disturbance may precede a tension headache. The pain — which may last for weeks, months, or even years — is dull, steady, and throbbing; the steady, pressing ache is almost like having on a hat that is too tight. Accompanying symptoms may include nausea, diarrhea, fatigue, loss of appetite, sleeplessness, inability to concentrate, ringing in the ears, dizziness, or runny eyes. In addition, the muscles of the jaws, neck, back of the head, and temples may become tense and tender.

Self-Care Treatment

To gain relief from a tension headache, massage the scalp and the back of the neck; apply hot packs (moist heat) to the head, and take hot baths. Get extra rest. Lie down with your eyes closed and your head supported; take aspirin with milk or food (to prevent stomach upset). Eliminate anything that may be causing stress or strain; change your activities often, and get as much fresh air as you can.

Headache in Children

Forty percent of all children have had a headache by the time they reach the age of seven; 4 percent of all seven-year-olds have frequent headaches. Three-fourths (75 percent) of all children have experienced a headache by the time they are fifteen. A child's headache should respond to the same kind of therapy as an adult's. Call a doctor if the child gets a stiff neck (is unable to touch the chin to the chest), or if the child experiences marked irritability, lethargy, severe pain, visual difficulty, repeated vomiting (more than twice), purple spotted rash, head injury in association with the headache, or unexplained fever, or if the headaches are recurrent or a single headache lasts longer than three days.

When to Call the Doctor

Regardless of the type of headache or its origin, call a doctor if you experience fever, paralysis, weakness, numbness, double vision, speech impairment, difficulty in using your arms or legs, or a stiff neck. You should also call a doctor if the headache persists for longer than two days, if the headaches are recurrent, if they are worse in the morning, if they rapidly increase in frequency and severity, or if they are associated with head injury.

INFECTIOUS MONONUCLEOSIS

Infectious mononucleosis — commonly known as the "kissing disease" — is believed to be caused by the Epstein-Barr (EB) virus and is spread through close physical contact with an infected person.

Signs and Symptoms

A blood disease, mono still has researchers baffled. It is not known how long a person is contagious, and the course of the disease depends on the general health of the victim. The illness develops slowly and may be mistaken for a number of other diseases — including strep throat, diphtheria, meningitis, appendicitis, rubella, cancer, or leukemia — before a diagnosis is finally made.

Symptoms of mono include general malaise, headache, fatigue, chilliness, fever, loss of appetite, puffy eyelids, swollen lymph glands in the neck and upper part of the body, sore throat, tonsillitis, difficulty in swallowing, bleeding gums, nausea, vomiting, and jaundice. The fever may go as high as 105° F. and can last as long as a week; the swollen glands are tender and firm and may last for several weeks; they range in size from a bean to a small egg. In some cases, no symptoms are present; others suffer from a wide range of severe symptoms.

Self-Care Treatment

Because there is no cure for the EB virus, treatment for infectious mononucleosis centers on relieving the symptoms. While most symptoms last for several weeks, they can last only a few days or can persist for months. (Children generally have only a mild case of mononucleosis that does not produce many symptoms and that lasts only a few days.)

You should avoid strenuous exercise, but if you are not tired, you should not confine yourself to bed. On the other hand, if you are tired and weak, rest in bed. In some cases, the spleen and liver become enlarged with mono; avoid lifting, straining, and engaging in competitive sports.

Take aspirin to reduce fever and to relieve the pain of headache, muscle ache, and joint pains. If you have a sore throat, gargle with salt water (one teaspoon of salt to eight ounces of warm water) every two hours, and suck on a throat lozenge or hard candy. Use a humidifier or vaporizer to keep the air in your home moist.

If you have an earache, take aspirin and apply heat to the affected ear (a heated juice glass or an electric heating pad are best).

When to Call the Doctor

You should see your doctor at the onset of mononucleosis symptoms so that he or she can use a blood test to diagnose the condition; since mono mimics so many other diseases — some of them serious — it is critical that you be diagnosed correctly so that you do not end up omitting treatment for another serious condition.

If you develop signs of a secondary infection — most notably a high fever after your initial fever has subsided, swollen lymph glands in the armpits or groin, redness and tenderness that begin anywhere in the body, or symptoms that arise midway through the disease (most symptoms that will accompany mono are present at the beginning of the disease, by the time you get a fever) — call your doctor immediately, since he or she will need to initiate antibiotic therapy.

A severe pain or tenderness in your abdomen could signal problems in the spleen or liver. Although it is not common, the spleen can rupture as a result of mono, and it represents a surgical emergency. Call your doctor immediately if you develop such pain, especially if it is accompanied by high fever.

INSOMNIA

Many people in the United States have sleeping problems. Some have difficulty falling asleep, some awaken early in the morning, some experience periods of wakefulness furing the night, and some do not feel that their sleep is satisfying enough.

Over-The-Counter Sleeping Pills

You should take the following measures before you choose a sleeping pill:

- Read the label carefully. The only thing you need in a sleeping pill is something to make you drowsy—an antihistamine. Choose a sleeping pill that has a single ingredient. Acquaint yourself with the possible side effects of antihistamines and discontinue use if you develop a side effect. The major antihistamine used in over-the-counter sleep aids is methapyrilene. Recent research has revealed that it may be a cancer-causing agent.
- Don't use a sleeping pill that does not clearly list all its ingredients. Don't use a sleeping pill if you are unsure about one of the ingredients or if you are confused about what one of the ingredients does.
- Don't use a sleeping pill that contains a bromide.
- Don't use sleeping pills that contain extra ingredients, such as aspirin, unless you need the aspirin for pain relief of a headache associated with the tension.
- Over-The-Counter sleeping pills are often ineffective. It is best to correct the cause of insomnia rather than use a sleeping pill.

You may wonder how much sleep a person needs to function efficiently and effectively. Some sources suggest that seven to eight hours during a twenty-four hour period is the norm; however, amount of sleep needed is purely an individual matter. Some people need nine to ten hours of sleep, while others may be able to get along with five to six hours of sleep a night.

Several factors may cause insomnia. Age is a factor in that if you are over sixty years of age, you will undoubtedly sleep less than when you were younger. Stress from life change can produce sleep loss. Physical illness and psychological problems (such as anxiety and depression) can also cause sleep difficulties. Some individuals are considered to be "night owls," but this may be because their bodies' inner clocks are set for sleep at later hours than "normal." Other sleep difficulties can occur as a result of rotation of work shifts and jet lag. Insomnia may result from repeated use of drugs (for medical purposes or otherwise) and alcohol.

Signs and Symptoms

Difficulty sleeping may result in irritability and a feeling of physical tiredness or weariness. Also, someone with sleeping problems may be unable to concentrate on work or other daily activities.

Self-Care Treatment

If your sleep problems are severe or prolonged, you may wish to consult your physician, who may prescribe some type of prescription sedative as a sleep aid. However, in using such sedative preparations, you should be aware of some adverse effects that may result:

- Sedatives may reduce essential dream time or may affect the nervous system such that sleep-disrupting dreams occur
- Repeated sedative use may cause tolerance to such medication
- Persons may become psychologically dependent upon sedatives for sleep induction

Before you ask your doctor for a prescription medication, or before you ask your pharmacist for an OTC sleep aid, you might consider some of the following suggestions:

1. Try to get as much exercise during the course of the day as is

reasonable and possible.
2. Wear comfortable night clothes.
3. Make sure that your sleeping conditions, such as your bed, are as comfortable as possible.
4. Learn to associate your bedroom with sleep.
5. Keep your bedroom dark and quiet.
6. Reading should be light and relaxing. Avoid vigorous mental stimulation before bed.
7. Avoid alcoholic beverages before bedtime, and avoid beverages that contain caffeine after lunchtime.
8. If you cannot sleep, don't worry about it — this will make you less able to fall asleep. Rather, get up and pursue some relaxing activity that you enjoy.
9. Avoid taking naps during the day, as this decreases your ability to sleep at night.

CHAPTER 6

COMMON SKIN COMPLAINTS

DANDRUFF

Dandruff — a common and simple problem — results from oily scales on the scalp. Dandruff can also appear at other places on the body — most usually the eyebrows — and often coexists with other problems of the scalp, including psoriasis.

While it is a common problem, dandruff is often stubborn, and treatment usually has to be repeated often to be effective. Although it is ugly, it is rarely dangerous; in some rare cases, it may make the scalp more susceptible to bacterial or yeast infection.

Signs and Symptoms

Fine, white, oily scales appear on the scalp and in the hair; these scales often fall from the hair onto the shoulders. In some cases, mild scalp redness may be present, but it is only slight. The scales are confined to the scalp and eyebrows.

Treatment

Most of the over-the-counter dandruff shampoos are helpful if your dandruff is mild or moderate. Follow package directions strictly, since incorrect usage may result in oiliness or yellow discoloration of the hair. In more stubborn cases, over-the-counter shampoo that contains selenium sulfide can be effective against dandruff; again, follow package instructions carefully.

When to Call the Doctor

If, despite your treatment efforts, your dandruff grows worse instead of improving over the course of several weeks, call your doctor; you may have psoriasis or some other problem in addition to dandruff.

ECZEMA

One of the most common skin conditions, and one of the most frustrating to treat, is eczema — a noncommunicable disease that generally occurs in families with a history of hay fever allergies. Eczema is a common allergic reaction among children, but it afflicts adolescents and adults as well and results because the skin is unable to retain adequate amounts of water.

Childhood eczema often begins in infancy; the rash first appears on the face as red, chapped cheeks. From there it progresses to the neck, folds of the elbows, and folds of the knees. It is due in most cases to dust, inhaled pollens, or foods such as nuts, chocolate, dairy products, eggs, and fish.

Signs and Symptoms

The oozing, moist, red, blistering lesions of eczema can be confined to skin folds and creases or can cover the entire surface of the body. The lesions almost always itch intensely, and the skin becomes scaly. As the eczema progresses, the skin becomes thick and leathery and is darker colored than the nonaffected flesh.

Self-Care Treatment

Eczema signifies that your skin won't take any abuse. Avoid drying

TYPES OF SKIN RASHES

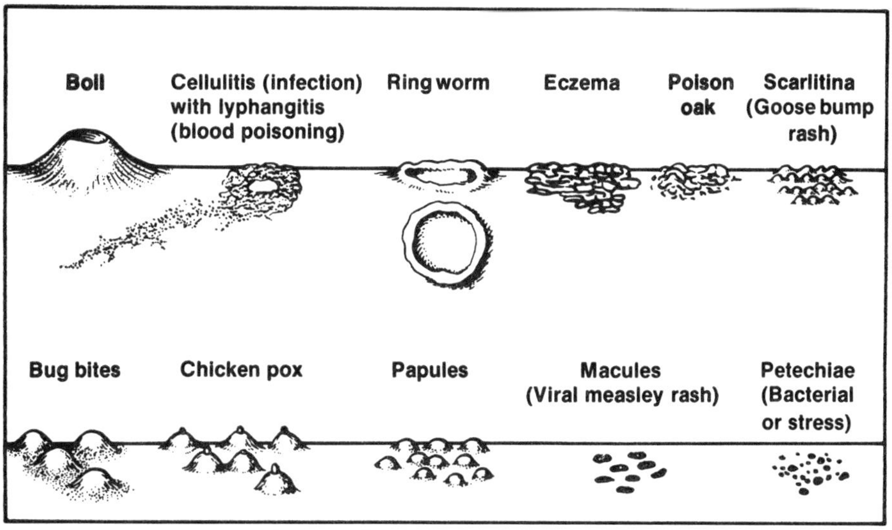

Figure 6-1

soaps, chemicals, and agents. Wash with a cleansing agent that also moisturizes; if your skin gets irritated from clothing, cover your skin with a thin layer of petroleum jelly and wear clothing styles that minimize irritation. Use rubber gloves if you work with soaps or detergents. Keep your fingernails cut short to avoid the temptation to scratch the lesions.

Keep bathing to a minimum; avoid overheating, which causes drying of the skin. Use calamine lotion to help curb itching. Compresses of salt water (one teaspoon of salt to a pint of cool water) applied for ten to thirty minutes three times a day will also help relieve itching.

Eczema in Children

To treat a child's eczema, avoid bathing him or her with soap, and cut down on the frequency of bathing. Avoid all skin preparations that contain oil or grease. Dress the child to promote healing: avoid wool or silk, tight elastic waistbands, and plastic pants, and avoid overdressing the child, since perspiration aggravates the eczema. Keep the child's nails trimmed short so that he or she cannot scratch at the lesions. Swimming in salt water can be soothing to the lesions, but swimming in fresh or chlorinated water can aggravate the eczema.

Eczema can result from food allergy, so stop all foods that you **started** feeding the child within one month of the time the rash first appeared. If no improvement occurs within three weeks, eliminate cow's milk, wheat flour products, eggs, citrus fruits (including juice), chocolate, nuts, peanut butter, fish, shellfish, tomatoes and tomato juice, tropical fruits, candies, ice cream, spices (not salt), corn, and berries from the child's diet until you notice improvement. Add the foods back, one at a time and gradually, until you are able to identify what causes the rash to reappear.

Give the child as much emotional support as you can — emotional tension tends to make eczema worse.

If the itching is worse at bedtime, give the child aspirin.

When to Call the Doctor

If any of the lesions start to crust, contact your doctor.

HIVES

A skin condition characterized by a sudden outbreak of itching and burning swellings or welts on the skin, hives are often caused by intense emotion, by mechanical irritation (such as the pressure created by a belt or collar), or by allergic reaction to medication or foods — common culprits include seafoods, eggs, chocolate, strawberries, nuts, penicillin, aspirin, and other medications. Hives may also result from jellyfish stings, from insect bites, from sensitivity to sunlight, from hepatitis, or from dust.

Signs and Symptoms

The large red patches that range in size from a dime to a half dollar can occur anywhere on the body; the welts, which may last from hours to weeks, appear as pink or white slightly raised bumps that itch. The hives, usually warm to the touch, can rise in one area of the body, subside, and then appear in another area of the body. Any welt that itches and rapidly changes appearance is a hive — no other rash reacts in that way. Hives that cause swelling of the eyes, mouth, or throat may interfere with breathing in serious cases.

Cold and Heat Treatment that can be Applied to the Skin

Application of Cold

Exposure to cold slows down the work in the cells, and the blood supply to a body part is decreased because the blood vessels narrow. Therefore, cold applications should be applied to any part of the body which is injured and may bleed, in order to narrow the blood vessels and prevent hemorrhage.

Cold applications also are indicated in persons with certain infections to prevent swelling and further damage that the swelling could cause. Thus, icecaps frequently are used when bleeding is highly possible, after an injury (as a blow to the lips or a sprained ankle) or in treating an infected area to prevent it from filling with blood and swelling.

Prolonged applications of cold, or exposure to excessive cold, may cause death of the body cells. Cold narrows the blood vessels so that the blood supply to the body part is cut off. Then, even though cellular activity is slowed down, the cells die because they are unable to take in food and oxygen or remove waste material. Signs of death of tissue include paleness, grayish-white appearance, or blueness (cyanosis) of the skin. Therefore the body part receiving a cold application must be watched as carefully as one receiving a hot application. The attendant should be on the alert for any signs that indicate tissue destruction.

Cold Eye Compresses

Cold, in the form of cold compresses, often is applied to an inflamed (reddened) eye to lower the blood flow to the eye. This reduces the bloodshot appearance of the eye and eases the pain caused by swelling.

Cold Moist Compresses

With any compress, warm or cold, care must be taken to show that the patient does not have an adverse reaction to the treatment. Cold moist compresses should be discontinued if the patient complains of numbness, or if the body part shows signs of paleness (either grayish-white or blue).

Application of Heat

Heat should be applied to a person's body when an infection is present, to increase circulation to a body part, help reduce congestion and inflammation, and relieve pain. In cases of abdominal pain or suspected appendicitis, NEVER APPLY HEAT — and contact a physician for directions.

When heat is applied to a person's body, these safety measures should be carried out:

- Test the water solution to be sure it is the exact temperature required. The following temperatures are guides only:
  Hot bath: 110° F (43.3° C).
  Warm bath: 95° F (35° C).
  Foot soak: 110° F (43.3° C).
  Hot wet dressing: 110° F (43.3° C).
  Hot water bottle: 115° F (46.1° C).

- Watch carefully for excessive redness on the patient's skin which may indicate that a burn is occurring.
- Apply the heat for the specified time.
- To prolong the effects of the treatment, keep the treated part warm, after the heat application is removed.
- To reheat the soak solution used on an arm or leg, *first remove the patient's limb from the container before adding the hot water* required to raise the solution to the desired temperature.

Self-Care Treatment

Calamine lotion, cornstarch baths, and cold applications can relieve itching. If you know what is causing the hives, avoid the cause. You may need to see a doctor to have a series of allergy tests conducted.

Hives in Children

In most cases, children get hives as a result of food allergy. Lamb and rice almost never cause hives, so restrict the child to this diet for two weeks. Gradually add foods, one at a time, to the child's diet until you find which is causing the hives to reappear.

When to Call the Doctor

See the doctor if hives cause shortness of breath, wheezing, dizziness, difficulty in breathing, difficulty in swallowing, cough, or fever. Call the doctor whenever you get hives on the tongue. Hives that do not respond to treatment or that cause a severe, prolonged itch should receive medical attention.

ACNE

While it most often strikes adolescents, acne can be a problem for people of all ages. More than 80 percent of all adolescents have acne at some time, and those who inherit oily skin have acne more severely than others.

The basic cause of acne is when a step-up in male and female hormones (androgen and estrogen) in maturing adolescents stimulates the secretion of sebum, an oily substance that works normally to keep the skin supple and soft. When combined with dirt, bacteria, and other factors, the sebum acts to clog the skin pores, resulting in blackheads (when lodged beneath plugs of dead skin) and whiteheads. Most often, acne forms at the base of hair follicles and in sweat glands.

Trapped beneath the plug of dead skin, the sebum breeds bacteria, and the resulting pus causes the pore to swell and form a pocket — called a cyst. In some severe cases, the cyst bursts and the infected mass is spilled into surrounding tissues.

Aggravating factors can include eating oily or greasy foods (although they are not as causative as once believed), menstruation (due to the release of hormones), emotional turmoil, and improper cleansing of the skin.

Signs and Symptoms

Pimples, blackheads, and whiteheads of acne range in size from a pinhead to a small pea; they most often appear on the face, neck, shoulders, upper chest, and upper back. Some of the acne lesions develop into cysts or abscesses, which may take months to finally burst and drain.

Nonprescription Acne Products

The table below lists many of the leading acne products that are available without a prescription, grouped by type. CU's comments are based on the FDA advisory panel's report on acne products and on the recommendations of our medical consultants.

Type	Products	Comments
BENZOYL PEROXIDE MEDICATIONS	*Benoxyl 5 Lotion (5% BP)* *Benoxyl 10 Lotion (10% BP)* *Clear By Design Gel (2.5% BP)* *Clearasil Lotion (5% BP)* *Clearasil Super-Strength Acne Treatment Cream (10% BP)*	Benzoyl peroxide is the most effective acne treatment ingredient available without a prescription. It helps prevent new lesions from forming. The gel form is considered more effective than lotions or creams.

	Dry and Clear Cream (10% BP) *Dry and Clear Lotion (5% BP)* *Fostex BPO Gel (5% BP)* *Oxy-5 Lotion (5% BP)* *Oxy-10 Lotion (10% BP)* *Topex Lotion (10% BP)*	Products with 10 percent benzoyl peroxide are not necessarily more effective than those with lower percentages but may be more irritating to the skin.
SULFUR MEDICATIONS	*Acnomel Acne Cream* *Fostril Medicated Drying Lotion* *Postacne* *Rezamid*	Sulfur medications help heal existing lesions by peeling and drying them out. But they're not considered useful in preventing new lesions from occurring. The flesh-colored tints in these products help mask pimples.
SALICYLIC ACID CLEANSERS	*Clearasil Medicated Cleanser* *Dry and Clear Cleanser* *Stri-Dex Medicated Pads* *Therapads Plus*	Salicylic acid cleansers may be of some help in unseating blackheads in mild acne, according to some of our medical consultants. As a cosmetic benefit, the alcohol in these products helps remove surface oil.
ALCOHOL CLEANSERS	*Noxzema Antiseptic Skin Cleanser* *Propa P.H. Super Cleanser* *Sea Breeze Antiseptic for the Skin* *Seba-Nil Cleanser* *Ten-O-Six Lotion*	Alcohol cleansers have no effect on acne. They help remove surface oil, but ordinary soap does that just as well.
SOAPS	*Betadine Skin Cleanser* *Clearasil Antibacterial Soap* *Fostex Medicated Skin Cleanser* *Fostex Wash* *Oxy Wash* *pHisoDerm*	Medicated soaps are no more effective against complexion problems than ordinary soaps. Many of the touted soaps contain benzoyl peroxide or sulfur, which are effective ingregients when left on the skin. But they're of little value in soaps, which are immediately washed away.
SCRUBS	*Buf-Puf Cleansing Sponge* *Epi-Clear Scrub Cleanser* *Komex Cleanser* *Listerex Scrub Lotion* *Loofah Sponges* *Multiscrub* *Oxy Scrub* *Pernox Scrub Cleanser*	Avoid scrubs; the abrasive particles in the cleansers and the rough surfaces of the sponges can irritate the skin and may make acne worse.

Consumers Union of United States, Inc., Mount Vernon, New York 10550. Reprinted by permission from *Consumer Reports*, August 1981.

Acne lesions that are severe or that are picked and squeezed can lead to pitting and scarring.

The skin that is affected by acne usually remains oily and is generally flabby and lacking in tone.

Self-Care Treatment

Basic to any acne treatment is a program of cleanliness. Wash your face at least once each day with soap and tepid water (not hot, since hot water aggravates oil production); dry it gently. A number of soaps are available over-the-counter that act to reduce oiliness. Keep your skin free of greasy makeup and lotion.

A number of over-the-counter lotions promote slight peeling of the top layer of skin, acting to loosen plugs of dead skin that trap sebum. Preparations containing benzoyl peroxide, sulfur, resorcinol, or vitamin A acid have proven useful.

Drink plenty of fluids, and get extra rest. Try to remove sources of tension and stress from your life. If you notice that a certain food aggravates your acne, avoid that food.

Natural sunlight or a sunlamp can be used sparingly to promote natural healing and peeling of the skin. Always use a sunlamp according to directions; keep it at least twelve inches from your skin, wear goggles (or place damp cotton balls over your eyes), use a timer to limit your exposure (start at thirty seconds, and increase each exposure by thirty seconds), and never read or sleep under a sunlamp.

When showering, use a back brush to scrub your back, and wash your upper chest and neck and shoulders carefully. You may need to apply a stronger peeling agent to those areas that you are able to wash less frequently than your face.

Never scratch or squeeze pimples, blackheads, or whiteheads — it leads to deeper scarring and the possibility of spreading the infection. To be effective, your acne treatment must continue twenty-four hours a day, seven days a week. Your acne will get worse during the first few weeks of treatment, since pimples started forming before you began treatment, and they will work their way to the surface; avoid the temptation to get discouraged and abandon treatment.

Other supplemental guidelines that may be helpful are as follows:

1. Avoid objects and clothing around the face that may aggravate acne such as rough clothing, musical instruments, masks, hats, or athletic equipment.

2. Wash your face after eating greasy foods that may leave residue around the chin and mouth.
3. If you work in a greasy environment, wash your face often.
4. Change pillowcases often, as they may be collectors of grease.
5. Avoid oil-based cosmetics and creams. They may clog pores.
6. Avoid using greasy sunscreens if you are in the sun for any length of time.

When to Call the Doctor

You should seek medical help for acne that does not respond to treatment, that leads to frequent infection, that is accompanied by low-grade fever, or that occurs in pre-pubescent children.

HERPES SIMPLEX (Cold Sore)

A recurrent condition that most commonly affects the lips, cold sores are caused by a virus that can lie dormant in your body for years before it flares up, often in association with other illness or infection. Herpes may appear with colds, fever, emotional stress, menstruation, gastrointestinal upset, injury to the lip (most common, biting), or overexposure to the sun. Herpes is highly contagious and usually lasts from one to three weeks.

Signs and Symptoms

Herpes usually appears on the lips but may occur elsewhere on the body. It begins with a single blister or cluster of blisters that breaks down to form a painful, irritated sore. The area may be hot to the touch and tender, but there is no fever and usually no swelling of the local lymph glands. After several days, the blisters dry up and form a yellowish crust. Remember: herpes is almost always painful. The more serious kinds of sores — those caused by syphilis and cancer — are usually painless.

Self-Care Treatment

No medication will prevent, dry up, or cure herpes, so treatment is aimed at simply relieving any discomfort. Don't scratch or rub the cold sore, or you will spread the infection.

When you feel a cold sore coming on, bathe the area with very hot water. Once the sore develops, tincture of benzoin, spirits of nitre, or camphorated lip ice will help dry the lesions. A combination of phenol and camphor or an antibacterial solution (such as *Neosporin* or *Bacitracin*) will help prevent the infection from spreading.

The blisters will generally clear up more quickly if you dab them gently with rubbing alcohol — it dries them. Apply zinc oxide to the crusts to speed healing. Cold milk, cornstarch paste, or cold compresses applied for five to ten minutes four to six times a day can be soothing to the pain.

Aspirin or throat lozenges containing mild analgesics can also relieve pain, as will saltwater gargles. A new drug for herpes simplex has recently been developed and is available by prescription from your doctor. The medication, in ointment form, is purported to prevent and cure cold sores.

Cold Sores in Children

Give a child who develops a cold sore a mild, bland diet, including pudding, milk, gelatin, and ice cream. While a very young child should not gargle with salt water, an older child can do so to relieve pain.

When to Call the Doctor

Cold sores that do not clear up within three weeks signal a problem, and you should seek medical attention.

POISON IVY AND POISON OAK

You won't get a rash the first time that you bump into poison ivy or poison oak — the rash is a form of contact dermatitis (an allergic reaction), and you have to encounter it at least once to the extent that your skin becomes sensitized to it. In subsequent encounters, if the plant oil stays on the skin for several hours, the characteristic rash appears within twelve to forty-eight hours of contact; the rash usually lasts about two weeks. Contact can be directly with the plant or can be with an indirect source — smoke, a pet, or contaminated clothing.

While many plants of the *Rhus* family cause the rash, poison ivy and poison oak are the two most common and well-known.

Signs and Symptoms

The rash that accompanies exposure to poison ivy or poison oak is a peppery, red, blistered rash that sometimes oozes and that itches intensely.

Self-Care Treatment

The best approach, of course, is to avoid contact with the plants; you should teach children what the plants look like, and you should be on the alert yourself.

If you do contact the plant, wash all of the plant oil from the skin as soon as you can with plenty of soap and water; repeat the washing three times, and use a lot of water to flush the soap from your skin. If soap is not available, alcohol-based disposable cleansing tissues can also be effective. If the oil has been on your skin for less than six hours, you can probably prevent the rash from developing.

Once lesions form, you can use an oatmeal bath (one cup of oatmeal to a tub full of water), calamine lotion, aspirin, or cool compresses of *Burow's Solution* to relieve the itch. Even if you are too late to prevent the rash, you should wash the affected skin thoroughly with soap and plenty of water, three times, to make sure that the plant oil is removed from your skin — or it will spread.

Because heat causes the skin to release the histamines responsible for itching, a hot bath or shower can provide relief. At first, the itching will be intense as the skin releases the histamines; slowly increase the temperature of the water until you can barely tolerate it. A hot bath is especially helpful if itching is intense at bedtime.

Don't scratch the lesions; scratching can lead to secondary infection. Once the oil has been absorbed by the skin or removed by washing, poison ivy cannot be spread to others; it is not contagious.

Poison Ivy in Children

Children benefit from the same treatment as adolescents and adults. You should trim their fingernails extremely short to prevent them from scratching the lesions.

When to Call the Doctor

You should call a doctor if the person cannot tolerate the lesions, if the lesions cover more than half of the body, if a secondary infection occurs (evidenced by puslike discharge from the rash), or if the poison ivy does not respond to treatment within two weeks.

HERPES ZOSTER (Shingles)

The painful viral infection commonly known as "shingles" appears as a large group of blisters along a sensory nerve path — usually on the skin of the abdomen under the ribs leading toward the navel. Shingles can occur at any age and often appears on people who have been exposed to chicken pox; it often accompanies other diseases, most commonly pneumonia and tuberculosis. It can also be triggered by emotional trauma or certain drugs. In some cases, it appears without apparent reason.

Signs and Symptoms

Before the onset of shingles, you may have mild, flulike symptoms. Shortly after such symptoms appear, a line will develop around your body at your neck, back, or chest; the line will become reddened, will start to burn, and will produce a sudden crop of painful small blisters. The area along the path of the blisters is red and tender to the touch. After several days, the blisters break and leave a sore, ulcerated area; the string of blisters is usually on only one side of the body. While shingles may itch in some cases, it is always acutely painful; the pain can be so severe that it seems like a heart attack. Local lymph glands are usually enlarged, and the sores are often moist and weeping. Within about three weeks, the sores get dry, become crusty, and disappear; in some cases, the pain may persist for months after the sores have disappeared. In some cases, shingles causes severe eye inflammation and possible destruction of the cornea.

Self-Care Treatment

Since there is no prevention or cure for shingles, treatment is aimed at relieving discomfort. Calamine lotion, benzoin, or other drying lotions can help dry the blisters; cortisone cream or ointment should never be used for shingles. Aspirin can help relieve pain.

When to Call the Doctor

You should seek medical help if the pain becomes too severe to tolerate and does not respond to treatment.

SUNBURN

Severe, prolonged exposure to the sun results in sunburn — a common, painful testimonial to too much sun. Depending on the degree of burn, the pain associated with sunburn can be mild or severe.

Signs and Symptoms

A general reddening of the exposed skin occurs within six hours after exposure; if the exposure is severe, the reddening may appear sooner. The pain associated with mild to moderate sunburn is most severe six to forty-eight hours following exposure to the sun. Three to ten days after exposure, the burned skin dries and peels. Rarely, sunburn results in blistering, a sign that second-degree burn has occurred.

Self-Care Treatment

The best treatment is prevention: limit your exposure to the sun by starting out with only fifteen minutes and gradually increasing your exposure time. Never go into the sun during the hottest hours of the day —between 11:00 A.M. and 2:00 P.M. — and use an effective sunscreen when you are in the sun (reapply after swimming and perspiring heavily).

To ease the pain of sunburn, bathe in a cool tub of water mixed with half a cup of baking soda. Cool compresses can also relieve pain and

Sunscreens

Sunscreens work by absorbing, reflecting, or scattering ultraviolet light, thus reducing the amount that reaches the skin. To help consumers select products that best suit their needs, labels rate the effectiveness of sunscreens — called the "sun protection factor" (SPF). The higher the SPF value, the more protection the product will give. For example, if you get red in ten minutes and a particular product would allow you to stay out for 150 minutes, then that product would rate a SPF 15 (150 divided by 10 = 15). Other ratings range from 6 to 12, 4 to 6 and 2 to 4.

What You Need to Protect Your Skin

SKIN TYPE I always burns, never tans	A product with a sun protective factor of 10 to 15
SKIN TYPE II burns easily, tans minimally	A product with a sun protective factor of 6 to 12
SKIN TYPE III burns moderately, tans gradually	A product with a sun protective factor of 4 to 6
SKIN TYPE IV burns minimally, tans well	A product with a sun protective factor of 2 to 4

burning, as can aspirin. Lubricants — such as *Vaseline* — can help relieve irritation but should not be used the first day, since they retain heat. Products that contain benzocaine may provide relief at first, but they prolong healing due to skin irritation.

When to Call the Doctor

You should seek medical help if you are dizzy, if you suffer abdominal cramps, if you develop a fever, if you develop visual difficulties, or if you develop blisters that get filled with fluid. You should see a doctor immediately if your temperature drops below 98.6° F.

IMPETIGO

A highly contagious bacterial infection limited to the outer skin layer, impetigo occurs most frequently in infants and children and is a result of contamination with a combination of staph or strep bacteria. Impetigo is spread by direct contact with the moist discharges of the sores; bacteria can lodge on clothing or under fingernails and can spread to other body parts or other people. If not properly treated, impetigo may lead to a systemic infection and can be serious or fatal to newborn infants.

Signs and Symptoms

Single sores or groups of sores appear suddenly, usually on the face, arms, or legs. The sores are mildly tender to the touch and itch or burn slightly. The skin surrounding the sores appears normal at first, but a ring of redness develops in a day or two. Within a few hours, impetigo develops into a blister, a pustule up to three inches in size, a raw glistening spot, or a crack in the skin.

As the condition progresses, healing may occur in the center of the lesion with a surrounding crust that may resemble ringworm. A small crop of blisters forms — usually around the mouth and nostrils — and they enlarge, finally breaking and oozing a straw-colored fluid.

Within a day or so an easily removable soft, yellow, or colorless soggy crust forms. An infected fever blister, hangnail, or insect bite, or a cut or burn at the same site or elsewhere on the body, may be the source of the bacterial infection. Often, though, there is no preceding infection. Impetigo heals without scarring, but it may leave a red or brown mark for approximately two weeks.

Impetigo is always worse in summer and in moist warm climates.

Self-Care Treatment

Only attempt to treat impetigo at home if there is no fever, there are only a few lesions, and the lesions are only on the arms and legs.

Clean the sores with antibacterial soap and water, and wipe the surrounding skin with alcohol. To remove the crusts, soak the affected area in a saline (salt) solution and apply an antibiotic salve (such as *Neosporin* or *Bacitracin*) to the sores. Completely wash your hands after working with the lesions, and keep all washcloths and towels separate. Keep the sores open and dry and exposed to the air as much as you can.

Wash clothing and underwear in hot water, and iron them to prevent spread of the infection.

If treatment works, don't stop until the sores have completely healed and the skin is smooth.

When to Call the Doctor

Any of the following signal danger and should be an indication for prompt medical treatment:

- Fever
- Presence of more than two lesions
- Sores anywhere on the body other than the arms and legs
- Sores that last longer than two weeks
- Sores that are covered with thick, dried pus
- The sores spread
- The patient is an infant
- The urine is dark cola-colored
- Severe headache
- General feelings of illness

ECTHYMA

Ecthyma, a staph or strep infection, is similar to impetigo except that it goes into the second layer of skin (the dermis) and heals with a scar. It occurs most frequently on the legs and begins as a large pustule that ruptures, leaving a pus-covered base with a ragged red margin. Ecthyma has a tough, hard brown or black crust that is difficult to remove. When the crust is removed, the raw base may bleed and then crust over again within a few hours. The raw ulcer is extremely painful to the touch.

Ecthyma should be treated in the same manner as impetigo.

BOILS

A furuncle, or boil, is a staph infection that occurs most often in areas where there is hair and irritation, such as on the neck, in the armpits, on the genitals, on the breasts, on the face, and on the buttocks. Boils occur most frequently on the neck or buttocks or at the base of a hair root but can develop wherever friction, irritation, or a scratch or break in the skin allows the bacteria on the surface of the skin to penetrate the outer layer. Poor hygiene, deodorant irritation, insect bites, excessive sweating, hot and humid weather, and infection elsewhere in the body can cause boils to appear.

A boil on the upper lip, above the upper lip, on the nose, on the scalp, or in the outer ear can be very dangerous, since infection in those areas has easy access to the brain. Other danger zones are the armpit, the groin, or the breast of a woman who is nursing.

Boils range from the size of a pea to the size of a walnut; some are even larger. The infection begins in the tissue beneath the skin; it develops into abscess pockets filled with pus. Eventually, the pus pocket points toward the skin surface, ruptures, and drains. Healing follows.

Signs and Symptoms

A high fever is often present with a boil; the patient is often tired (due to toxicity in the blood). At first there may be only a red lump; the inflamed area is hard, dark red, swollen, hot, tender, and quite painful. Within a few days, a yellow "head" develops on the skin surface. Instead of growing out on the skin as impetigo does, the boil forms a deep pocket filled with pus; it feels soft to the touch at that stage. Marked folding of the skin occurs, with severe local pain, tenderness, and fever; the local lymph glands are usually tender and inflamed.

Eventually, the boil ruptures, spilling pus, blood, and a plug of dead tissue (the core). The boil drains — small boils heal without a scar.

Self-Care Treatment

Handle a boil extremely gently — squeezing it may force infection deeper into the tissue. Never attempt to squeeze or lance a boil yourself.

Apply warm, moist compresses made of two teaspoons of salt to a quart of water, for twenty to thirty minutes three or four times a day, to speed the development of the pocket of pus and to soften the skin for the eventual rupture and draining. Get plenty of rest, and eat well-balanced meals. Leave the boil area unbandaged, and keep it clean with frequent soapings.

After the boil has come to a good head and has ruptured on its own, continue to apply warm compresses to maintain good drainage and to allow the boil to heal from the inside out. The more drainage that occurs, the better it is. Never squeeze pus from the boil — you could drive it deeper into the tissue and spread the infection. Apply alcohol and antibiotic salve to the area to keep the infection from spreading. Once the boil has drained, cover it with a sterile dressing until healing is complete.

When to Call the Doctor

Seek medical attention if the infection is extensive, if red streaks extend from the boil, if lumps or swelling occur in other body parts, if the boil is on the face, if there is fever, if a general sensation of illness accompanies the boil, if the boil shrinks instead of coming to a point, if the boil contains fluid but does not rupture or drain, if the infected person is an infant or an elderly person, or if the boils do not respond to self-treatment. A **carbuncle** — a group of interconnected boils — must always be treated by a doctor.

RINGWORM

Carried by humans or animals (usually cats, dogs, or horses), ringworm is the popular name for a fungus infection of the skin that is **not** caused by a worm and that is **not** always shaped like a ring.

Most fungus infection, especially in children, can be traced to exposure to infected pets, combs, towels, or other children.

Signs and Symptoms

The infection begins as an itching, red patch on the skin, with no local pain or tenderness. The patch grows outward in all directions, and the center begins to heal, leaving a clear area in the middle surrounded by a ring of infection. When ringworm is on the scalp, patchy hair loss accompanies local inflammation.

The round, red, scaling lesions attack the scalp and all other exposed areas of the body, particularly the arms and legs. The infections appear as reddish patches, often scaly or blistered, and may cause destruction of the hair shaft. Tiny pustules and severe itching accompany the sudden onset of the infection. If the pustules are scratched open, the bacteria invade the skin, resulting in secondary infection. On hairy areas, the fungus may grow into the hair follicles and cause pustules or small boils.

Ringworm is contagious and can be spread to other people and to other areas of the body.

Self-Care Treatment

Tinactin cream, solution, and powder are available over-the-counter and are effective in treating ringworm. *Selsun Blue* shampoo is also effective in treating ringworm of the scalp and as a cream in treating ringworm located on other areas of the body. Only a small amount should be used.

Cleanliness is important in preventing fungal infections. Wash all body parts with soap and water each day, especially hairy areas and body folds where perspiration is likely to collect. Fungi thrive in warm, damp climates, so thorough drying is essential.

When to Call the Doctor

If the scalp gets infected with ringworm or if ringworm infection does not respond to home treatment within a week, see a doctor.

ATHLETE'S FOOT

Athlete's foot, the most common fungal infection, is persistent and can be a difficult problem if it involves toenails. A fungus is usually responsible only for getting things started; bacteria and moisture aggravate the infection and worsen the condition. Infection with athlete's foot is almost impossible to prevent if you share a locker room or showers. The fungus that causes athlete's foot is abundant in the environment — even outside locker rooms and showers!

Signs and Symptoms

Athlete's foot normally involves only the area between the toes but may in some cases spread to involve the soles of the feet and the toenails. The area between the toes gets red and scaly; there is usually intense itching, and in most cases redness and small blisters appear. The skin between the toes usually cracks, leading to pain and more severe itching.

Self-Care Treatment

In many cases, it is possible without drugs to clear up athlete's foot by exercising scrupulous hygiene. Twice each day, wash the feet with soap, water, and a cloth; pay special attention to the area between the toes. Dry the entire area carefully with a dry towel — especially between the toes —despite the pain. Athlete's foot fungus thrives on moisture, so it is critical that the feet are kept dry. Put on a clean pair of socks and a pair of dry shoes. Friction and moisture act together to encourage fungus growth, so

---

Over-The-Counter Athlete's Foot Medications

Over-the-counter athlete's foot preparations generally come in several forms of delivery such as creams, liquids, gels, ointments, powders, and sprays. Generally, you should avoid using oil-base creams or ointments because they often complicate healing and may produce secondary bacterial infections. Even though powders are widely used, they tend to deliver their ingredients with less certainty than products that are used in the forms of liquids, gels, or sprays.

Athlete's foot products contain three general types of ingredients:

- *Fungicides:* These products control and, in some cases eliminate, fungus infections and the spores they produce. Probably the most effective compound in fungicides is tolnaftate. The following brand names contain fungicides in one form or another: *Campho-Phenique, Compounded Undecylenic Acid, Desenex, Foot-Guard, Fungacetin, Fungi-Spray, NP 27 Aerosol, Quinsana, Solvex, Sporonal, Tinactin, and Ting.*
- *Keratolytics:* Keratolytics are skin-peeling agents. They are an important form of treatment since the tissue most often affected by the athlete's foot fungus is shed when the external skin layers peel off. The most common chemicals included in keratolytics are salicylic and benzoic acids. *NP 27 Aerosol* and *Ting* contain keratolytic agents as well as fungicidal products.
- *Other ingredients:* Other ingredients are often added to athlete's foot products: various alcohols, astringents, surface anesthetics, absorbents, detergents, and antibacterial agents. These products serve to cool, relieve itch, desensitize, dry, or prevent secondary infections that may arise.

---

choose shoes that are loose and comfortable and that allow the feet to air out — sandals or canvas sneakers are best. Change shoes regularly to make sure that they have a chance to air out completley.

Sprinkling powder on the feet and between the toes can help prevent reinfection; an over-the-counter preparation, such as *Tinactin,* is effective in killing the fungus and drying the feet.

JOCK ITCH

A fungus infection of the pubic region, jock itch does not involve the penis or scrotum and never spreads beyond the groin area. Like athlete's foot, it is aggravated by moisture and friction. It is almost exclusively a male condition and is usually intensified by athletic supporters that get moldy in lockers.

Signs and Symptoms

Lesions are present only on the thighs and in the groin area; the penis and scrotum are not involved. There is intense itching, and lesions often ooze. The skin surrounding the lesions is red and scaling.

Self-Care Treatment

Jock itch can be effectively treated by removing the contributing factors, friction and moisture:

1. Wear boxer shorts instead of jockey shorts.
2. Change soiled and sweaty underwear often.
3. Wear only clean, dry underwear; make sure that athletic supporters are clean and dry.
4. Dry the groin area thoroughly after bathing, and sprinkle a powder over the area to keep it dry; *Tinactin* will also work to kill the fungus.

Jock itch will generally clear up in two weeks with regular treatment. The problem will return if treatment is not thorough and if prevention is not exercised.

PUBIC LOUSE (Crabs)

The pubic louse or "crab" usually lives in the hair of the pubic region but may be found occasionally in hair located elsewhere on the body. The pubic louse lays its eggs on the shaft of the hair, and the lice, which are larger than other lice, can be seen easily with the naked eye. Pubic lice are transmitted through sexual intercourse, from infected toilet seats, by wearing crab-infested clothing, or from contact with infested bedding.

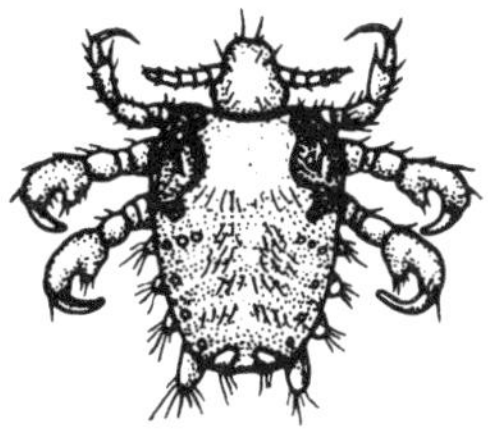

Figure 6-2
Pubic louse.

Signs and Symptoms

The main symptom of crabs is itching — fingernail scratch marks are often found on the skin where the crabs are located (usually the pubic region, but also on the lower abdomen, in the armpits, on the chest, or even in the eyebrows). Pale blue-gray bite marks can be seen on the skin, and the eggs appear as gray or white sacs attached to the skin at the base of the pubic hairs. The tiny, dark lice are visible and move violently when pulled off the hair or the skin.

If infestation is extreme, the condition may result in the patient being tired and irritable and experiencing a rash similar to that found with measles.

Self-Care Treatment

Over-the-counter preparations effective against lice are available and should be left on for twenty-four hours. The application should be repeated after one week and again after two weeks.

You can prevent infestation by frequent bathing, thorough drying, and frequent changing of clothes. If you are exposed to pubic lice, bathe thoroughly and dust your groin area with pesticide powder. Thoroughly dust all contaminated clothing and bedding with pesticide powder. Check with your pharmacist to make sure that the pesticide powder you have chosen is safe for this use.

BODY LOUSE

The body louse lives and lays eggs on the seams of a person's clothing and feeds on his or her skin. It lives on human blood and dies in a short time if denied food. The adult body louse has six legs; the female attaches its eggs to fibers of clothing, ususally along the seams, and the eggs (nits) mature in three to fourteen days.

Signs and Symptoms

Nits (clusters of eggs) appear as small gray or white sacs that are seen in the seams of clothing. On examination, scratch marks and bite marks

Figure 6-3
Human louse and bedbug.

HUMAN LOUSE

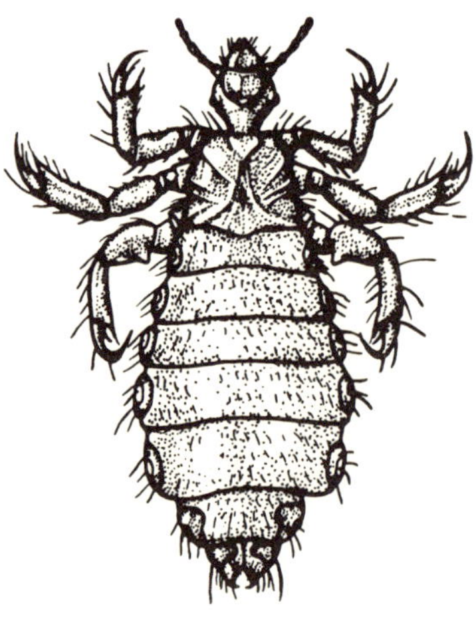

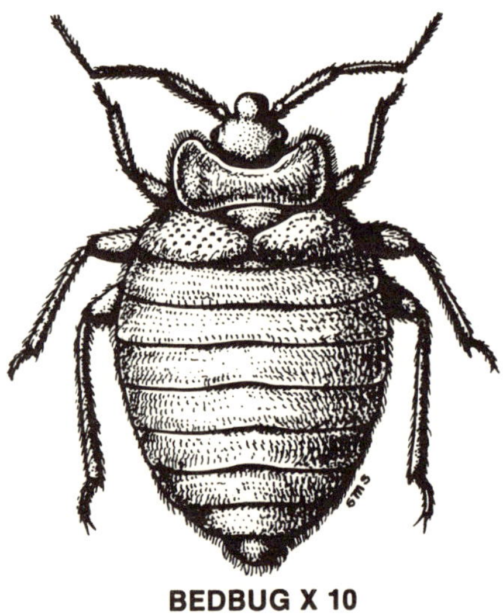

BEDBUG X 10

—which appear as tiny punctures with encircling redness — can be seen on the skin. Lesions are located mostly on areas where the clothing comes in close contact with the skin — the shoulders, the chest, around the waist, and on the buttocks. There is severe itching, and the louse is visible to the naked eye. Lymph nodes in the area occasionally swell.

Body louse infestation may be especially dangerous because the body louse carries a number of diseases — including relapse fever, trench fever, and typhus.

Self-Care Treatment

Treat the infested areas of your body with pesticide powder (check with a pharmacist to ascertain safety of the pesticide powder). Also, dust the seams of your clothing thoroughly and the other areas of clothing lightly. You can further decontaminate your clothing by having it dry-cleaned or by boiling it for at least ten minutes; ironing the seams with a hot iron kills the nits. Make sure that you change your bedding and clothing simultaneously to prevent cross-contamination.

HEAD LOUSE

Less than one-eighth of an inch long, the head louse is a grayish-white, transparent louse that lays its nits in silvery, oval-shaped envelopes that attach to hair shafts; milk-white, the nits often look like dandruff. Because it causes intense itching that leads to scratching, the head louse may cause secondary infections. It is passed easily on combs and hats.

Signs and Symptoms

A victim of head lice often looks like he or she has severe dandruff. There is a red, scaly rash on the back of the neck at the hairline and an itching, scaling scalp. The nits are visible and resemble flakes of dandruff.

Self-Care Treatment

Apply a mild vinegar solution to the scalp, and comb the hair with a fine-toothed comb to remove the nits. Apply a shampoo of 1 percent benzene hexachloride (*Lindane*) in a cream or shampoo by shampooing the cream into dry hair, working it into a lather, leaving it on for four minutes, and rinsing. Apply the shampoo only two times.

Boiling your pillowcases and ironing them with a hot iron will kill any lice that infest your bedding.

TICKS AND CHIGGERS

Ticks and chiggers are the most common of the small, disease-bearing insects that feed on human blood. Ticks are easily seen; about one-quarter of an inch long, the tick buries its head and crablike pincers beneath the

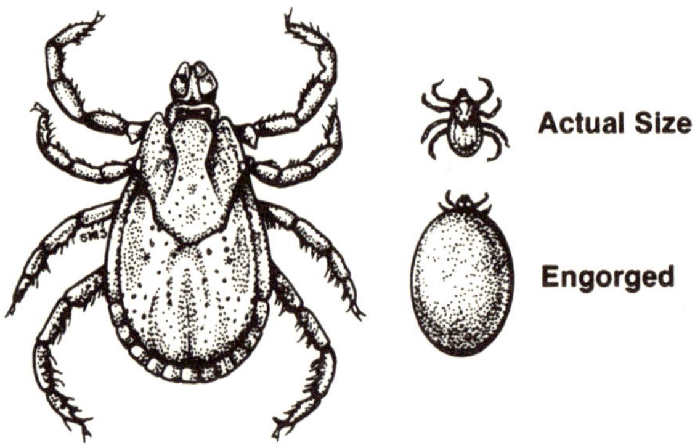

Figure 6-4
The tick.

skin, with its body and legs protruding above the skin surface. If a pregnant tick is left to feed for several days, she can secrete a toxin that results in partial paralysis of the victim; the paralysis clears up shortly after the tick is removed. Ticks attack animals as well as people and may be passed to people from animals.

Chiggers, small red mites, are sometimes called redbugs. Their bite causes an intense itch due to a chemical that eats away at the skin. Chiggers deposit tiny red larvae at the bite site.

Signs and Symptoms

Because the tick buries its head in the skin but leaves the body and legs protruding above the skin surface, it is easy to see the tick at the bite site. Occasionally, the tick may become completely buried in the skin but still remain visible; in other cases, the tick may appear to be swollen and attached to the skin. The tick can become buried in the skin of the scalp or other hairy areas, so you should inspect those, too.

Chigger bites almost always occur around the belt line or at other openings in the clothing. The itching red sores are round and small, and the larvae (red) or the chigger bites are visible in the centers of the sores.

Self-Care Treatment

The trick to getting rid of a tick is getting it to let go of its hold. Make the tick uncomfortable by applying heat (a heated paperclip is good to use), acetone, oil, or alcohol; when the tick starts to wiggle its legs and begins to withdraw, grasp it firmly and remove it with a quick twisting motion. If the head is left under the skin, soak the bite gently with warm water twice daily until it heals.

Chigger bites itch intensely — often for several weeks — and the itch persists even after the larvae have been killed. Keep the sores clean; soak them with warm water twice daily. The larvae can be killed by applying *A200* or *Cuprex* during the first few days. To prevent chigger bites, wear clothing that fits tightly around the cuffs, sleeves, neck, and waist; use insect repellent, and be sure to spray it around the openings of your clothing. Bathe thoroughly if the suspect that you have been exposed to chiggers.

Inspect yourself closely after hiking in the mountains or camping out in fields where tall grasses and weeds may harbor ticks or chiggers.

When to Call the Doctor

Call the doctor if you develop a fever, rash, or headache within two weeks after a tick bite — they may signal the onset of Rocky Mountain spotted fever, a disease commonly transmitted by ticks.

SCABIES

Extremely contagious, scabies is caused by a mite that is barely visible with the naked eye. Occurring where hygiene is poor, the mite is easily transmitted from person to person on clothing or bedding; its incidence has recently been on the rise in the United States.

The female mite burrows under the skin to lay eggs, leaving a wavy line. It usually begins burrowing between the fingers or toes. As the mite burrows, it leaves pimples, blisters, and wavy lines (the burrowing causes intense itching, so as the victim scratches, the wavy lines may not be so obvious). Scratching often causes secondary infections. The eggs hatch in four to eight days.

The areas of the body most affected are the webs of the hands, the elbows, the skin folds, the genitals, the buttocks, and the underarms. Scabies rarely appears on the face.

Signs and Symptoms

A pimple or blister appears at the point of entrance. Itching is intense, and the marks from scratching may cover up other signs. Pimples, blisters, and gray lines (up to three-eighths of an inch long) appear on the affected areas.

Self-Care Treatment

Follow this procedure to treat scabies:

1. Take a prolonged bath. Scrub yourself thoroughly with a nail brush and soap so that the burrows are uncovered.
2. After the bath, take cool soaks to relieve the itching, since the warmth from the bath will make the itching worse.
3. Cover your entire body with sulfur ointment; repeat the application every eight to twelve hours.
4. Apply calamine lotion to the affected areas to relieve the itch.
5. Take aspirin to relieve the pain.
6. Change bedding and clothing simultaneously and daily. Launder bedding and clothing thoroughly, and iron them with a hot iron.

The condition should clear up within seventy-two hours if you follow a strict treatment regime.

When to Call the Doctor

If the condition does not clear up within seventy-two hours, despite your treatment attempts, call your doctor.

PSORIASIS

Psoriasis is a chronic, recurrent, erratic, and distressing skin condition common in adults. It seems to occur in families with a previous history of the disease and may be hereditary. It is not contagious and does not pose a threat to life. The cause of psoriasis is unknown.

Signs and Symptoms

Psoriasis is marked by bright red patches covered with silvery scales. The sores appear most often on the knees, elbows, and scalp; the chest, abdomen, backs of arms and legs, palms of hands, and soles of feet are also often affected. When fingernails are involved, the condition begins as dot-shaped marks on the nails; the nails become split, cracked, discolored, pitted, and separated from the beds.

As the disease advances, large, raised, thickened, scaling patches develop on various parts of the body; they may itch, and a tiny bleeding spot appears under the scale if it is removed. Lesions generally heal without scarring.

If the scalp is involved, patchy hair loss may accompany the condition.

Self-Care Treatment

At present, there is no cure for psoriasis, but the condition is controllable; over half of the disease remissions occur in summer, and 20 percent of the cases experience remission at one time or another.

Treatment is aimed at control. Use warm baths, a soothing lotion, and an antidandruff shampoo to counter sudden attacks. Expose your full body to the sun or to ultraviolet light on a regular basis. A warm climate and freedom from anxiety seem to help in control of psoriasis.

When to Call the Doctor

A case of psoriasis that does not respond to home treatment or that worsens instead of improving should be referred to a doctor; a number of cortisone-containing ointments are available for use with a prescription.

WARTS

Ranging in size from a pinhead to a small bean, warts are irregular, firm, rough skin growths caused by a virus. Usually less than a quarter of an inch in diameter, warts often occur at sites exposed to friction, trauma, or abrasion. Highly contagious, they are common among children.

Signs and Symptoms

Commonly found on the hands, feet, forearms, and face, warts usually do not cause itching or pain; repeated trauma to the wart, however, can cause it to bleed.

Warts may be flat or raised, dry or moist. Usually, they have a rough and pitted surface that is either flesh-colored or darker than the surrounding skin. Plantar warts, which occur on the soles of the feet, are very sensitive because of pressure. Anal warts cause itching. A wart usually develops between one and eight months after the virus is lodged in the skin. The virus is spread by scratching, rubbing, and slight razor cuts.

Self-Care Treatment

Many warts resolve themselves over a period of time and do not require treatment. You should leave a wart alone if it is individual and not bothersome. While 50 percent of all warts will disappear without treatment, others will remain for years. Self-treatment by cutting, scraping, or use of acids and patent medicines may cause bacterial infection, scarring, and other harm without eliminating the warts. Even surgery is not completely successful.

Warts in Children

Warts in children are more common than they are in any other age group. You should have a child's warts removed early (by a physician, who will use a combination of heat, chemicals, and freezing), because warts are easily spread by scratching and other childhood activities.

When to Call the Doctor

Call your doctor if a wart enlarges, gets red or tender, interferes with daily activities, or is accompanied by a fever.

MOLES AND BIRTHMARKS

Birthmarks — such as strawberry marks and port-wine stains — are completely harmless, almost never lead to complications, and do not require treatment. If they are particularly disfiguring, sometimes cosmetic surgery is effective. A new laser treatment is also being used.

Moles are either acquired during early childhood or are present at birth. Rarely, moles can lead to a rare form of cancer called melanoma.

Signs and Symptoms

Moles have a great range in size and shape, and range in color from pale (almost skin-colored) to dark brown and black. They may be flat, raised, smooth, warty, or hairy.

Self-Care Treatment

No home treatment is available for moles.

When to Call the Doctor

You should consult a doctor immediately if a mole suddenly begins to grow (unless you are pregnant, since many moles increase in size during pregnancy), suddenly begins to ulcerate, begins to itch or bleed, or suddenly develops a halo of color or nodules around its base. In such cases, the surrounding lymph glands swell or harden — another danger sign.

You should also call your doctor to arrange for surgical removal of moles if they are situated in areas of chronic irritation — such as under the arms or under the breast, or on the waist where clothing will irritate them repeatedly.

CORNS

Usually caused by tight shoes, a corn is a horny, thickened mass of skin that is caused by friction and pressure. It forms a cone-shaped mass that extends down into the deep layers of the skin; when the corn is pressed inward against the nerve endings, pain results. The longer the pressure and friction persist, the greater the reaction in the skin, and the thicker the corn will become. The condition may precipate a bunion (see below).

Figure 6-5
A bunion is a thickened swelling that usually occurs on the side of the foot at the joint of the big toe. Because there may be a deformed joint, bunions should be seen by a physician.

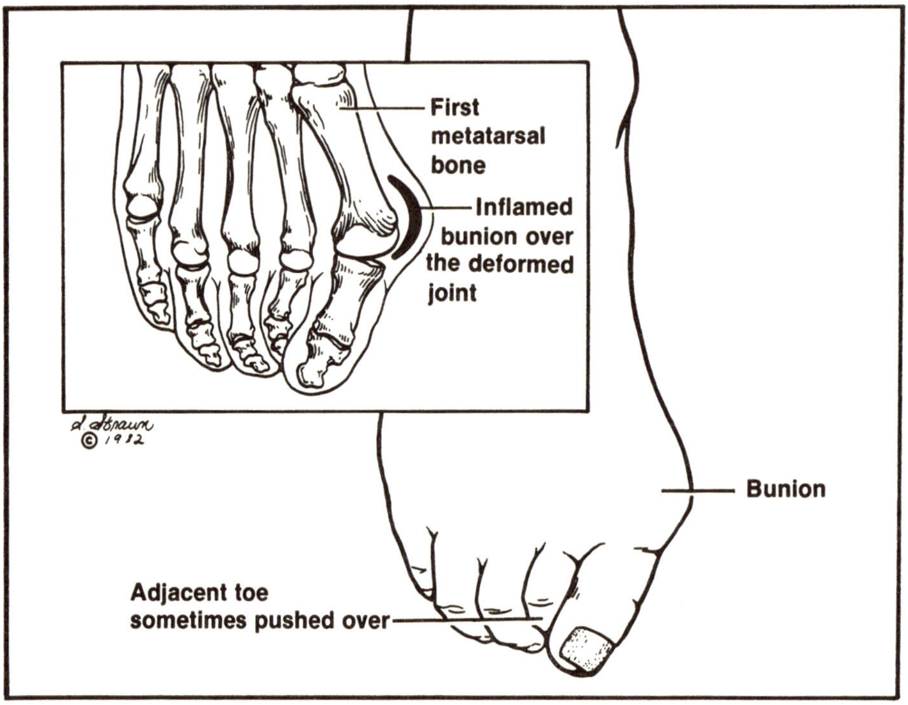

Signs and Symptoms

In addition to the thickened corn on the skin, often appearing as a bump or lump, there is usually a bony bump underlying a corn that has persisted for a long period of time.

Self-Care Treatment

To remove a corn, soak your foot in warm water, apply mineral oil, and rub the corn with an emery board or pumice stone. To soften a corn in preparation for removal, soak the foot in warm water for at least fifteen minutes, and apply a lubricant or mineral oil to the corn; cover it with a corn pad for four days. At the end of four days, the corn will come out easily when soaked again.

Bathroom surgery can be dangerous. Never cut a corn with scissors or a razor blade; infections of the feet that result can be quite serious. Use commercial preparations with great caution — the acid contained in them can cause a chemical breakdown of the skin and can result in infection.

Any cure for a corn must be centered around relieving the friction and pressure on the corn site; use corn pads to relive pressure, and discard tight-fitting shoes.

When to Call the Doctor

Never attempt to treat your own feet if you are diabetic. Under any condition, call a doctor if the corn does not respond to home treatment and if it becomes painful enough to cause debilitation.

INGROWN TOENAIL

Ingrown toenails can be caused by wearing shoes that are too tight or that constrict the toes, but by far the most prevalent cause is improper cutting of toenails. Ingrown toenails most frequently affect the big toe. Besides improper trimming of toenails and shoes that fit improperly, an ingrown toenail can be caused by stretch stockings that push the skin up over the toenails.

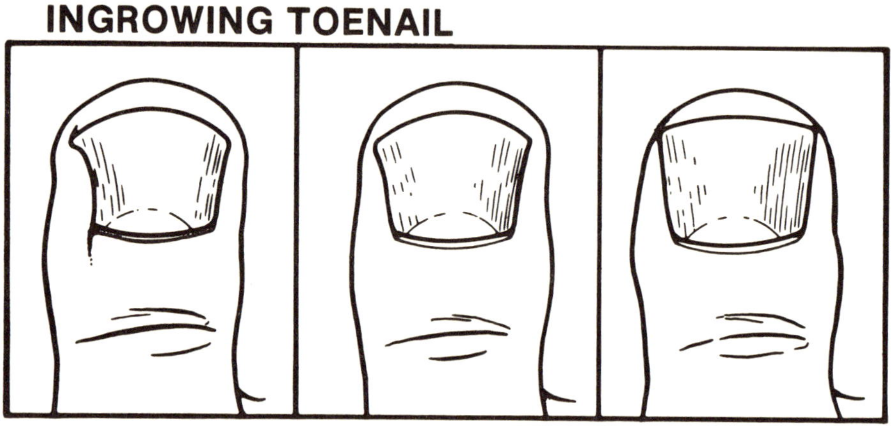

Nail growing into skin fold

Incorrect cutting - too short and curved

Correct cutting - straight across, not too short

Figure 6-6

Signs and Symptoms

The edges of the toenails begin to dig into the surrounding flesh, and the edges of the nail become overgrown with tissue. Pus may form in the area. The skin over the nail becomes infected and painful.

Self-Care Treatment

1. Soak the affected foot frequently in hot water to relieve the pain; use an antibiotic salve to prevent further infection.
2. A wisp of cotton soaked in castor oil should be placed under the corner of the nail to keep it pointing outward and upward.
3. Place a cotton pad over the nail tip to protect it from pressure.
4. Remove any dead tissue with scissors; be extremely careful not to cut into live tissue.
5. Probe the ingrown part of the toenail with gentian violet (available over-the-counter) in a 1 percent solution.
6. If pain becomes extreme, wear shoes with the toes cut out.

Ingrown Toenail in Children

Ingrown toenails, while not common among children, are extremely painful and debilitating. While most adults get ingrown toenails only on the big toes, a baby — whose toes are pushed against the crib mattress for hours at a time — can develop ingrown toenails in any or all of the toes.

Wipe an infant's toes with rubbing alcohol several times a day; the nails are so delicate that they often heal with this treatment.

For a child, soak the affected foot in a solution of one cup of Epsom salts to one quart of water. Soak a bandage in the same solution, and encase the foot in a plastic bag for several hours (overnight, if possible). After the soaking, gently cut out the spur, and apply antibiotic salve to the toe.

When to Call the Doctor

If pain becomes debilitating or the toe shows signs of infection (redness, tenderness, hot to the touch, with accompanying fever or puslike discharge), call your doctor.

BLISTERS

Resulting from excessive friction or continuous pressure on the skin, blisters are common on the feet from wearing poorly fitting shoes or stockings and on the hands from using unfamiliar tools. Blisters are an elevation of the outer skin layers, and they contain watery fluid. They become infected easily.

Self-Care Treatment

Unless a blister is being irritated by pressure, you should leave it unbroken. If you do need to break a blister, do so with the following technique:

1. Wash the blister and the surrounding skin with soap and water.
2. Sterilize a needle by heating it in a flame until it turns red.
3. Insert the needle gently at the lower edge of the blister, and apply gentle, steady pressure to drain the fluid.

4. Protect the blister with a sterile bandage until healing is complete. Avoid any further pressure or friction to the area.

If a blister breaks on its own, treat it like a minor skin wound; watch for signs of infection.

CHAPTER 7

COMMON MUSCLE AND JOINT COMPLAINTS

ARTHRITIS

Arthritis, or inflammation of the joints, results when one bone moves against another at the surface of the joint. Arthritis can strike anyone at any age, although it occurs less frequently in those under the age of twenty-five. Certain kinds of arthritis are caused by infection (bacterial) that is carried to the joints from other sites in the body. Rheumatoid arthritis involves chronic inflammation of the synovial membrane that cushions and surrounds the joints. Almost anyone who lives beyond middle age develops some kind of degeneration of the joints.

Signs and Symptoms

Pain, swelling, and stiffness in the joints are the characteristic symptoms of arthritis. Some joint deformity develops in some cases. Due to scarring of joint surfaces, joints may become permanently stiff with limitation of motion. Other symptoms include infection elsewhere in the body, redness of the joints, and a low-grade fever.

Gout, a form of arthritis that is confined to one joint and that results from excessive acid levels in the blood, occurs in the big toe in 90 percent of the cases, although the joints of the ankle, wrist, and thumb may also be involved. The toe becomes red to purplish red, shiny, swollen, and so excruciating that the pressure of even the lightest shoes or stockings cannot be tolerated. While arthritis produces a pain that is deep and aching, gout produces a sharp, agonizing pain. The first attack usually lasts from one to four days; subsequent attacks are usually not as intense, but they tend to last longer. Attacks become more frequent with time.

Self-Care Treatment

Treatment for gout consists of regular, daily, consistent exercise. Keep the affected joint wrapped in cotton and immobile when not active. Avoid foods that tend to produce large amounts of uric acid in the blood — among them liver and kidney — and drink plenty of water to help wash the excess acid from your system.

To treat other forms of arthritis, take aspirin with meals to relieve pain; check with your doctor if you want to take the aspirin for longer than two weeks. Rest your joints; an elastic bandage can provide some support and ease pain. Heat is usually helpful; try using a hot water bottle, an electric heating pad, or hot soaks.

Arthritis in Children

If you suspect that your child has arthritis, get a doctor's diagnosis —joint or muscle pain in children usually is **not** arthritis. Most arthritis in children is caused by infection, and prompt treatment by a doctor can arrest the infection and prevent long-term joint deformity.

When to Call the Doctor

Call your doctor if you suspect arthritis in your child, or if any of the following occur:

- Swelling in a joint
- Redness in a joint

- Warmth in a joint
- Limitation of joint movement
- Rash
- Abdominal pain
- Vomiting
- Fever not accompanied by a cold or the flu
- Joint pain that lasts longer than seven days
- Pain that is severe and limited to one joint
- Pain that results from an injury to the joint
- Limitation of movement (even slight) that persists for six weeks

Call the doctor whenever joint pain is preceded by a sore throat.

OSTEOARTHRITIS

Most people over the age of fifty have osteoarthritis to some extent; 5 percent of those are disabled by the disease. Osteoarthritis is considered a common and natural part of aging and involves the progressive deterioration of joints due to normal wear and tear, excessive use, or injury. The exact cause is unknown, but overweight hastens the development of the condition, and continued joint injury tends to lead to osteoarthritis.

Signs and Symptoms

The weight-bearing joints — those of the hands, feet, and knees — are most commonly affected by osteoarthritis; the hips, spine, and ankles are also common sites for the disease. Joints become red, swollen, and stiff and may feel hot to the touch or may creak with use. Pain is more pronounced after vigorous exercise, is worse in the morning, and is pronounced during inclement weather. The amount of pain varies; pain can be moderate to severe and can travel from one joint to another. Bony, knobby lumps sometimes develop under the skin around the finger joints (most frequently in women) but are usually not painful.

Self-Care Treatment

The aching of osteoarthritis is worse in cold, damp weather and improves in warm, dry weather. Weight reduction is essential to treatment, especially if the osteoarthritis involves the knees, ankles, or feet.

Apply hot compresses to the affected joints to relieve pain; aspirin is also helpful. Massaging the muscles around the affected joints may help bring some relief.

Participate in **moderate** exercise to keep the joints from getting stiff and to keep the muscles stretched and strong. Be moderately active, but rest for at least thirty minutes every four hours.

To relieve the nodes that develop under the skin of the fingers, soak your hands in alternate hot and cold baths; each should be about four minutes.

Provide extra warmth during inclement weather by wearing nylon or synthetic gloves under wool mittens and by wearing knitted wool covers over your knees. If you suffer extreme pain in the knees, try wrapping an elastic bandage in a figure eight around your knee, and use a cane to walk to relieve the pressure.

When to Call the Doctor

If aspirin makes you dizzy, causes ringing in your ears, or gives you indigestion, heartburn, or constipation, consult your doctor. Call your doctor if you are taking medication for high blood pressure, if your pain is confined to one joint, if you have a family history of osteoarthritis, or if you experience an increase in general fatigue and weakness. It is best to consult a physician if you even suspect osteoarthritis.

SHIN SPLINTS

Shin splints — pain in the tibia (front of the lower leg) or the surrounding soft tissue — most often occur in a competitive athlete or jogger but can occur in anyone who engages in a physical activity. Shin splints are caused by repetitive running on hard surfaces or forcible, extensive use of the foot flexor muscles.

Signs and Symptoms

The pain, usually most intense at the beginning of exercise, tends to decrease during the warmup in milder cases; it is a burning, sharp pain that occurs in the shin area (between the knee and the ankle). It is usually self-limiting, although it may appear after the exercise period is over and may cause considerable pain.

Self-Care Treatment

Mild shin splints can be relieved with ice, heat, taping the legs, or wearing arch supports and cushioned soles. If shin pain is serious enough to interfere with your physical performance, rest the leg until the pain disappears.

Avoid excessive early training on hard surfaces such as concrete. Make sure that the shoes you wear during exercise and sports are well-fitted and cushioned — especially important early in the season.

RHEUMATIC FEVER

Rheumatic fever is an allergic response to strep infection; it often develops as a complication of the same infection that causes strep throat, tonsillitis, scarlet fever, or ear infection. It is common, occurring mostly among children between the ages of five and fifteen. It may affect only the joints or may include the heart and the nervous system. The onset of the disease may be gradual or sudden; initial symptoms usually appear from one to four weeks after the initial strep infection has occurred. After one occurrence, there is a tendency for recurrence of the disease.

Signs and Symptoms

Initial symptoms include slight fever, tiredness, vague pain in the limbs, and nosebleed. In sudden onset, the fever may reach 104° F. by the second day and may continue for several weeks.

The joint involvement is usually migratory; one or two joints may become swollen or feverish for a few days. The pain will then disappear and will appear in another joint. If the heart is involved, a murmur may result; involuntary muscle movement may result if the nervous system gets involved.

Self-Care Treatment

You **must** see a doctor immediately if you suspect that rheumatic fever has developed, since antibiotic treatment is essential to controlling the disease.

Home treatment, after consultation with a doctor, centers on relieving symptoms. Take aspirin to reduce pain and fever. Bed rest is important, especially if the heart has been affected by the disease.

BURSITIS

Bursitis is an inflammation of the bursae — the fluid-filled sacs located in joint areas over the bone tips that allow the muscles to move smoothly over the bones. Bursitis may be caused by anything that irritates bursae — repeated trauma, excessive joint use, chilling of the joint, calcium deposits, or infection. The most common sites are the shoulder (most frequent), the knee, the elbow, and the hip.

Signs and Symptoms

Bursitis is signalled by localized tenderness or hot swelling over a bursa. Sudden onset is accompanied by severe pain and limitation of motion in the affected joint; when the shoulder is affected, elevation of the arm may be limited. Some redness may accompany fluid accumulation.

Self-Care Treatment

Rest the joint in a sling, and apply moist heat frequently. Take aspirin for pain. Cold packs may relieve pain if the hot packs are ineffective.

When to Call the Doctor

Consult your doctor if the bursitis persists and does not respond to home treatment.

SCIATICA

Sciatica — an inflammation of the longest nerve in the body — the sciatic nerve — affects men more often than women, mainly between the ages of thirty and fifty. The most common cause of sciatica — which causes inflammation from the buttocks down the leg to the foot — is pressure at the root of the nerve in the spine, a common result of arthritis in the spine, a slipped disc, or a ruptured disc. Anything that presses against the nerve outlet — heavy bowels (due to constipation or tumor), infection of a nearby organ, or engorged blood vessels — can trigger sciatica. Occasionally, sciatica is caused by the prolonged inactivity of driving a car for long distances or by the twisting involved in lifting a heavy object the wrong way.

Sciatica is made worse by dampness, cold, and excessive muscle strain during the period of inflammation; poor posture increases the pain.

Signs and Symptoms

The most characteristic symptom is an agonizing and torturous pain that begins at the buttocks and continues down the leg to the foot. The pain sometimes disappears but almost always returns.

The pain of sciatica is made worse by straining during bowel movements, coughing, sneezing, or any other strain. The pain that results from back injury or from lifting a heavy object improperly is sharp and jabbing.

When the leg is straightened, a sharp jab of pain occurs in the buttocks. The pain from sciatica can be intense enough to limit the motion of the leg.

Self-Care Treatment

To relieve the pain of sciatica, take aspirin and apply heat — a hot water bottle or an electric heating pad, or take a hot bath. Rest on a firm mattress (insert a sheet of plywood between your mattress and box springs) with a pillow under the knee of the affected leg. You may need to immobilize your back to gain relief from the pain.

You can prevent sciatica by sitting and standing properly. Keep your

Figure 7-1
To prevent sciatica, avoid lifting heavy objects improperly. Bend your knees and squat, using your body weight in lifting.

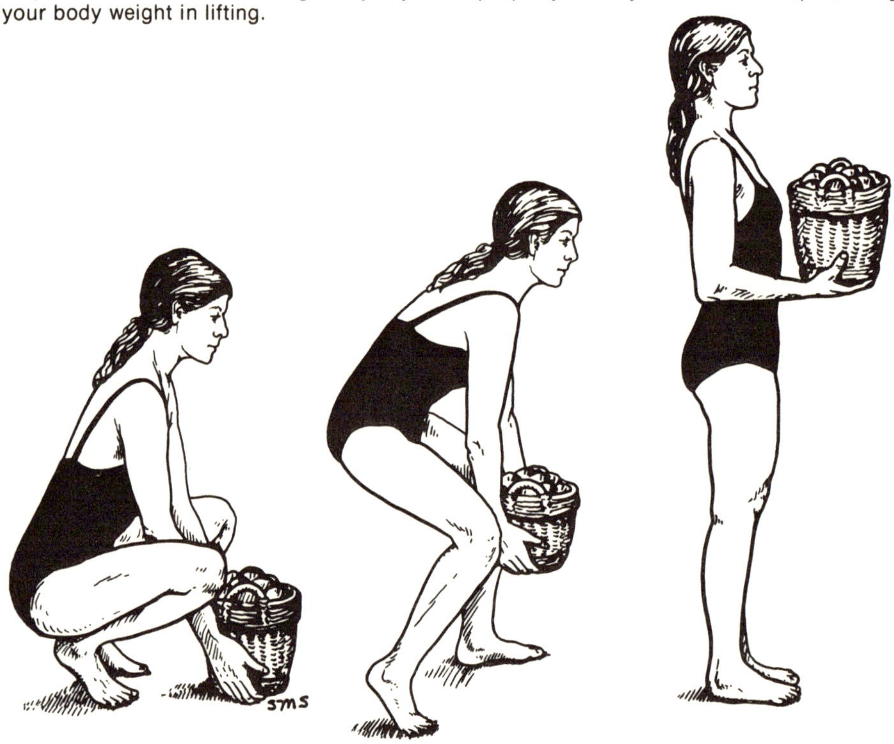

back straight and aligned, and never sit on one buttocks or on the edge of a chair. Avoid lifting heavy objects improperly; bend your knees and squat, using your body weight in lifting.

When to Call the Doctor

If you suspect that the sciatica is the result of a back injury — such as a slipped disc, ruptured disc, or spinal arthritis — you should see your doctor so that the underlying cause can be treated.

LOW BACK PAIN

Usually involving a spasm of the large, supportive muscles next to the spine, low back pain can be sudden and violent or low-keyed and chronic and is usually due to the lifting of heavy objects.

Low back pain is more common in tall people, people with poor flexibility, and obese people. It can be caused by tension, menstruation, pregnancy, kidney infection, prostate gland problems, rectal disorders, arthritis, a slipped disc, the flu, and poor posture, or by having a sedentary occupation.

Signs and Symptoms

Low back pain may be chronic, or it may occur only once. Its onset may be sudden or gradual. Pain in the lower back is usually most severe when the patient stands erect.

Self-Care Treatment

Resting the muscles is essential in treating low back pain. When the pain first appears, rest flat on your back for at least twenty-four hours on a firm mattress (use a sheet of plywood between your mattress and box springs) or a waterbed; sleep without a pillow. Follow the period of rest with a gradual increase in activity; avoid strenuous activity of any kind for about six weeks.

To relieve pain, lie on your back with an electric heating pad under the most painful area. Take two to three aspirin every three hours. Soaking in a hot tub can also help relieve pain. Knotted muscles can be relaxed by gentle back massage around the affected area.

Begin an exercise program of mild stretching and strengthening of the back muscles; increasing the strength of your abdominal muscles can also help relieve low back pain. Use good posture when sitting and standing.

EXERCISES TO STRENGTHEN BACK MUSCLES

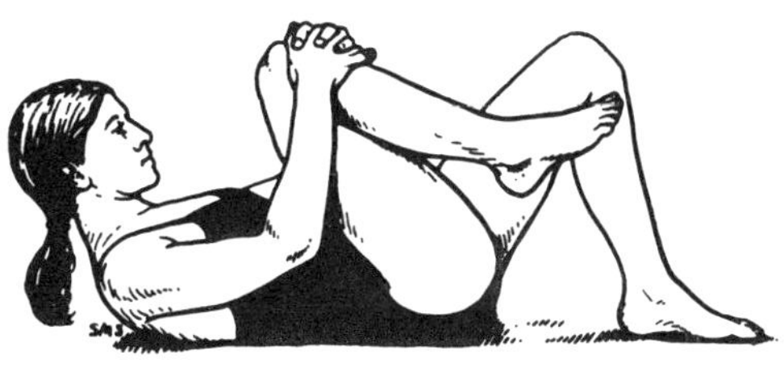

Figure 7-2
Pull your knee toward your chest with one hand; lift your head and shoulders forward at the same time. Hold for 6 seconds. Repeat with the other leg.

Figure 7-3

Modified push-up. Begin by lying on your stomach, elbows bent. Push your upper body up, then lower.

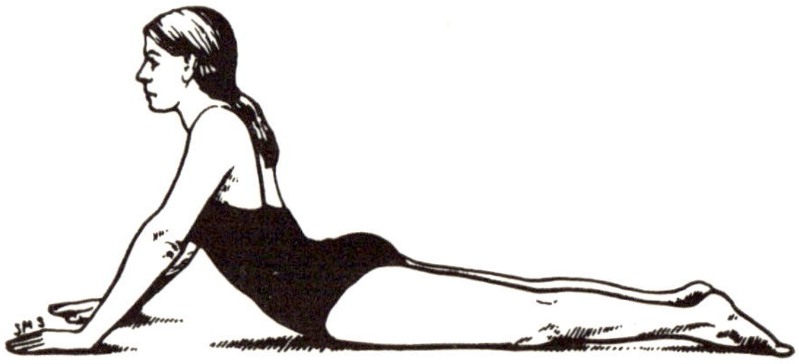

Figure 7-4

Leg raises. Lie on your stomach, and raise one leg completely off the floor. Hold for a while, keeping your leg straight. Lower, and repeat with the other leg. When you have completed this exercise, roll onto your back and pull the knees to the chest.

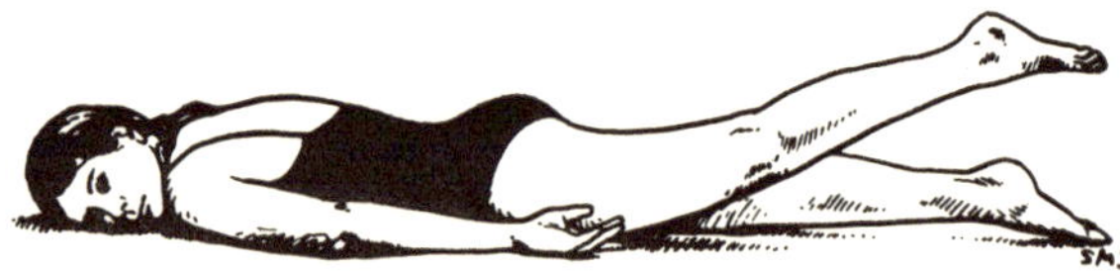

Figure 7-5

Lie on your back with your arms at your side. Slowly raise both legs. Hold your legs about 6 inches off the floor for a few seconds. Return to original position. Then pull your knees to your chest.

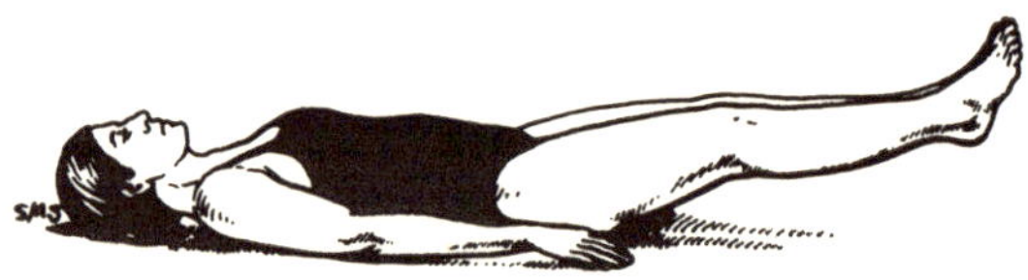

Figure 7-6

Modified sit-up. Begin on your back. Slowly lift your head and shoulders off the floor, reaching for your knees. Hold for 6 seconds, then lower your back one vertebra at a time.

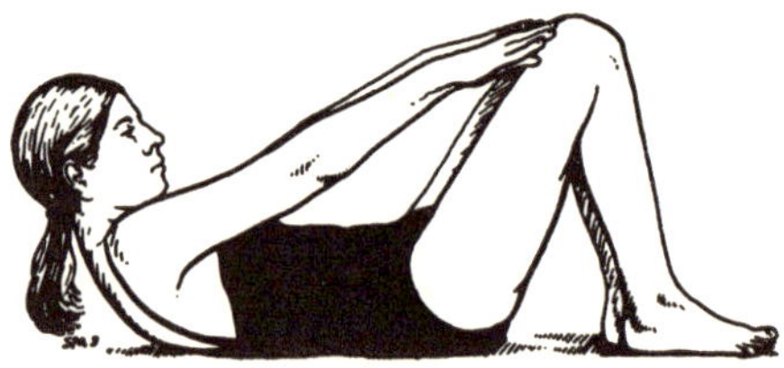

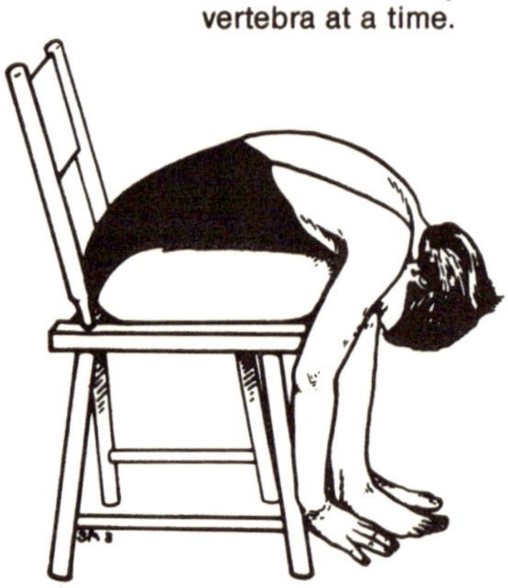

Figure 7-7

To stretch the back gently, sit on a hard chair, feet flat on the floor. Slowly roll forward from your waist and reach your hands to the floor. Hold your position for a few seconds, then return to an upright position.

Figure 7-8

Pelvic tilt. Lie on your back, knees bent and hands folded behind your head. Inhale and exhale while you tighten your buttocks to press your lower back against the floor. Hold for 6 seconds, then relax.

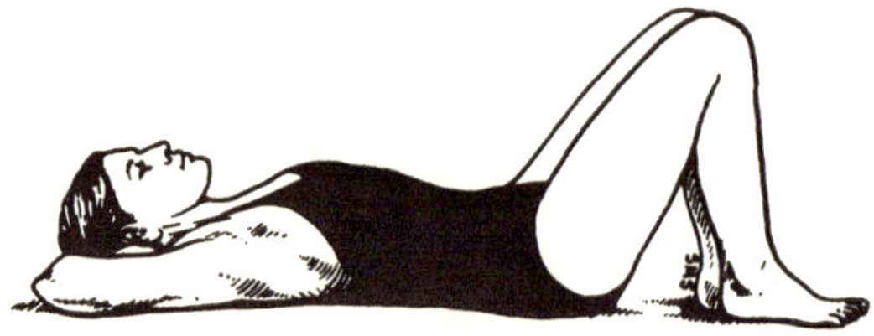

Some of the following may help prevent and relieve backache:

1. Sitting can be taxing on the back. To avoid backache, sit in a chair that provides firm support. Keep the feet slightly elevated if possible. If you sit all day, take frequent breaks to relax and stretch.

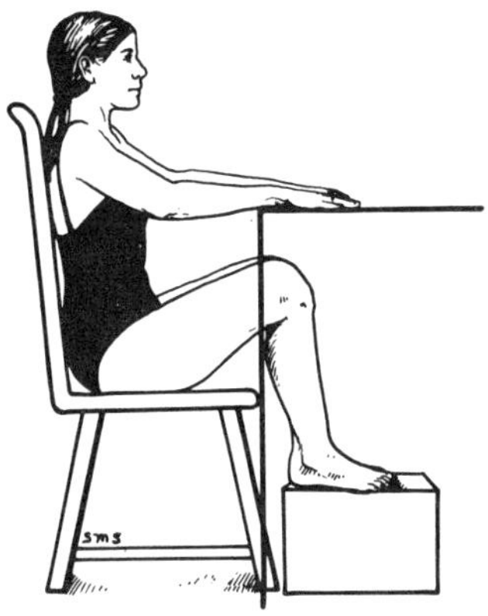

Figure 7-9
Proper way to sit at a desk.

2. Prolonged standing may not only be dull, but it may put undue pressure on the spinal column. If your occupation requires that you stand for long periods of time, shift your weight often from one foot to the other. It is also helpful to move around.
3. Poor sleep posture may irritate or cause backache. The best position for sleeping is on the side with the knees slightly bent. Lying on the stomach causes a sort of swayback position that may aggravate back problems. Using a firm mattress will also help correct abnormal back conditions associated with sleep.

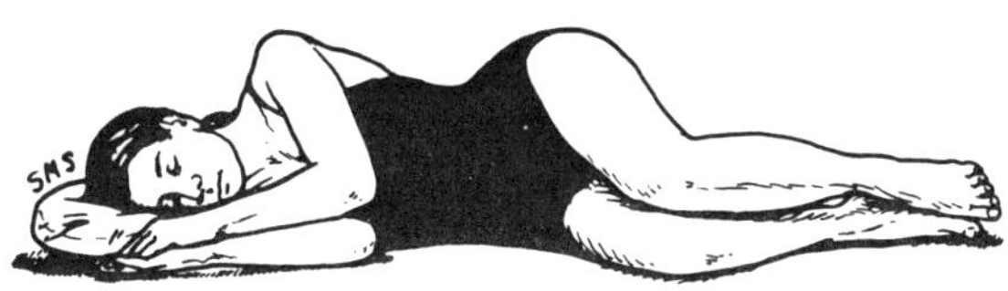

Figure 7-10
Two good ways to sleep: (1) On your side, using a pillow only large enough to keep your back straight; (2) On your back, with your head on a pillow and your knees draped over another pillow.

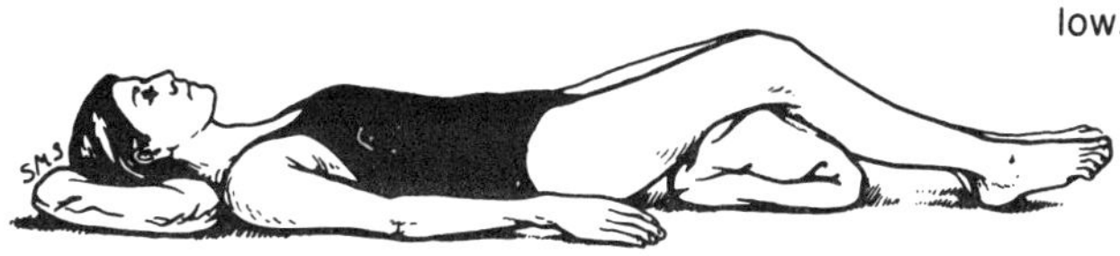

4. High-heeled shoes throw the spine out of alignment and tilt the pelvis. Wearing lower heeled shoes may help relieve back pain.

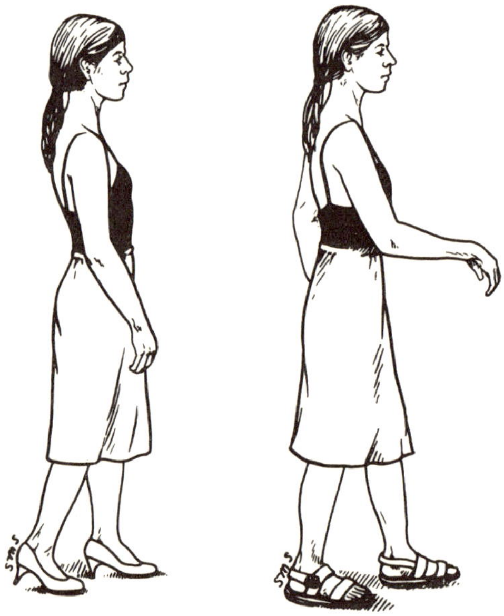

Figure 7-11
Avoid wearing high-heeled shoes if possible.

5. Carrying shoulder bags or attache' cases may aggravate back conditions, especially if the objects are heavy. Balancing weight on both shoulders or in both hands is helpful. If weight cannot be evenly distributed, change packages or objects from hand to hand frequently.
6. Wearing girdles or skintight jeans may weaken the abdominal muscles. These muscles are a key prop for the spine, and when they are weak, the chances of back injury are increased. Avoid wearing such apparel for any length of time.
7. If you must drive for some length of time, get out of the car every hour and walk around. Placing a pillow behind the back may help relieve

Figure 7-12

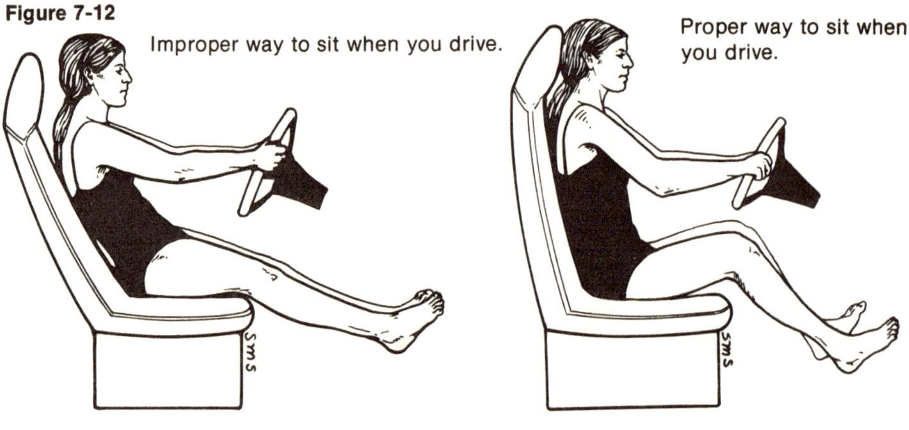

Improper way to sit when you drive.

Proper way to sit when you drive.

strain, and tilting the seat to different angles periodically (providing your car seat tilts, of course) can be helpful. It is also wise to have the car seat forward enough so that your knees are slightly bent.

8. Rather than bending from the waist to pick up a heavy object, squat and keep the back straight. Use the large thigh muscles to do the lifting.

Low Back Pain in Children

Low back pain is an uncommon complaint prior to adolescence; sometimes it accompanies hip injury or deformity, and the child will limp in such cases.

Treat a child much the same as you would yourself — have him or her rest on a firm, flat mattress and sleep without a pillow. Administer aspirin and heat to relieve pain. Allow a gradual increase in activity; complete recovery takes about six weeks.

When to Call the Doctor

Call the doctor if you suffer fever, weakness or numbness in the legs, pain that travels down one or both legs to below the knee, or low back pain that is associated with injury.

BACKACHE

Acute backache is usually caused by trauma from lifting heavy objects, a blow or a fall or jump from a height that injures the back, or sudden twisting or lifting that strains muscles that are already fatigued or out of condition. Acute backache can also result from meningitis, encephalitis, prostatitis, kidney or bladder infections, localized infections around the vertebral column, and kidney stones.

Signs and Symptoms

Acute backache results from strain that is localized in the spinal area, and it is aggravated by motion of the spine. There is severe, direct tenderness over localized back infections. The pain from kidney stones is severe, often radiating down into the groin and the inner sides of the thigh on the affected side. An individual with acute backache walks very cautiously, stooped forward so that he or she does not jar the spine.

Self-Care Treatment

Mild to moderate back strain usually improves with time and rest. Take aspirin for pain, and apply heat — hot wet towels, a hot water bottle, or an electric heating pad, or soak in a hot tub — for relief of tension and pain.

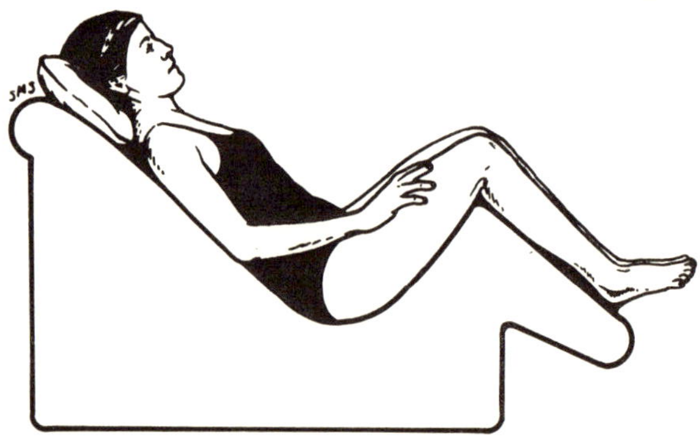

Figure 7-13
This position in a recliner will help your back to relax and feel better.

Backache in Children

Backache is as common in children as in adults and is frequent among adolescents. Most of it results from strenuous activities encountered in play or sports competition, but it can also be caused by kidney infection or abnormalities, abnormalities of the spine, defects of the growth plates of the vertebrae, compression fracture of the vertebrae, or arthritis in the spine.

To treat a child with backache, place a piece of plywood between the mattress and box springs, and see that the patient gets plenty of bed rest. Have the child soak in a tepid bath, and give aspirin for pain. An electric heating pad can also relieve pain. Watch the child to make sure that he or she avoids strenuous activities until the back is healed.

When to Call the Doctor

Call the doctor if your own backache results in persistent, severe pain. See your doctor if your child's backache is accompanied by visible deformity, fever, sharply localized pain, one-sided pain, burning or frequent urination, discoloration of urine, or curvature of the spine.

STIFF NECK

Pain and stiffness in the neck can result from a number of factors, most common among them getting chilled, sleeping in a cramped position, unaccustomed exercise, sudden twisting of the neck, or simple muscle strain. Some disease conditions — tonsillitis, meningitis, flu, fever, arthritis, and others — can also result in pain and stiffness in the neck. A pinched nerve in the neck can result from arthritis.

Signs and Symptoms

It may feel like there is a "crick" in the neck; it may be painful to turn the head from side to side, and the pain and stiffness in the neck may result in headache. In severe cases, the neck is so stiff that the victim cannot touch the chin to the chest. If arthritis pinches a nerve, the pain may extend down the arm, the pain will be only on one side, neck stiffness will not be prominent, and there may be numbness or tingling sensations in the arm or hand.

Self-Care Treatment

Neck pain that is caused by muscle strain instead of disease can be successfully treated at home with hot wet packs and hot showers. Take aspirin for pain, and have someone gently massage the muscles of the neck.

If you experience neck pain in the morning, sleep on a firm, hard surface without a pillow (try putting a sheet of plywood between your mattress and box springs).

Neck pain, like back pain, takes a long time to improve. Try folding a bath towel lengthwise into a long four-inch-wide strip, wrapping it around your neck and pinning it in place with safety pins before you go to bed. It will keep you from sleeping in a cramped position and may provide great relief from neck pain.

When to Call the Doctor

Call the doctor if you cannot touch your chin to your chest, if fever and headache are present, if you experience numbness or tingling in the arm, or if the pain travels down one arm. Stiff neck that results from disease must be cared for by aiming treatment at the underlying cause.

FLAT FEET

Some people get concerned about flat feet that aren't flat at all. Infants have *fat* feet — but the pad of fat disappears as the child begins to walk and the muscles of the feet develop. Arches do not appear in the normal child until he or she is three to four years old, when the muscles have had an adequate chance to develop.

Flat feet can be caused by forcing an infant to wear shoes too soon, by putting ill-fitting shoes on an infant or small child, or by outfitting children in shoes that do not have proper arches (sneakers, sandals, and tennis shoes are common culprits).

Signs and Symptoms

With true flat feet, there is no arch when the individual stands. Flat feet cause the shoes to wear in a unique pattern: the tops of the shoes break down from the inside, and the inner edges of the heels and soles wear out more quickly than the rest of the shoe.

In some cases, there is no pain, but in most cases, foot pain and fatigue occur after even moderate exercise. The pain, originating in the arch area, can radiate to the calf of the leg and even up to the lower back. Many victims experience night cramping of the legs and feet.

Self-Care Treatment

The best treatment for flat feet is exercising the muscles that enable the arch to develop. A child between the ages of three and six should walk on tiptoe five to ten minutes each day; from six to eight years of age, the child should walk on the edge of his or her foot (barefooted) with the toes clenched for ten minutes each day.

Don't give your child walking shoes until he or she is able to walk unaided on hard surfaces — sometimes as late as three years of age.

Adults can exercise the arch and strengthen muscles by daily picking up marbles with toes, picking peanuts and pencils up off the floor with the feet, walking on the outer rims of the feet for ten minutes, standing and walking on tiptoe during the day, bending the feet sharply upward while sitting, walking barefoot, and walking long distances across sand. You might want to try any or all of these exercises if your feet are flat.

If you suffer from aching or painful feet following walking or exercise, alternate hot and cold foot baths, and rest your feet following exercise. Gentle massage of the foot muscles can help relieve pain.

To prevent the development of flat feet, allow your children to go barefoot as long as possible, and correct bad posture habits as soon as they begin to develop. If you are overweight, reduce your weight to a reasonable level to avoid putting strain on your feet.

When to Call the Doctor

Consult your doctor if your feet or your child's feet are extemely painful and do not respond to home treatment. You should not attempt to use orthopedic shoes, arch supports, or other mechanical devices without your doctor's prescription or instruction.

CHAPTER 8

COMMON EYE COMPLAINTS

All potentially serious eye conditions require prompt medical care, preferably by an ophthalmologist. Delay in proper treatment of a relatively minor eye injury or disease can cause loss of vision. Without exception, the following eye conditions should be referred to a physician or ophthalmologist:

- Serious infections or injuries of the eye or the immediately adjacent structures
- Foreign bodies lodged on the eyeball that cannot be flushed off by gentle irrigation
- All cases of foreign objects in the eye when multiple objects are involved, even if all are flushed from the eye
- The feeling that a foreign object is still in the eye, even after one has been removed
- A foreign body in the eye that cannot be located
- A loss of vision or a sudden change in vision

IMPAIRED VISION

Refractive Errors

The most common complaints of vision impairment involve refractive errors. Shortening or lengthening of the eyeball causes the lens to focus the image not on the retina, but behind it or in front of it. Nearsightedness occurs when the eyeball is too long; the eye is adapted for close work but cannot adjust for distant vision. Farsightedness occurs when the eyeball is too short; distant vision is clear, but near vision is blurred, so eyes are adapted best for vision at long distances. Presbyopia, a form of farsightedness, begins in middle age and progresses to the fifties and sixties as the lens loses elasticity with age. Astigmatism occurs with an irregularity in the curvature of the cornea or lens; light rays are focused on the retina in an irregular pattern, and a distorted image is received.

Options Available to Correct Refractive Errors

Type of Lens	Comments
Hard Contacts	These are the least expensive of the contact lenses. However, they are difficult to adjust to, and some never get used to them. They can be worn for years and can correct astigmatism. They are made of rigid plastic and can easily pop out.
Soft Contacts	They are more comfortable than hard contacts. They are made of water absorbent plastic and contain 35-45 percent water. They conform to the surface of the cornea and are excellent for sports and outdoor activities because they rarely pop out. However, they are easily torn and require daily disinfecting to keep bacteria from growing on them.
Gas-Permeable Contacts	These are rigid like hard lenses but allow oxygen to pass through and reach the cornea, and they can be worn for longer periods of time without discomfort. They are more flexible than the hard lenses and correct vision better than the soft and are more durable.
Bifocal Contacts	Presently available only in hard lenses. They help in focusing on nearby objects but are difficult to fit and quite expensive.
Extended-Wear Contacts	These can be worn continuously for weeks and even months because of very high water (70 to 80%) content and high oxygen permeability. They are very thin and soft and easily damaged, and can be more easily contaminated with bacteria or a buildup of protein deposits.
Toric Soft Lenses	These are a new refinement of soft lenses designed to correct moderate astigmatism. They must be individually fitted and custom made.
Intraocular Lenses	These are designed for those who undergo cataract surgery and are plastic lenses that are implanted inside the eye. They give excellent vision.
Eyeglasses	Glasses are less expensive than hard or soft contact lenses and require no daily upkeep. However, there are problems with weight, activities, peripheral vision, and blind spots.

Self-Care Treatment

All cases of impaired vision due to refractive errors should be treated by a trained ophthalmologist or optometrist. Eyeglasses or contact lenses are usually needed and cannot be obtained without a prescription.

STRABISMUS

Eyes that are crossed or eyes that are not properly aligned characterize strabismus, a condition caused by weaknesses in some of the muscles that control movement of the eyeball. Strabismus usually apears at an early age, and if it goes uncorrected, it can impair vision and mar the appearance of one eye. The eye that is not used can, over a period of time, deteriorate.

Any case of strabismus should be referred to an ophthalmologist; he or she will prescribe treatment that you can carry out under his or her direction, including eye exercises, wearing of a patch, and use of eyeglasses and eyedrops.

In extreme cases, surgery may be needed.

EYESTRAIN

In the absence of disease, eyestrain can be due to refractive errors, muscle imbalance, poor illumination, exposure to excessive glare, poor general health associated with prolonged use of the eyes, or intolerance for fluorescent light. Eyestrain is seldom present upon awakening but comes on after some degree of visual effort—especially reading, watching television or movies, or at the end of the day. Some people develop eyestrain after prolonged visual effort despite optimal visual conditions.

Signs and Symptoms

Signs and symptoms of eyestrain include arching of the eyes, headache in the frontal region, dizziness, a hot scratchy feeling in the eyelids, eye ache, poor vision, blurred or dim vision, nausea, or other functional and/or emotional effects.

Self-Care Treatment

To soothe the burning and aching of eyestrain, rest in bed in a darkened room for fifteen to twenty minutes. Apply cool compresses to your eyes for fifteen minutes (cotton balls soaked in cool water work well). Change to an incandescent light if you need to continue working or reading under light. Take aspirin for the pain or if you have a headache. Eye drops may give some minor relief.

When to Call the Doctor

If eyestrain becomes a recurrent, persistent problem, you should see an ophthalmologist for a complete eye examination so that the doctor can rule out any possibility of other eye disorders or disease.

DACRYOCYSTITIS

Dacryocystitis is an infection of the sac that collects and contains the tears; it is generally a result of a blockage of one of the tear canals that lead into the nose and is commonly associated with sinus infection or other infection of the nasal passages or sinuses. It is common in infants and in those over forty years of age.

If it is not treated, dacryocystitis can lead to infection of the cornea and permanent blockage of the tear ducts.

Signs and Symptoms

Profuse tearing with purulent discharge is normal with dacryocystitis; there is usually pain below the eyeball, with redness and swelling below the eye. The redness and swelling from the dacryocystitis infection often spread to the eyeball, resulting in conjunctivitis.

Self-Care Treatment

In some cases, the infection from dacryocystitis disappears on its own. Frequent application of hot compresses may help relieve the pain.

When to Call the Doctor

You should always call the doctor in cases of dacryocystitis, since antibiotic treatment is generally necessary. When the condition flares up due to some underlying cause (such as nasal polyps), the doctor will need to remove the aggravating cause.

CONJUNCTIVITIS

Often called "pink eye," conjunctivitis can be acute or chronic and is common in children. The membrane that covers the front of the eyeball and that lines the eyelids becomes inflamed as a result of bacterial infection, viral infection, smoke or dust, exposure to wind, foreign bodies in the eye, intense light, or allergies. A common aggravating cause of pink eye is a foreign object in the eyeball.

Signs and Symptoms

Conjunctivitis is usually characterized by itching, burning, or smarting and the feeling of "sand in the eye." Redness, pain, swelling, tearing, and a purulent discharge accompany some degree of blurring of vision that results from the abnormal secretions over the cornea. The eyelids generally get swollen, and the eyes are usually sensitive to light. Pink or beefy red streaks run across the surface of the eye—hence, "pink eye."

Characteristically, the eyelids stick together in the morning, and it may be necessary to soak the eyes before they can be opened.

Self-Care Treatment

Initially, examine the eye carefully to see if any foreign body is embedded in the eyeball or the eyelid; even a tiny sliver can cause pink eye.

Flush the eye thoroughly with sterile water if you can. Wear sunglasses to cut down on eye irritation, and take aspirin for pain.

If no burning, itching, or pain occur, apply warm wet compresses to your eye for fifteen minutes at a time, three or four times a day; soak your eye with warm compresses if the eyelid is stuck closed in the morning. If you have allergies or if burning, itching, or pain accompany the conjunctivitis, use cool, wet compresses. Avoid rubbing or wiping your eye.

To avoid spreading infection to your other eye and to others in your family, wash your hands frequently while you have pink eye, and wash them thoroughly each time you touch your eye. Make sure that no one else uses your washcloth or towel, and change to a fresh washcloth and towel several times a day. Carefully dispose of any handkerchiefs or tissues that you use on your eye.

When to Call the Doctor

Call your doctor if there is no improvement after twenty-four hours of treatment. You should also contact your doctor if you experience pain in your eye that radiates to the temple, a change in your ability to see (other than the slight blurring due to secretions on the cornea), difference in the size of your pupils, or an inability to adapt to light change.

STYE

A stye is an acute localized inflammation followed by an abscessed formation on an eyelid. Usually caused by a staph infection of the glands at the base of the eyelashes, styes are frequently associated with a lowered body resistance in general and often follow other illnesses and infections because the body resistance is lower.

Signs and Symptoms

At first, a stye may manifest itself as a burning, smarting sensation of the eye, as if something were in the eye; there is generally tearing and tenderness. A small, hard, red boil at the base of an eyelash eventually comes to a head, ruptures, and discharges pus. The small lump may remain for several weeks after the stye has drained and the infection has cleared up.

Self-Care Treatment

Styes are highly contagious, so handle your eye with caution. Wash your hands carefully after touching the stye, and change your towel and washcloth frequently.

Never squeeze a stye. To promote draining and rupture, apply hot wet compresses to the eye for fifteen or twenty minutes at a time, three or four times daily.

When to Call the Doctor

A stye that does not rupture and drain spontaneously after twenty-four to forty-eight hours of treatment with hot compresses should be seen by a doctor. Contact your doctor if you have recurrent styes.

CONTUSIONS (Black Eye)

A variety of nonpenetrating eye injuries can result from a blow directly to the eyeball, to the bony structure around the eye, or from air blasts or explosions. A contusion can produce a small, insignificant hemorrhage of the eyelids—as in the case of a simple black eye—or can result in blindness due to serious disruption of the contents within the eyeball.

Signs and Symptoms

Common signs and symptoms of black eye include bleeding into the loose tissues of the area around the eye, which produces discoloration of the lids and surrounding skin, and swelling.

Self-Care Treatment

Always let a doctor see a black eye within a short period of time after the injury occurred so that it can be checked for a detached retina or bleeding inside the eyeball. You should not attempt to treat black eye until it has been seen by a doctor.

Once you have been assured that the black eye is a simple one, apply ice packs to the eye area immediately following the injury and at intervals during the first twenty-four hours. After the first twenty-four hours, apply warm, moist packs at fifteen-minute intervals throughout the day until all blood has been absorbed by the tissues.

FOREIGN OBJECTS IN THE EYE

Any type or size of foreign material may adhere to or become embedded in the cornea or other parts of the eye, causing considerable pain, tears, and sensitivity to light. The amount of damage done to the eye depends on the extent of penetration, the duration of the irritation, and the degree of bacterial contamination that results. Slivers of iron or steel present a unique problem: they rust. The rust ring that surrounds such a sliver after about two days must be removed along with the sliver.

Common foreign bodies in the eyes include eyelashes, powder, sand, cinders, and insects; as the eye blinks, the object can scratch and irritate the lining of the eyelid.

Signs and Symptoms

You can generally tell if a foreign body is present in your eye. Your eye (or part of it) may get red, and usually the eye will tear profusely. You may be unable to open your eye because it is sensitive to light. Even tiny dust specks can cause considerable pain.

Self-Care Treatment

Before you touch or examine your eye, be sure to wash your hands thoroughly with soap and water.

Roll back your upper and lower lids gently to expose the eyeball and the lining of the lids; if you can see a speck of any kind, remove it carefully with the tip of a cotton swab that has been moistened with warm water.

If you cannot see a speck, bring your upper eyelid down over your lower lid, hold it there for a few seconds, and roll your eyeball upward (as if you were looking up). This procedure causes tears to flow, and the tears will often wash out the particle naturally.

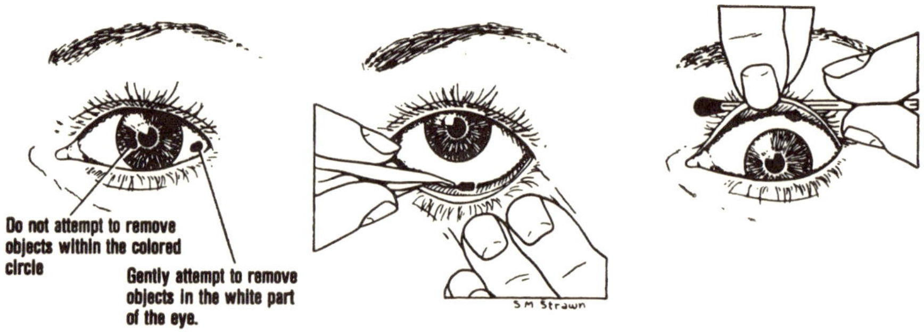

Figure 8-1
Gently attempt to remove objects in the white part of the eye. Using two fingers, gently pull down the lower eyelid while the patient looks up. Carefully pull up the upper eyelid as the person looks down. A matchstick can help you to grip the lid as shown.

If you still are not successful, carefully place your index and middle fingers just below your lower eyelid, and gently pull down on your lower eyelid; examine the inside of the lower lid. If you see an object, carefully lift it out with the corner of a clean handkerchief that has been moistened with warm water (or use a cotton swab moistened with warm water).

Check your eye from the front and the side to make sure that the foreign particle has been removed; use a good light and several mirrors. Pay particular attention to the cornea, the colorless membrane that covers the iris and the pupil. If you have gotten rid of the particle, make an eye patch of several layers of sterile gauze, and keep it over the eye for twenty-four hours. Wear sunglasses to protect the eye from strong sunlight. Do not rub the eye.

If you still are unable to dislodge the foreign particle, irrigate your eye with copious amounts of clear sterile water. Turn your head to one side, and pour water from the corner of your eye closest to your nose to the corner of your eye closest to your temple. (This way, water doesn't run toward the other eye.) Use plenty of water, and be sure to flush out the inside corner of the eye, where dust and chemicals collect.

Never try to remove any particle that is actually embedded in the eyeball.

When to Call the Doctor

Call your doctor if you cannot locate the foreign body, if you cannot remove it with any of the procedures described above, if the body is actually embedded in the eyeball, if your vision is impaired in any way, if there is blood in your eye, or if you sustained an injury that could have penetrated your eyeball.

CHAPTER 9

COMMON EAR, NOSE, AND THROAT COMPLAINTS

BLOCKED EAR (Excessive Wax)

Excessive ear wax—the most common cause of conductive hearing loss—is not a disease but may be a contributing factor in deafness and infection. Wax is normally produced in the auditory canal and is eventually excreted from the ear; excessive amounts may act as a medium for bacteria growth or may partially or completely block the ear canal—resulting in a decrease in hearing or a sensation of fullness or pressure in the ear. Accumulated water in the ear after swimming or bathing can make the wax swell and can cause the sudden onset of symptoms.

Signs and Symptoms

Unless a bacterial infection has settled in the external ear canal, there is no pain. There may, however, be a sensation of uncomfortable fullness or pressure. You may notice a decrease in hearing ability. As stated above, these symptoms may occur suddenly following swimming or bathing.

Self-Care Treatment

Never try to remove ear wax by poking at the wax with cotton swabs, fingers, rings, bobby pins, or any other device. Such efforts will only compact the wax against the eardrum. You should not use ear drops without your doctor's prescription and instruction, since they could be dangerous in case of a perforated eardrum.

When to Call the Doctor

A doctor should be consulted for every case of excess ear wax; the doctor is equipped to remove the wax safely and effectively and to cleanse the ear canal.

PERFORATED EARDRUM

The eardrum—the tiny, thin membrane responsible for the vibration that enables you to hear—is located much closer to the outside of the body than most people suspect. Perforation of the eardrum is quite common and can occur without too much trouble—usually from careless use of cotton swabs, use of toothpicks or bobby pins to clean the ear, a blow to the side of the head (even a playful slap with an open palm can rupture the eardrum), or insertion of the tip of the tongue during a passionate kiss (the suction created as the tongue is withdrawn causes the rupture). The eardrum may also rupture if infection in the middle ear causes pressure due to pus buildup. The eardrum frequently ruptures at its weakest point—the center—which is also the point that sometimes does not heal. (A small surgical incision in the eardrum can allow the pus from a middle ear infection to drain safely without rupturing the eardrum; the incision heals rapidly and without scarring.)

Signs and Symptoms

The pain that accompanies rupture of the eardrum is usually severe and agonizing. A loss of hearing and a hollow reverberation in the head occur, accompanied by dizziness, nausea, and vomiting. There is usually blood in the ear canal.

Self-Care Treatment

Always see a doctor for possible eardrum perforation. If nothing is draining from the ear canal (fluid, pus, or blood), insert a small piece of clean, dry cotton loosely in the end of the ear canal to prevent infection from entering the ear. While some cases of small perforations may heal spontaneously, drugs and medical care are necessary to treat larger involvements.

EARACHE

Earache results from ear infection, usually infection of the middle ear, and is usually secondary to a common cold or sore throat. An earache may result when violent nose blowing forces infected mucus into the ear canals leading to the inner ear, or may result when there is a blockage of the canals that does not permit proper drainage from the ears. Earaches are common in children, because their eustachian tubes (the canals connecting the throat to the middle and inner ear) are narrow and do not permit proper drainage.

While earaches usually result from bacterial infection, the infection may in some cases be viral.

Signs and Symptoms

Pain, of course, is the primary symptom of earache; the pain is throbbing, sharp, penetrating, and constant. (Pain may be absent in some serious cases, with only other symptoms present.) Usually, impaired hearing, a feeling of fullness in the ears, ringing in the ears, and dizziness occur. Infants who have an earache usually tug at their ear, rub their ear, or roll their head with a drilling motion; they usually cry with agonizing shrieks.

Self-Care Treatment

Never probe into your ear with cotton swabs, bobby pins, or other instruments. Apply heat for pain relief; use a hot water bottle, an electric heating pad, or heated glass (heat a juice glass under hot, running water, place several paper towels saturated with hot water in the glass, and hold the bottom of the glass against the ear; make sure not to invert the glass over the ear, because hot water from the paper towels will run into the ear). If you have your doctor's permission, use warm eardrops in an ear that has no discharge.

If you have a fever, rest. Take oral decongestants, and use nose drops four times daily for two days. Use a vaporizer to keep the air moist. Unless your doctor specifically tells you to, you should not take aspirin; it may mask important pain that serves as an indicator of the progression of infection in the ear.

When to Call the Doctor

Call your doctor if you experience an increase in pain or headache despite your treatment; if you experience drainage from the ear canal or the symptoms of a perforated eardrum; if you have a fever higher than 102° F.; if you develop convulsive twitching of the facial muscles; or if you are dizzy. Always consult a doctor if the person is under the age of three.

EAR DRAINAGE

The only substance that normally comes from the ear canal is ear wax: normally brown, but sometimes yellowish or beige when mixed with water during bathing or swimming. Normal ear wax contains no blood, never flows out of the ear canal in abundance, and has only a mild odor.

Any other kind of discharge is symptomatic of something wrong—usually a foreign body in the ear canal, a perforated eardrum, a boil in the ear canal, swimmer's ear, a middle ear infection, or tumor of the middle ear. Some disease conditions—including eczema and some fungus infections—can result in a chronic slight discharge, but this is not common.

Signs and Symptoms

Abnormal drainage from the ear canal is usually thin, watery, and

How to Apply Ear, Nose, and Eye Drops

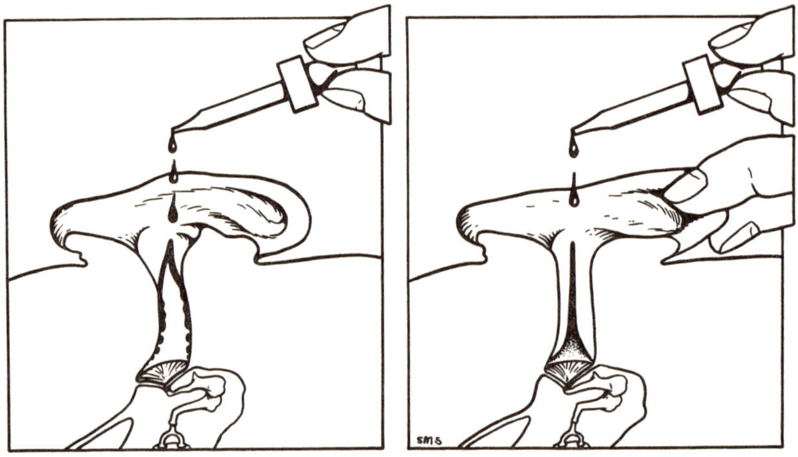

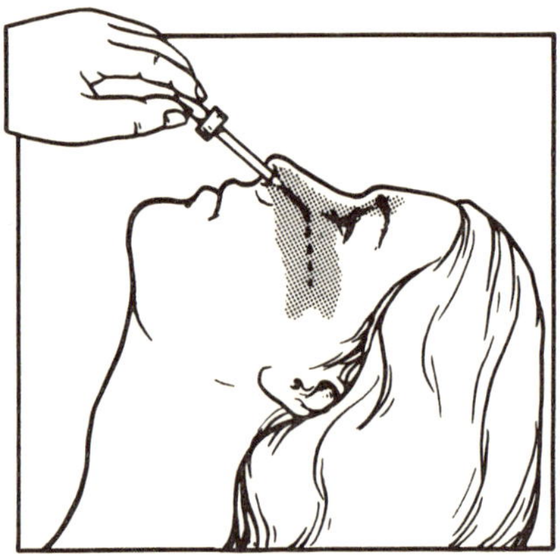

Figure 9-1

To apply eye drops, tilt your head back and toward the eye to be treated. Pull down the lower lid with one finger. Looking up, squeeze the drops into the pouch. Blink to move the drop around the eye.

To straighten the ear canal when applying ear drops (the ear canal has a curvature), lie on your side, with the ear to be treated up, and gently pull the top of the ear up and toward the back of your head.

To apply nose drops, sit upright, tilt your head backward, and push up on the tip of your nose to open the nasal passage. Insert the dropper about 1/3 inch. Apply the drops, and keep your head tilted for a few moments.

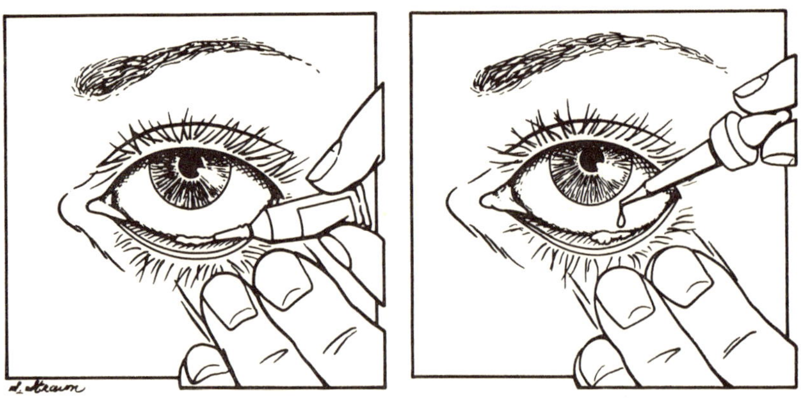

bloody and may be green, yellow, or white. It may be cheesy and resemble pus. It usually has a strong odor. Typically, earache, slight loss of hearing, fever, and a feeling of fullness or pressure in the ear occur.

Self-Care Treatment

All cases of ear discharge should be seen promptly by a doctor. Do not take aspirin, and never put cotton plugs in your ear—they force the drainage back into the middle ear. Don't try to remove the drainage from the ear canal with a cotton swab, and don't wash out the ear. Get to a doctor within twelve hours.

SWIMMER'S EAR

Swimmer's ear, a bacterial or fungal infection of the lining of the outer ear canal, is the most common cause of ear pain in adults and is common among children. Ear wax usually provides a certain degree of protection against bacteria in the ear canal; when that ear wax is absent (due to too-vigorous cleaning with cotton swabs), when too much bacteria is present (due to drainage of infected pus from the middle ear during infection), or when the climate is moist and conducive to bacterial growth (due to the ear's inability to dry out following swimming or bathing), the normal balance is disturbed and the outer ear canal gets infected. Other causes can include injury to the ear canal, boils in the ear canal, eczema, infectious dermatitis, and other skin eruptions (such as herpes zoster).

Signs and Symptoms

Swimmer's ear produces inflammation and acute tenderness at the ear opening (external); pain results from movement of the ear or movement of the jaw in talking, chewing, or other activities. The swelling can cause partial loss of hearing; pain is moderate to severe, and sometimes a fever is present. The external ear canal is red, swollen, and tender and itches severely. Some discharge may accompany the condition.

Self-Care Treatment

Avoid scratching the ear canal with cotton swabs or bobby pins; keep all devices out of the ear canal to prevent further aggravation of the infection. Take aspirin for pain, and apply a hot water bottle or heated juice glass to the ear to relieve discomfort.

Gently cleanse away any drainage or crust from the external ear with water and zinc oxide. Cleanse away only what drains out of the ear canal; don't cleanse the ear canal itself.

Keep your ears dry to promote healing and prevent further infection. Wear loose earplugs while bathing, and avoid swimming until the infection subsides. You may want to place a few drops of rubbing alcohol into your ear canals following immersion in water to dry the canals and prevent reinfection.

Swimmer's Ear in Children

Swimmer's ear is common in children and manifests the same symptoms as it does in adults. A child may often experience swollen glands with swimmer's ear. Take the child to the doctor if there is sudden, acute, severe pain (evidenced by sharp crying and insistent rubbing or tugging at the ear); if the ear starts to drain; if the child screams when you touch the ear; or if the child runs a fever or at least 101° F. for twenty-four hours.

Use a few drops of rubbing alcohol in the ear canal after the child swims or bathes as a preventive measure if the swimmer's ear recurs frequently.

FOREIGN OBJECTS IN THE EAR

Various objects—such as insects, seeds, stones, broken toothpicks, matchsticks, cotton, and others—can become lodged in the external ear canal.

Signs and Symptoms

A foreign body in the external ear canal results in a fluttering or itching in the ear canal. If the object is sharp and is lodged in the canal or against the eardrum, pain will result. If the object is lodged deeply enough, it may rupture the eardrum.

Self-Care Treatment

Never probe the ear with an instrument. If you can see an object easily at the ear opening, remove it gently with your fingers or a pair of tweezers; do not force it.

If the object is an insect (evidenced by fluttering of wings or buzzing sounds), shine a bright flashlight into the ear; insects are attracted to light and will crawl out of the ear. If the light does not attract the insect, place three drops of 3 percent hydrogen peroxide or baby oil into the ear, and lift the insect out when it floats to the ear opening.

Never put moisture into the ear if the object is a seed, wood, or anything else that will swell if it gets wet.

When to Call the Doctor

Consult your doctor if you cannot remove a foreign object that you can see, if you have to use force to remove the object, or if you cannot see the foreign object. Also call the doctor if you suspect that the object punctured your eardrum or broke skin in the external ear canal.

VERTIGO (Dizziness)

Vertigo itself is not a disease, but it is a symptom common to many diseases and disorders—among them excess wax in the ear, perforation of the eardrum, blockage of the ear canal or eustachian tube, swimmer's ear, middle ear infection, drug overdose (including too much aspirin or alcohol), high blood pressure, congestive heart failure, stroke, or a sudden change of position. Vertigo results when the equilibrium of the inner ear is disturbed, and it ranges from a simple feeling of "lightheadedness" to a fainting sensation where objects seem to move or rotate or where the individual himself seems to spin around.

Signs and Symptoms

Loss of balance is the most characteristic sign of vertigo; others include fainting, nausea, vomiting, sweating, change in pupil size, abdominal cramps, diarrhea, excessive thirst, confusion, collapse, intense itching, and chest pain.

Self-Care Treatment

Vertigo is common among children, and you should treat a child as you would an adult. Rest in a quiet, dim room in whatever position is most comfortable.

When to Call the Doctor

Contact a doctor if the vertigo is persistent, if it is recurrent, if the dizziness interferes with daily activities (including school for a child), or if it is accompanied by fever, nausea, and vomiting.

MOTION SICKNESS

As a result of shifting of the fluid in the canals of the inner ear (due to motion), the equilibrium of the inner ear is disturbed and a disorder known as motion sickness results. The disorder is caused by motion—why some people get it and others don't is not fully understood. Certain factors can aggravate motion sickness, including riding backwards, riding in a hot and stuffy vehicle, hearing strange or loud sounds, watching the horizon go up and down, or seeing or hearing another passenger vomit. People with sinus infections, chronic infection of the eustachian tube, chronic infection of the ears, or inner ear infection are much more likely to develop motion sickness.

Some people get motion sickness only on certain kinds of vehicles; others get motion sick on every kind of vehicle (including boats, cars, trains, buses, and planes).

Signs and Symptoms

The most characteristic signs of motion sickness are nausea and vomiting; these often come in recurrent waves. The motion sickness may also cause cold sweating, difficulty in breathing, dizziness, and a greenish pallor to the skin. Because motion sickness is so intensely unpleasant, a person who gets motion sick easily may develop intense anxiety when presented with the prospect of riding in a vehicle.

Self-Care Treatment

If motion sickness is a recurrent problem for you or a child, contact your doctor and get antinausea medication. Take the medication **before** starting out on a trip, and take it as instructed; don't wait to get nauseated first.

At the first signs of motion sickness, lie down and try to keep your head still. Don't try to read, work on a crafts project, or watch the passing scenery; especially avoid watching the horizon going up and down if you are in a boat. Avoid drinking any alcohol; you may be able to sip small amounts of cola drinks, ginger ale, or fruit juice to settle your stomach. Sucking ice can help. It often helps relieve the feeling of nausea if you can roll down a window and get some fresh air.

Avoid riding so that you are facing backward. Take frequent rest breaks so that you can get out of the car and walk around.

Self-Care Treatment for Children

Make sure that the child gets plenty of sleep before departure; don't take a sick child on a trip. Feed the child a light meal before leaving, and have the child eat light meals during the trip. Keep the inside of the vehicle cool. If you can, get the child to lie down with his or her eyes closed; if not, keep him or her preoccupied with a game. Try to keep the child from looking out the windows at the passing scenery. Roll down the window to get some fresh air into the vehicle.

If your doctor has prescribed an antinauseant, give the child one an hour before you start out, and repeat the dosage every four hours, even if the child is feeling well.

When to Call the Doctor

Stop traveling immediately and get to a doctor if vomiting persists for a period of several hours, if the vomit starts to contain blood, or if signs of dehydration appear (scanty urine, refusal of liquids, parched appearance, fever). Often, rest and avoidance of travel overnight will help.

You may want to stop traveling if one of the members of your party gets motion sickness—the sight, sound, and smell of the vomiting can trigger motion sickness in the other members of the party who had been previously unaffected.

TINNITUS (Ringing in the Ears)

Tinnitus refers to a ringing, buzzing, hissing, thumping, whistling, or roaring noise in the ear or head; the intensity of the condition and the volume of the noises change from day to day. Sometimes the sound is so loud that it can be heard by a doctor who is examining the victim. It is often accompanied by deafness and vertigo.

Tinnitus is most commonly caused by reaction to medication (often to aspirin), reaction to disease conditions (commonly high blood pressure), a shotgun blast, or sudden or loud noises (including loud music).

Always contact a doctor in cases of tinnitus. While you are waiting to see the doctor, treat tinnitus as you would treat vertigo.

NOSEBLEED

Commom in children and adults, most nosebleeds are caused by irritation of the blood vessels in front of the nose; almost always, the blood comes from a vessel located in the lower portion of the nose. Nosebleed can be caused by injury, underlying disease, acute infectious diseases, high blood pressure, kidney and liver conditions, heart problems, picking the nose, rubbing the nose, lack of moisture in the air, certain blood disorders, allergies, blowing the nose, foreign bodies in the nose, chronic nasal infection, acute colds, extremes of heat and cold, malignant growths in the nose, anemia, high altitudes, and strenuous activity.

Many nosebleeds in children occur at night, when the child unconsciously picks at a scab or crusty lesion that results from the common cold.

Almost all nosebleeds are associated with the common cold or with minor injury to the nose; they are more common in the winter and can be prevented by keeping the air cool and moist.

Self-Care Treatment

One of the most important aspects of treatment for nosebleed is to keep calm — you're not losing as much blood as it appears.

1. Sit up straight, or lean slightly forward. **Don't** tilt your head back or lie down — it can cause the blood to run down your throat and can lead to indigestion, vomiting, or choking. **Gently** blow your nose to remove any clots that have lodged there or that have formed.
2. Just below the hard cartilage of the nose, where the tissue is soft, pinch your nostrils together between your thumb and forefinger. Maintain a firm pressure for at least five minutes.
3. Release the pressure gently. If bleeding continues, gently insert a small wad of cotton into the nostril, but leave part of the gauze or cotton wad extending from the nose so that you can remove it easily. If you can, soak the cotton wad in hydrogen peroxide, nasal decongestant, or cool water before inserting it into the nostril (wring out the excess fluid first). Again, press your nostrils firmly together, and maintain firm pressure for another five minutes.
4. Slowly and gently release the pressure and remove the cotton wad from the nostril. If the bleeding has not stopped, remain in an erect, seated position and apply cold compresses and ice to the nose, lips, and back of the neck.
5. Once the nose stops bleeding, stay in a sitting position, leaning slightly forward. Keep quiet, and don't put any strain on your nose — don't blow your nose, talk, or laugh; don't bend over. If you have to sneeze, do it through your mouth. For a few days, keep the inside of your nostrils moistened with *Vaseline* or slightly salty water.

When to Call the Doctor

Call your doctor immediately if you have sustained a serious injury to your nose or if you have high blood pressure. If your nosebleeds have increased in frequency and if they are not associated with the common cold or with injury, make an appointment to see your doctor on a nonurgent basis. Your doctor should examine your nose at a time when it has not been bleeding so that he or she can see the tissues without causing the nose to start bleeding again.

THE COMMON COLD

While over 100 different viruses can cause the common cold, about 45 percent of all colds are caused by the same virus (a rhinovirus). Over half of the population in the United States has at least one cold during the winter months. The common cold is the most frequent of all nasal complaints, and it is highly contagious — spread by breathing droplets in the air or handling contaminated objects.

Most people suffer full-blown symptoms for about three days; those symptoms then greatly subside, and the cold usually runs its course in about seven days.

The uncomplicated cold requires only treatment for symptoms, but in some cases the common cold can lead to secondary infections —including ear infections, sinusitis, conjunctivitis, laryngitis, bronchitis, or pneumonia — that require vigorous treatment. A number of diseases start out with symptoms that mimic the common cold, and it is only later in the course of the disease as other symptoms develop that the disease can be identified —among them are the flu, diphtheria, strep infections, measles, mumps, and chicken pox.

Signs and Symptoms

The common cold comes on suddenly. All colds are not identical because they are caused by different viruses and because each individual reacts differently to the virus that causes the cold. Typically, the victim experiences a runny nose, sneezing, a stuffy feeling in the head, slight headache, watering of the eyes, general aching and listlessness, inability to concentrate, and a slight fever. Often, the inflammation spreads to the throat, causing a sore throat and a cough. The sense of smell and taste are blunted so that the individual hardly knows or cares what he or she is

Facts and Fancies about Catching Colds

Careful scientific investigation has debunked many firmly held beliefs about the causes of colds—fatigue, wet and chill, for example, seem to have no effect. But some of grandmother's cautions have been upheld, such as the advisability of covering sneezes and coughs. Below is a selection of presumed facts, some true, some false and some still in doubt.

Children catch more colds than anyone else.
True. Not only do young children suffer more colds, but parents with young children get more colds than other people their age.

Kissing is a sure way to spread a cold.
False. Colds are rather difficult to catch by way of the mouth. University of Wisconsin researchers tested couples, asking that in each couple, the cold-stricken partner kiss the unafflicted one for 90 seconds. Only one caught cold.

Adults tend to get fewer colds as they grow older.
True. The older a person is, the more likely it is that he already has had a particular cold virus and has some immunity to it.

Smokers catch more colds than nonsmokers.
False. Several studies have shown that both groups are equally susceptible. However, their symptoms differ. Smokers develop coughs more often than nonsmokers, and the cough persists longer, nonsmokers more often have a sore, scratchy throat.

Adults whose tonsils were removed in childhood get worse colds than those who still have their tonsils.
False. Laboratory experiements with volunteers given virus-laden nose drops showed that a tonsillectomy affected neither susceptibility to colds nor the severity of colds that were contracted.

Hay-fever sufferers get particularly bad colds.
True. Experiments on those afflicted with this allergy indicated that their colds were more severe than those of other people.

Introverts suffer worse colds than outgoing, extroverted personality types.
Probably true. When volunteers at Britain's Common Cold Unit were rated with standard psychological tests, scientists found introverts did indeed get worse cold symptoms than extroverts. Introverts also spread more virus particles, another indication that their infections were more severe.

Ongoing stress, such as a high-pressure job, increases vulnerability to colds.
Probably false. Studies at the Common Cold Unit found that sudden psychological jolts, rather than continuing stress, heightened susceptibility to colds. The true culprit seems to be the stress associated with change itself, whether the change is positive or negative; thus any major disruption of routine—even a pleasant diversion such as a vacation—increases the risk of a cold.

Source: Library of Health—Coping with the Common Cold, by Wendy Murphy. Editors of Time-Life books.© 1981, Time-Life Books, Inc.

eating. The person has no energy or ambition. The voice is weak and husky; the nasal membranes are swollen, and the discharge is a thick, yellowish mucus.

Self-Care Treatment

If you take a common cold seriously from the beginning, you will shorten its course and largely prevent secondary infections and complications.

Many people can recognize the earliest symptoms of a cold — a slight throat tickle, tightness or dryness in the nose or throat, loss of appetite, and a slight out-of-sorts feeling (including tension and physical uncoordination). When you feel these symptoms coming on, slow your pace; reduce your workload, alleviate tension, and walk in a slow, relaxed manner. Step up your intake of fluids, especially fruit juices. Eat a light meal at dinner time, and go to bed early. Making even these small changes can give your body the extra energy it needs to heal the cold more quickly.

There is no cure for the common cold, so treatment centers on providing comfort and alleviating discomfort. Treat each of your symptoms separately. If you are fatigued and aching or if you have a fever, go to bed and stay there until you feel like getting up; bed rest isn't necessary if you aren't running a fever and if you have the energy or the interest to be doing other things. Do get extra rest, avoid getting chilled, and avoid changing temperatures. Keep as warm as you can.

It's important to keep your body nourished. Eat nourishing foods — it's better to eat a few more meals with a smaller amount of food at each meal when you have a cold. Drink plenty of fluids — fruit juices are good, because they are nutritious. Set a goal of drinking at least eight ounces of liquid every two hours.

Take aspirin to relieve aches and to keep fever in check. You should take aspirin with milk or food to avoid stomach upset.

To relieve nasal congestion, use a vaporizer to keep the air moist. You can use nose drops or spray no more frequently than three times a day and for no longer than three days. Drinking hot teas and eating hot soups helps keep the mucus thin and breaks up the mucus in both the sinuses and the throat.

Gargle with saltwater to soothe a sore throat; do not use aspirin gargles, since they irritate inflamed throat tissues. Hot teas and soups soothe the throat by breaking up mucus; sucking on throat lozenges or hard candy can also provide relief. Stop smoking — it irritates the nasal and throat linings and provokes the common cold.

How to Choose a Cough/Cold Medicine

If you are suffering from	Choose a product with a(n)	Look for one of these on the package label
Nasal congestion, "stuffy" nose, "plugged" ears	Decongestant	Desoxyephedrine Ephedrine Methoxyphenamine HCl Naphazoline HCl Oxymetazoline HCl Phenylephrine HCl Phenylpropranolamine HCl Pseudoephedrine HCl Tetrahydrozoline HCl Xylometazoline HCL
Sneezing, runny nose, watery and itchy eyes	Antihistamine	Brompheniramine maleate Chlorcyclizine HCl Chlorpheniramine maleate Phenindamine tartrate Pheniramine maleate Phenyltoloxamine citrate Pyrilamine maleate Thenyldiamine HCl Thonzylamine HCl
	Anticholinergic	Atropine sulfate Belladonna alkaloids Hyoscyamine
Dry, hacking cough	Antitussive	Codeine Dextromethorphan
	Expectorant	Ammonium chloride Guaifenesin (glyceryl guaiacolate) Ipecac Potassium citrate Potassium iodide Terpin hydrate
Muscle aches	Anti-inflammatory agent	Aspirin Salicylamide
Headache	Analgesic (painkiller)	Acetaminophen Aspirin Salicylamide
Fever	Antipyretic agent	Acetaminophen Aspirin Salicylamide

Source: *Drug Therapy*, October 1980, p. 75.

Stay away from others — your cold is contagious. Once you have recovered, stay out of crowded places where you might pick up another cold, and stay away from those who you know have a cold.

When to Call the Doctor

Your cold may be leading to a secondary infection if any of the following appear: prolonged chills, an increase in throat pain, white or yellow spots on the throat, a fever above 101° F., earache, chest pain, shortness of breath, aching of the face, coughing up of blood-streaked or rust-colored sputum, or persistent hoarseness, or if a sore throat is your primary symptom. Call a doctor if you run a fever for longer than a week or if your cold persists for more than fourteen days.

The Common Cold in Children

Of primary importance in dealing with common colds in children is preventing spread of the cold — usually, a child is contagious for only two to three days before symptoms appear, but in some cases the child may continue to be contagious throughout the entire course of the cold. To be on the safe side, isolate an ill child from other children in the family until the symptoms have completely disappeared. Especially keep a child with a cold away from infants.

See that the child gets extra rest, but you probably won't need to confine him or her to bed: most children don't feel well and will restrict themselves. Don't force a child to eat if he or she is not hungry or does not want the food, but make sure that the patient drinks plenty of fluids —vary them to add interest.

Call the doctor if the child develops any of the following: marked irritability, rapid breathing, ear pain, sore throat, puslike discharge from the eyes or ears, puslike discharge from the nose, large red and tender neck glands, difficulty in breathing, chest pain, severe headache, stiff neck (can't touch chin to chest), vomiting, or shaking chills. The doctor should also be notified if the cold does not improve within five days.

Caution: There has been some recent concern about giving infants and children aspirin for fevers caused by some viruses. It may induce Reye's syndrome, which may cause symptoms ranging from vomiting to brain damage. Consult your physician concerning aspirin use in these cases.

ALLERGIC RHINITIS (Hay Fever)

Hay fever, an acute temporary obstruction of the nose, affects 10 percent of the population and is caused by allergy to airborne pollen (ragweed is the most common offender), household dust, chemicals, soaps, animal dander, feathers, or foods. Emotional stress can produce nasal inflammation that closely resembles an allergic reaction.

Attacks are most common in the spring, late summer, and fall, when pollen and seeds are in the air.

Signs and Symptoms

Common signs and symptoms of hay fever include recurrent nasal obstruction accompanied by profuse watery discharge from the nose, sneezing, itching (involving the throat, nose, and roof of the mouth), excessive tearing of the eyes, sensitivity to light, sore throat, inflamed eyelids, loss of appetite, loss of smell and taste, intermittent frontal headaches, and occasionally a nonproductive, hacking cough.

Other symptoms may include irritability, depression, insomnia, wheezing, and snorting.

You can differentiate between hay fever and a common cold in several ways. The nasal discharge from hay fever is thin, clear, and watery; nasal discharge from the common cold is thick, mucousy, and yellowish. The eyes itch and burn with hay fever; they don't with the common cold. The nose itches with hay fever but doesn't itch with the cold.

Self-Care Treatment

The best form of treatment, of course, is to remove the allergen that is causing the reaction. Antihistamines, taken three times a day, improve or relieve 70 to 90 percent of the cases. To be most effective, they should be taken before the attack begins. You can use nasal drops or sprays sparingly — no more than three times a day for three days. Get extra rest.

Wash your hands frequently during the allergy-prone times of year, and avoid touching your eyes, nose, or mouth. Stay inside on windy days; keep your sleeping room as free of dust as you can. Wear a protective mask over your nose and mouth while dusting, doing other housework, or gardening and mowing the lawn.

Increase your fluid intake, and stop smoking. Avoid drinking alcohol while you have hay fever symptoms.

When to Call the Doctor

If your hay fever gets worse over the course of the years or if it is severe and completely unresponsive to treatment, contact your doctor. He or she can run allergy tests that will help identify the allergen causing your misery; in some cases, the doctor may be able to give you allergy shots that will help prevent allergic reactions.

SINUSITIS

More than 50 percent of all cases of sinusitis — an inflammation of the nasal sinuses that accompanies upper respiratory infection — are caused by bacteria. The sinuses affected by infection include those above the eyes, inside each cheekbone, behind the bridge of the nose, and in the upper nose.

When the mucous membranes of the sinus become inflamed and swollen, the openings that lead from each sinus into the nasal passages are partially or wholly blocked. The mucus that accumulates in the sealed-off sinus causes pressure on the sinus walls, resulting in discomfort, fever, pain, and difficulty in breathing. Bacterial and viral microorganisms breed easily and profusely in the blocked sinuses.

Because the sinuses do not develop fully until adolescence, sinus infection is rarely seen in children.

Infection from upper respiratory infections and other infections can be spread to the sinuses by a deviated septum, excessively strong blowing of the nose, deep swimming, diving, tooth infection, allergy, certain infectious diseases (such as pneumonia and measles), air pollution, nasal allergies, and nasal polyps.

Signs and Symptoms

The most common symptom of sinusitis is headache or tenderness in

Figure 9-2

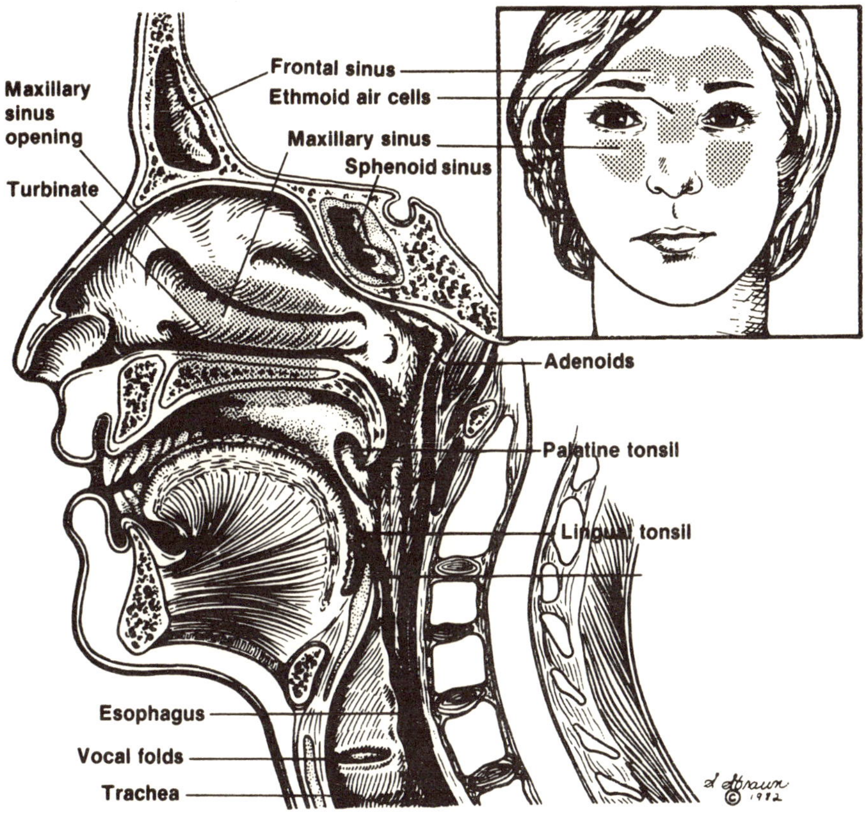

the cheekbones on one side of the face; the degree of blockage determines the intensity of the headache. The headache can be either constant or recurrent and is worse when you bend over. Common additional complaints include sore throat, chills, fever, loss of smell, dizziness, vomiting, mental sluggishness, postnasal discharge (thick mucus), nasal obstruction, pressure pain around the nose and eyes, toothache in the upper jaw, tenderness over the affected sinuses, and general weakness and discomfort.

Swelling around the eyes is a serious sign.

Untreated, sinusitis can lead to asthma, bronchitis, pharyngitis, laryngitis, pneumonia, or other respiratory disorders.

Self-Care Treatment

If you can, identify and remove any allergens that may be causing reaction. Get plenty of sleep and rest; avoid smoke, dust, and other irritants to the nasal passages. Stop smoking entirely.

To relieve the pain of sinusitis, alternate hot and cold compresses every three to four hours, applied locally over the tender or painful sinuses. Inhale steam from a vaporizer, tea kettle, or hot shower. An electric heating pad or hot water bottle applied for ten minutes every two hours can also relieve the pain and tenderness in the sinuses. Aspirin is also effective in pain relief.

Do not blow the nose forcefully. Be gentle; blow only one nostril at a time, and keep your mouth open. Take oral decongestants three times daily, and avoid sudden changes in temperature. Increase your fluid intake to keep the mucus thin; set a goal of one eight-ounce glass of fluid every two hours.

Complete convalescence requires about four weeks of treatment and rest.

When to Call the Doctor

Seek medical attention if you run a fever of over 101° F., if your nose bleeds, if you have a severe headache that does not respond to home treatment, if there is swelling in your face, if your vision blurs, if your nasal discharge increases in amount, or if your mucous discharge is blood-stained. You should also report sinusitis that does not respond to treatment and that does not begin to improve within seven to eight days.

SORE THROAT (Pharyngitis)

A sore throat — usually an extension of the common cold, tonsillitis, adenoiditis, or sinusitis — is the most common complication of the common cold. Eighty percent of all colds are caused by irritants or viruses; strep throat is caused by bacteria.

Sore throat can result from prolonged irritation to the throat, overindulgence in alcohol, overuse of the voice, exposure to irritating smoke, bacterial infection, fungal infection, viral infection, postnasal discharge, shouting, swallowing irritating foods, or diseases like measles or acute tonsillitis.

An acute sore throat should run its course within a few days to a few weeks.

Signs and Symptoms

Common signs and symptoms include itching, scratching, tickling, dryness, acute sharp or burning pain, the feeling of a lump in the throat, pain and difficulty in swallowing, stiff neck, fatigue, mild fever, harsh cough, a persistent urge to clear the throat, chills, difficulty in speaking, thick mucus in the throat, nausea, vomiting, gagging, stuffy nose, and swollen glands.

A strep throat is characterized by yellow or white mucous spots on the throat, swollen glands in the neck, and a fever over 101° F.

Self-Care Treatment

While you are running a fever, you should stay in bed; take two aspirin every four hours. Even after you have recovered from a fever, rest frequently in a cool room. Keep the home — and especially your sleeping room — humid with the use of a vaporizer. Rest your voice as much as you can.

To relieve throat pain, gargle with a solution of one teaspoon of salt in eight ounces of hot water (not to exceed 120° F.) every two hours. Frequent sips of hot liquids (at least six eight-ounce glasses a day) can help to break up mucus in the throat and relieve throat pain. Sucking on a throat lozenge, a cough drop, or a hard candy can keep the throat moist and the mucus moving.

If it is painful to swallow, drink as many fluids as you can, and eat a soft diet. Stop smoking, and avoid smoke-filled rooms.

When to Call the Doctor

Call a doctor if your throat is fiery red and raw, if your tonsils are red or enlarged or covered with a whitish material, if you run a fever over 101° F., if you experience a severe headache, if you develop chest pains, if your sore throat lasts longer than fourteen days, if you develop earache, if you experience abdominal pain, if you have a history of kidney infections, if you experience shortness of breath, if you develop a cough, if a skin rash develops, if you see white or yellow patches on the throat, or if someone in your family has been exposed to a strep infection.

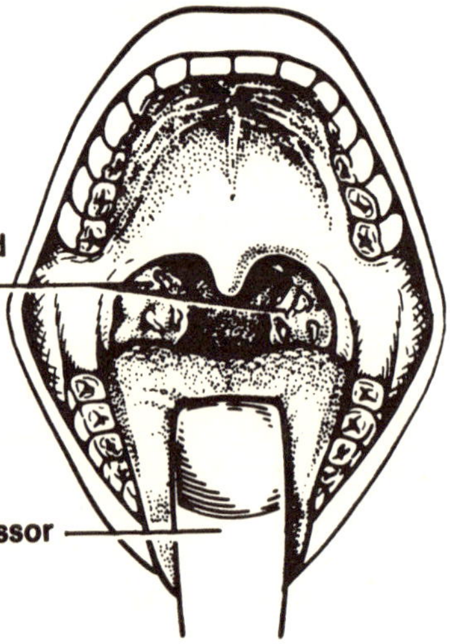

Figure 9-3
A sore throat may reflect the occurrence of tonsillitis. This occurs most often in children. Typically, the child will complain of a sore throat, and he or she will have a high fever. If the fever does not go away after two days rest, he or she may need to see a physician for penicillin treatment.

Sore Throat in Children

Sore throat is one of the most common complaints of childhood; strep throat is even more common in children than in adults and is highly contagious.

To treat a child's sore throat, give the child a bland diet consisting of soft foods such as pudding, jello, popsicles, and other mild foods. Push fluids — the child should drink at least eight eight-ounce glasses of water, fruit juice, or tonic a day. Also give the child soothing, coating substances such as honey in tea or karo syrup.

Keep the child's sleeping room cool and humid (use a vaporizer), but make sure that the child stays warm.

Give the child aspirin for pain as directed by your doctor. To relieve pain further, have the child gargle with hot saltwater (one teaspoon of salt to eight ounces of water, not to exceed 120° F.) every few hours; the gargling cleans the mouth, tonsils, and throat, kills some germs, heats and relaxes the throat muscles, reduces soreness, and increases the blood supply to the throat to speed healing. Some sore throat is worsened by spasms caused by swollen lymph glands; to soothe muscle spasms in the throat, wrap a warm towel around the neck.

You should take the child to the doctor if he or she loses his or her appetite for more than a day or two, if the lymph glands are swollen, if there are white patches on the throat or palate, if there is pus on the tonsils, if the child has a temperature of over 102° F., or if any of the following occur: body rash (red, like sandpaper, and covering the body), skin

ASSESSMENT
Chapter 3

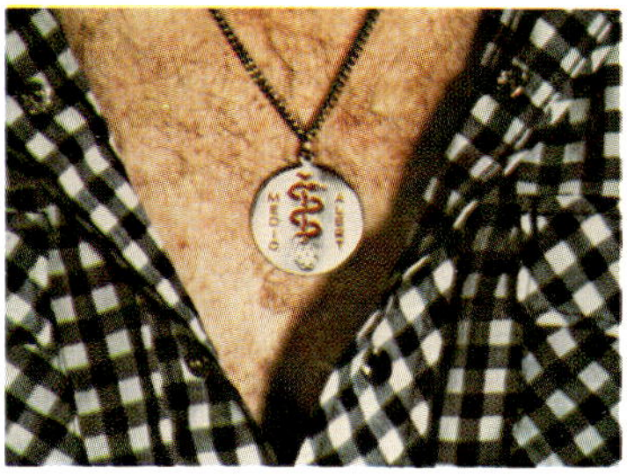

Medic Alert Necklace
Indicates Health Problems
for Emergency Use

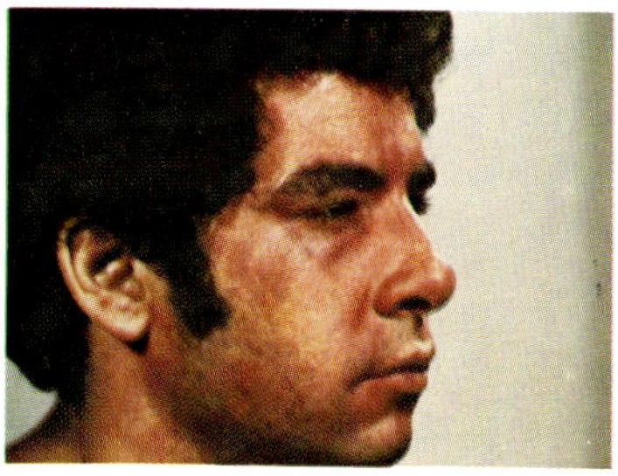

Blotchy Skin
Allergic Reaction

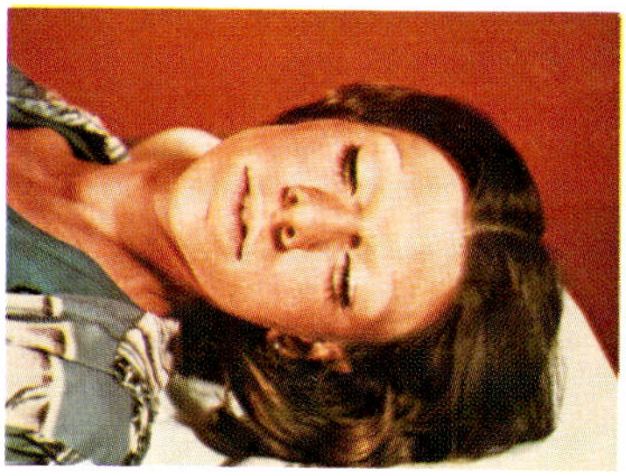

Red Flush Skin

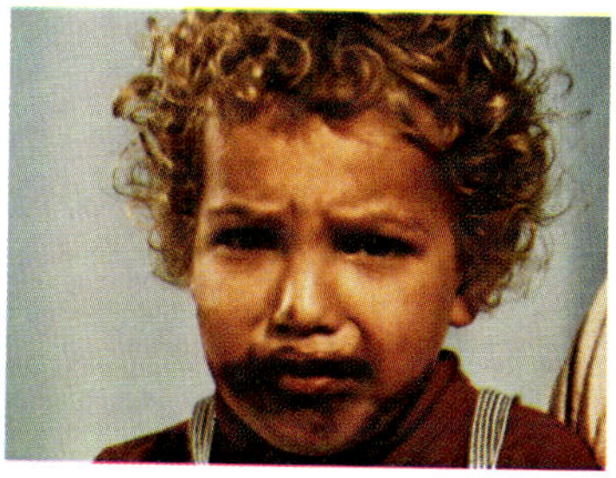

Skin Discoloration
Possible Poisoning

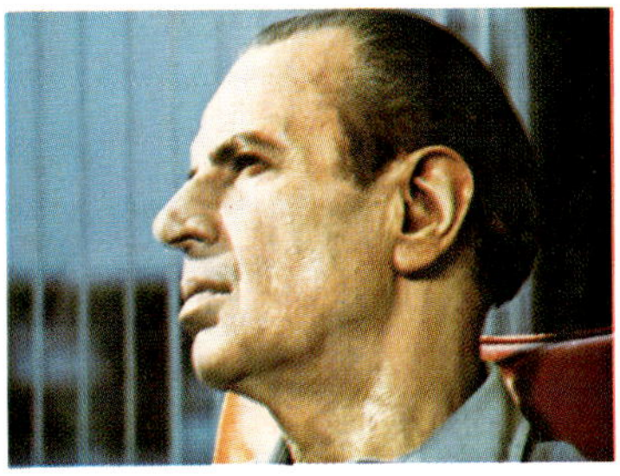

Pale Moist Skin

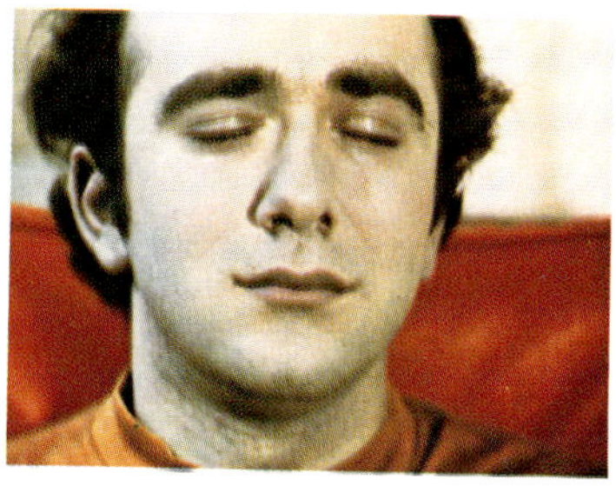

Bluish Skin
(Cyanosis)

EXAMINING THE EARDRUM

Chapter 3

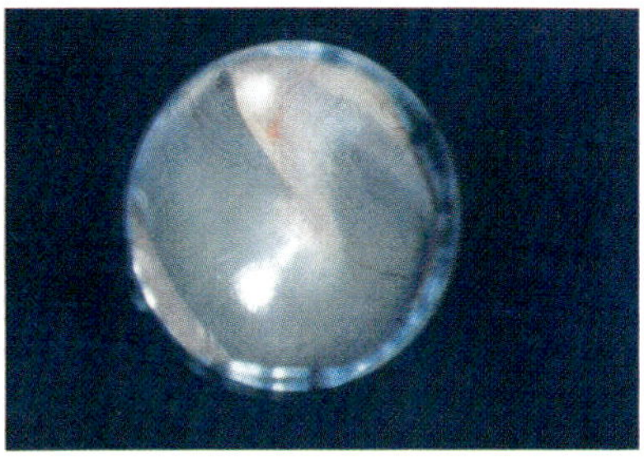

Normal Eardrum (Tympanic Membrane)

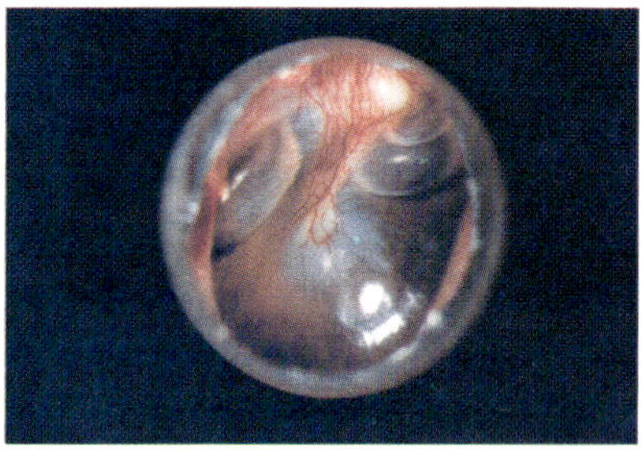

Buildup of Air Fluid Levels
in Upper Middle Ear

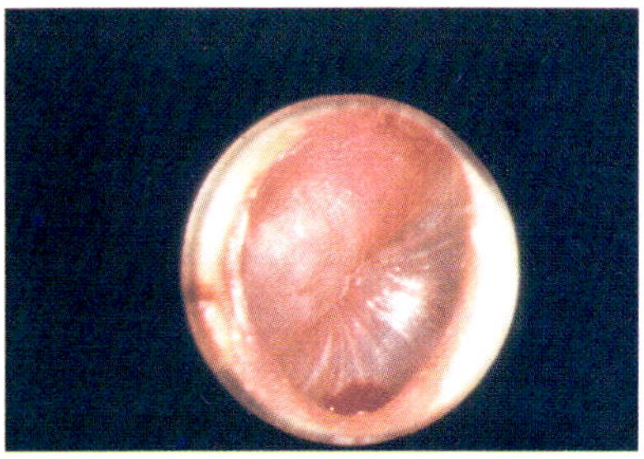

Inflammation of Middle Ear (Otitis Media)

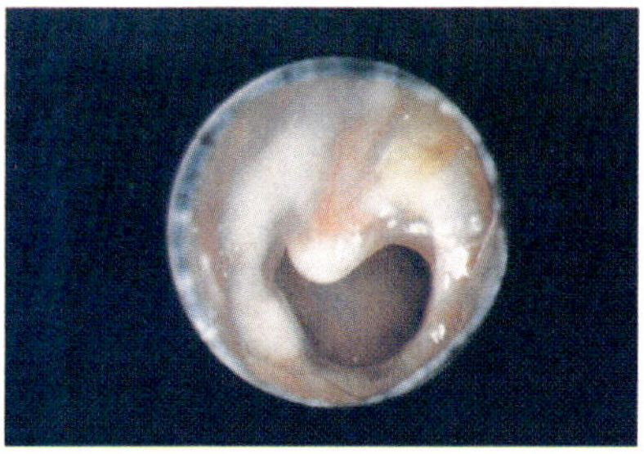

Perforation of Eardrum with Fluid
Discharge in Middle Ear

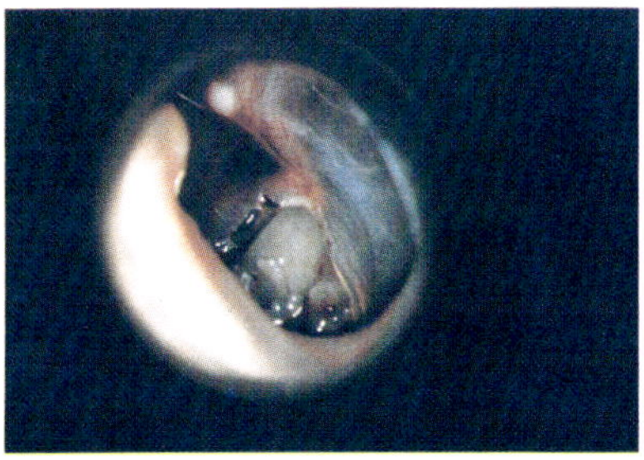

Perforation of Eardrum

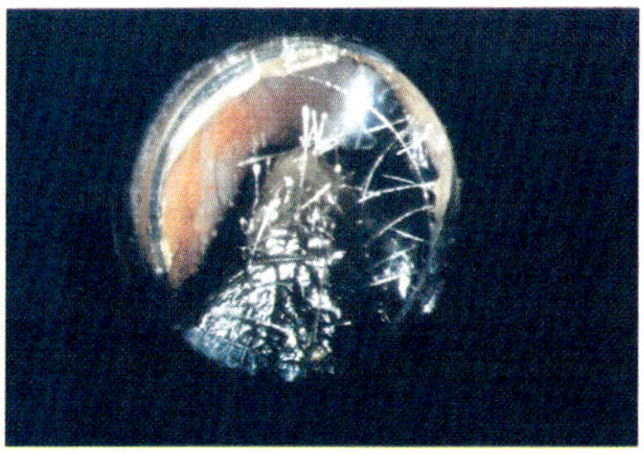

External Ear Partially Blocked with Ear Wax

Courtesy Dr. Richard A. Buckingham, Clinical Professor, Otolaryngology,
Abraham Lincoln School of Medicine, University of Illinois, Chicago, Illinois.

EMERGENCIES AND COMMON COMPLAINTS

Chapter 5

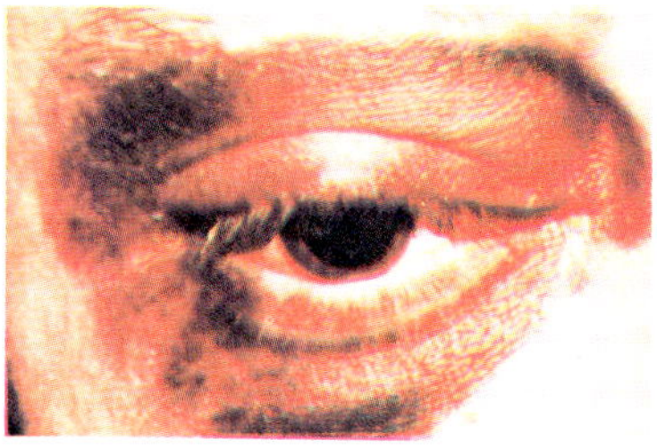

Contusion

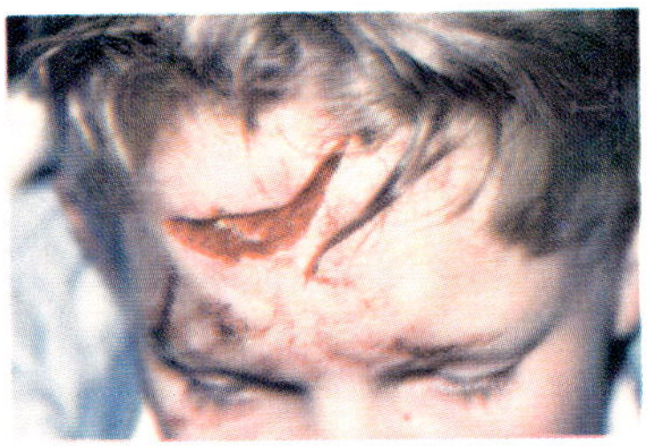

Laceration

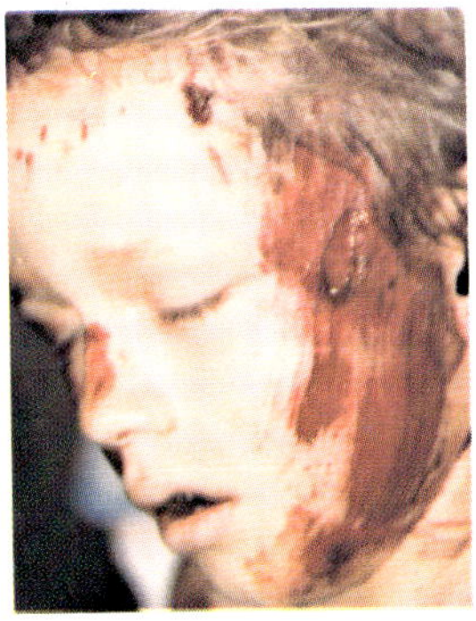

Abrasion

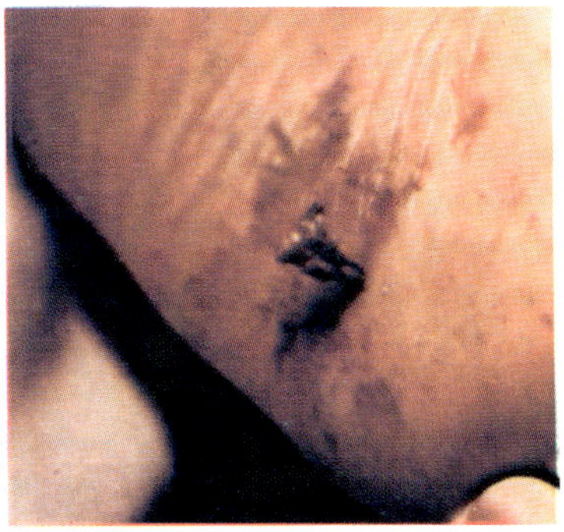

Puncture Wound

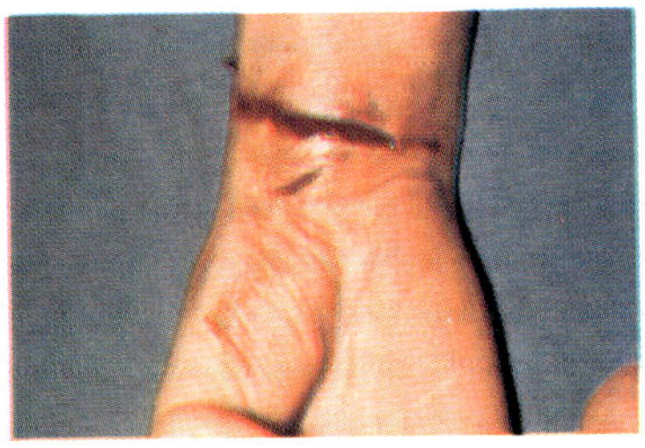

Incision

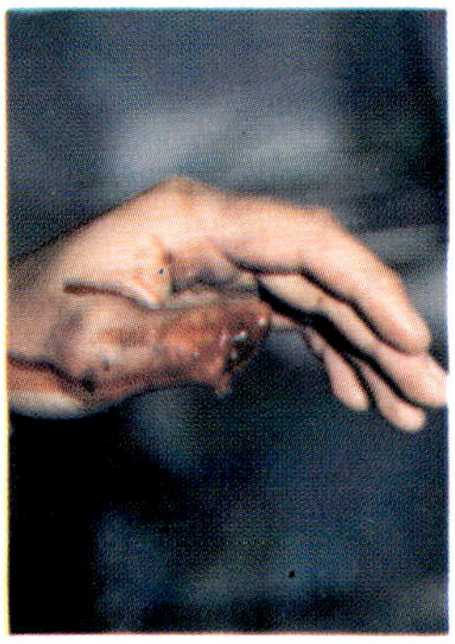

Avulsion

Courtesy Blayne Hirsche, M.D.

EMERGENCIES AND COMMON COMPLAINTS

Chapter 5

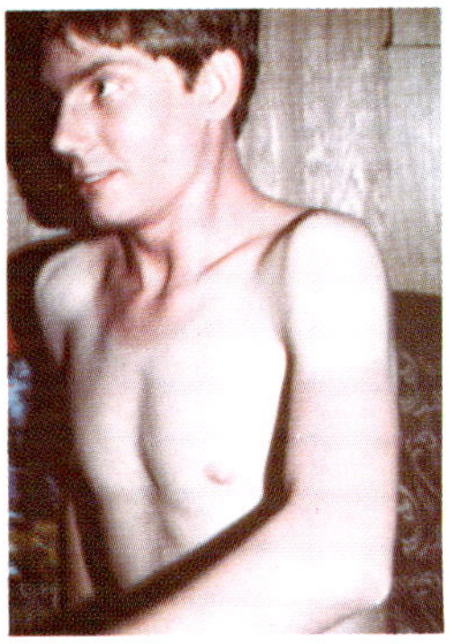

First Degree Burn

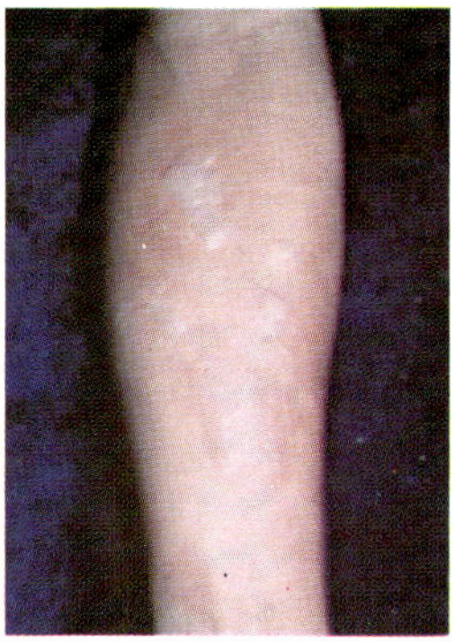

Second Degree Burn

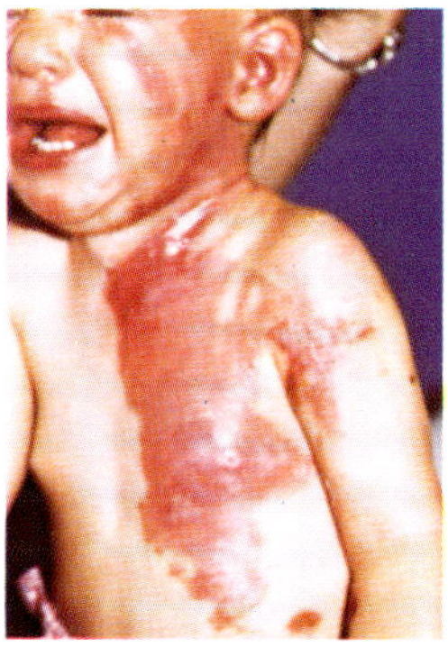

Third Degree Scald Burn

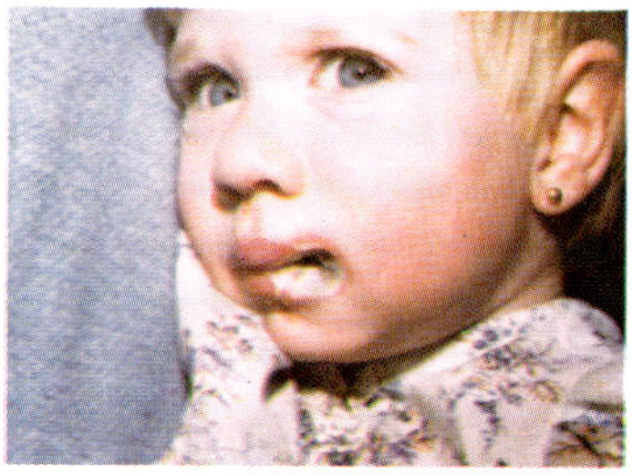

Electrical Burn
Chewing on Electrical Cord

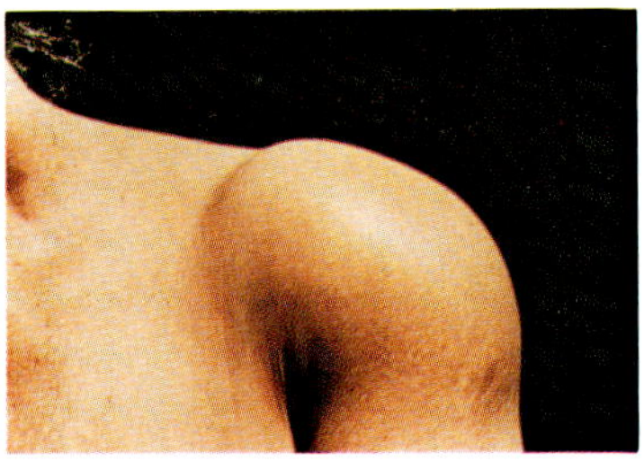

Dislocated Shoulder

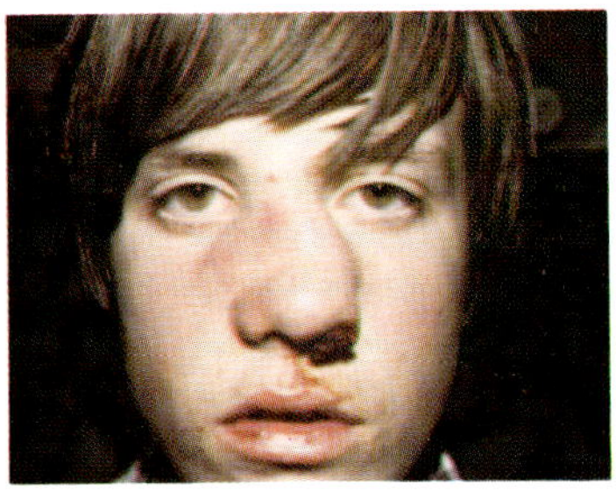

Fractured Nose

Courtesy Blayne Hirsche, M.D.

EMERGENCIES AND COMMON COMPLAINTS

Chapter 5

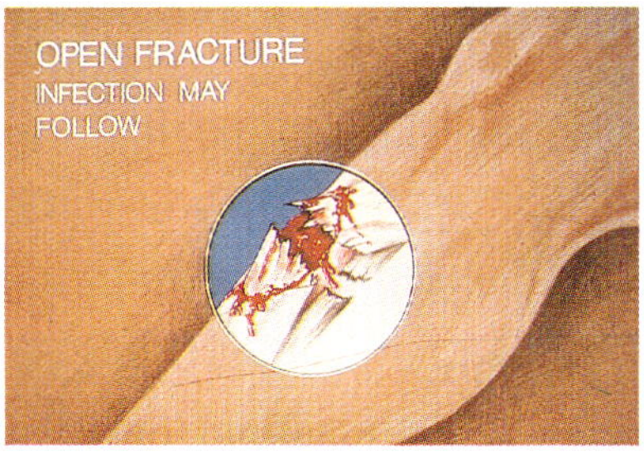

Open Fracture

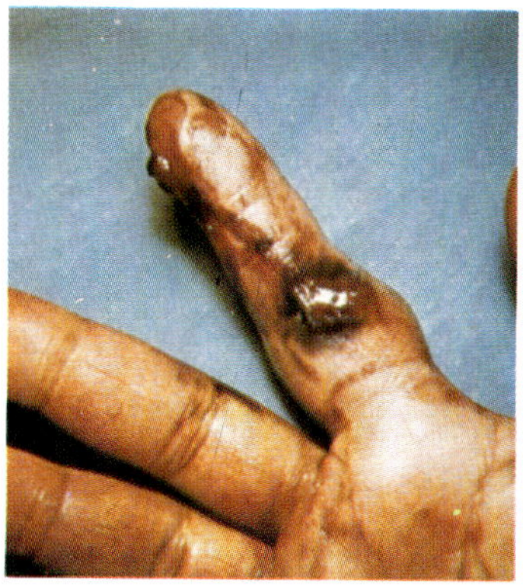

Open Finger Fracture

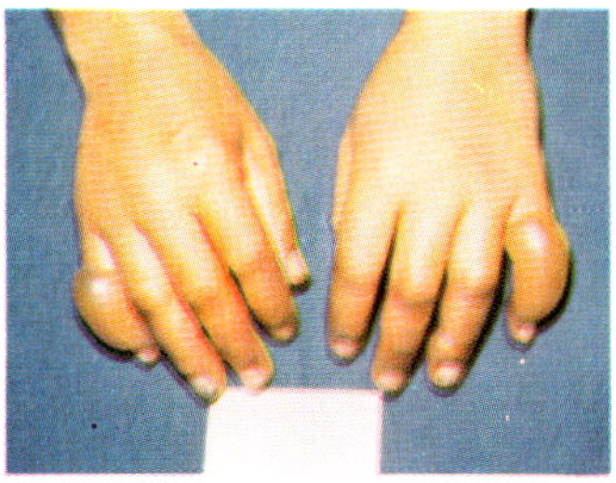

Frostbite

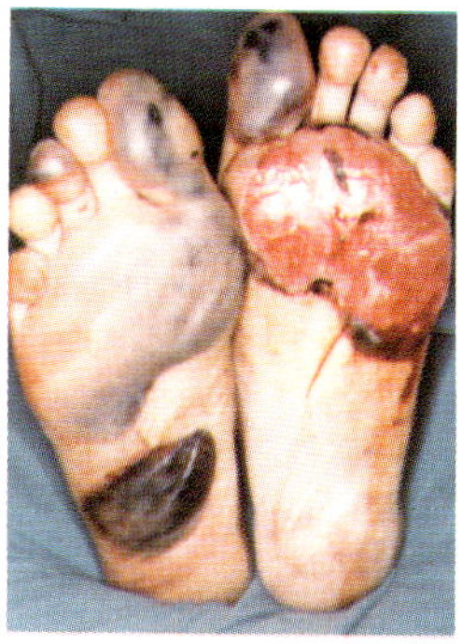

Frostbite

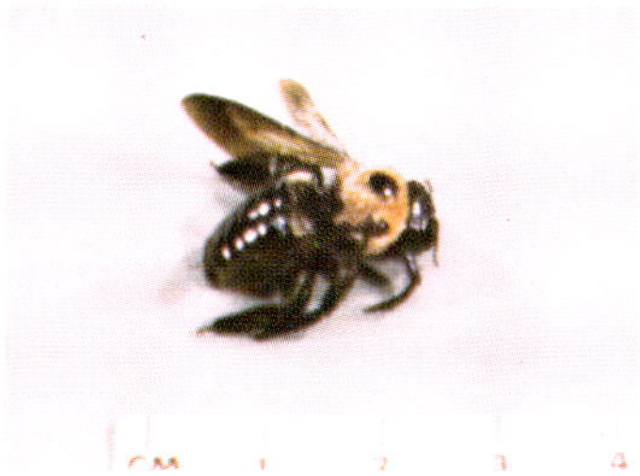

Bumble Bee

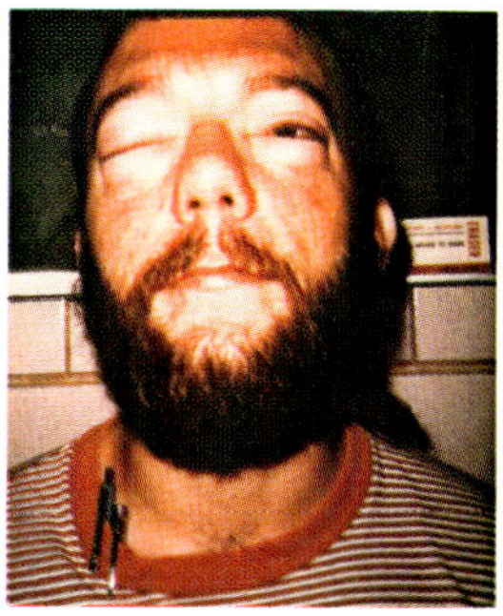

Allergic Reaction
Bee Sting

Courtesy of Spenco Medical Corporation, Waco, Texas
and John A. Boswick Jr., M.D.

EMERGENCIES AND COMMON COMPLAINTS

Chapter 5

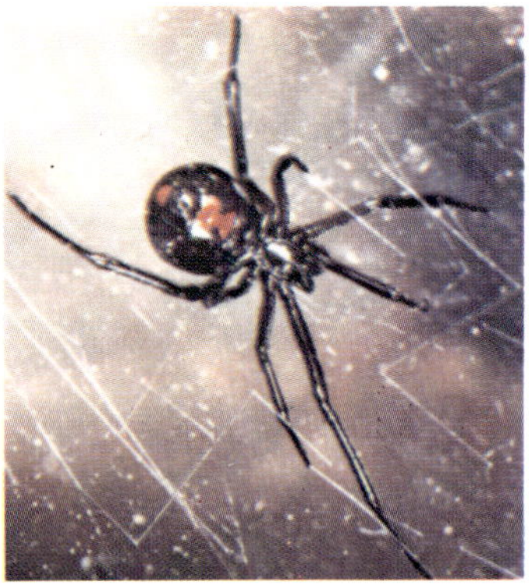

Black Widow Spider

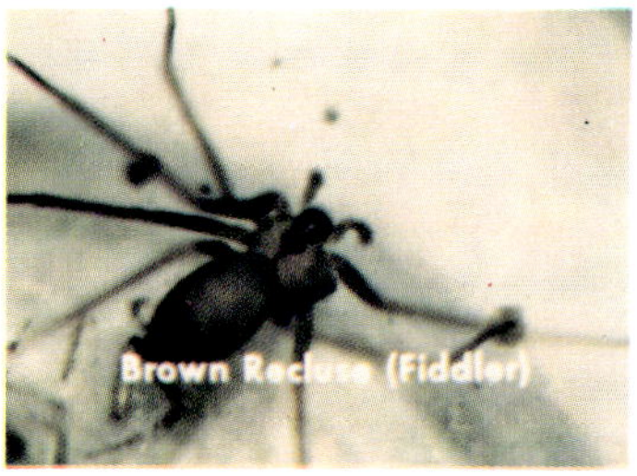

Brown Recluse Spider

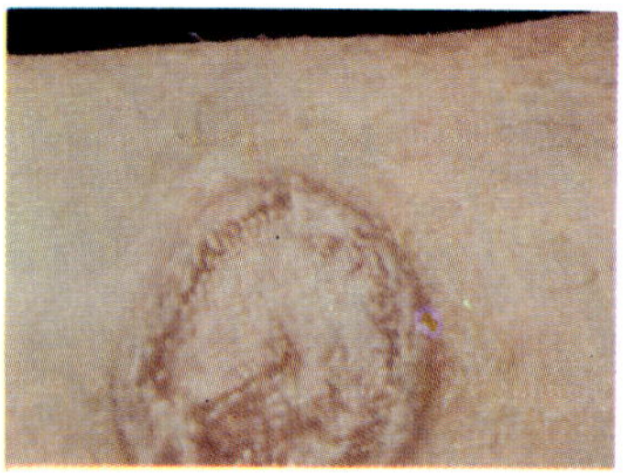

Brown Recluse Spider Bite
2 weeks later

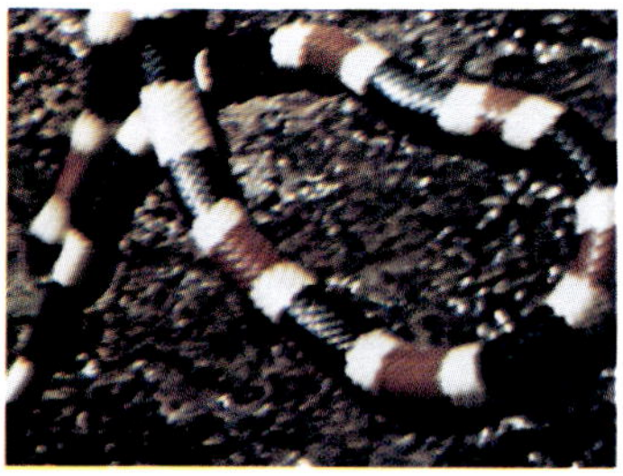

Coral Snake

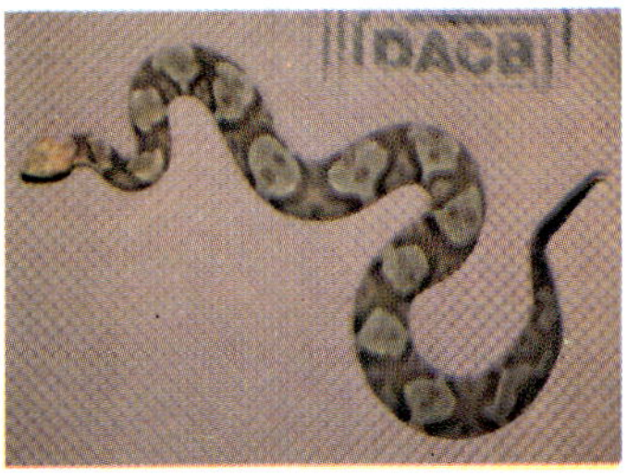

Copperhead

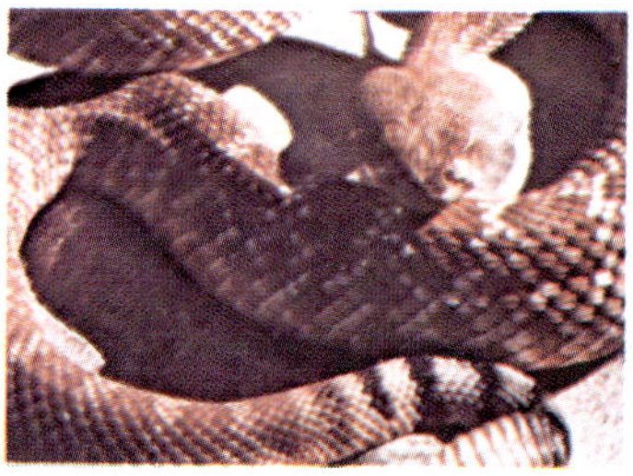

Diamondback Rattler

EMERGENCIES AND COMMON COMPLAINTS
Chapter 5

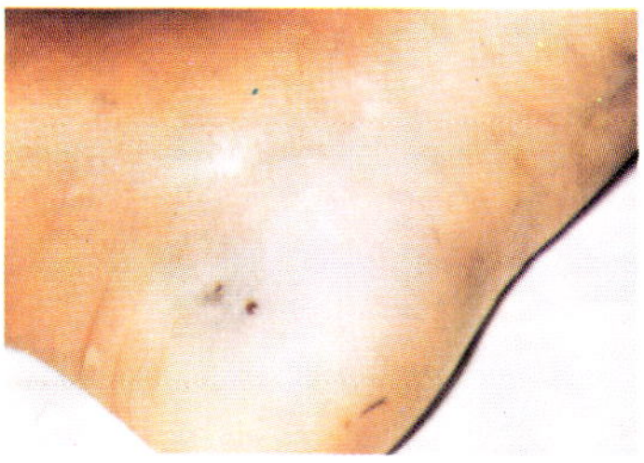

Recent Rattlesnake Bite

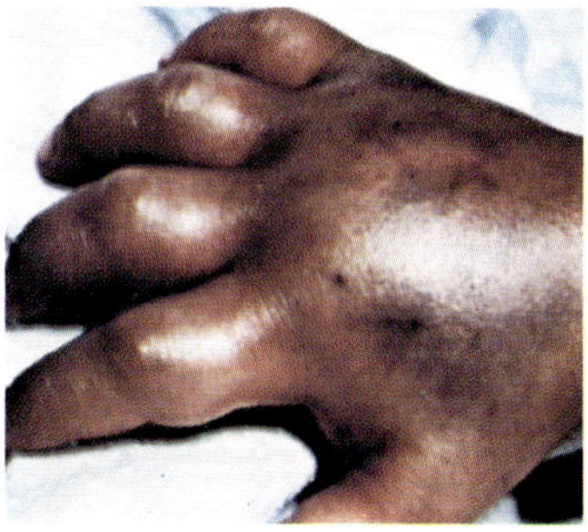

Rattlesnake Bite
Six Hours after

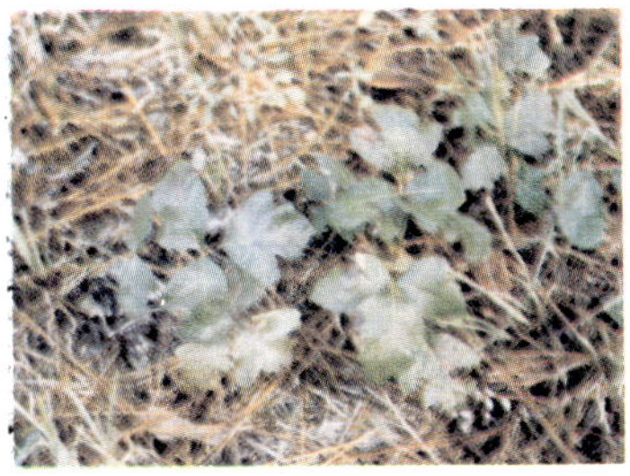

Poison Oak

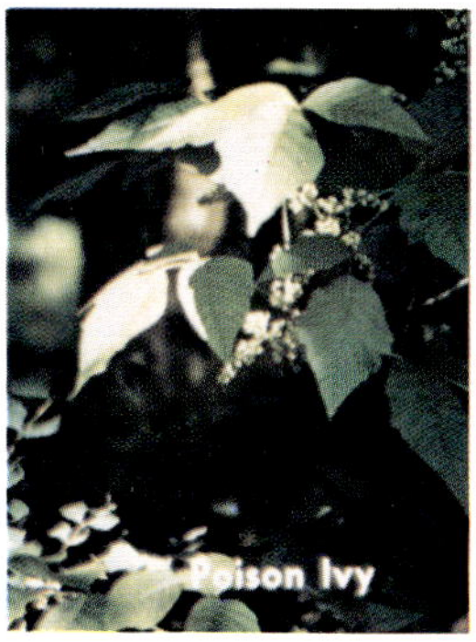

Poison Ivy

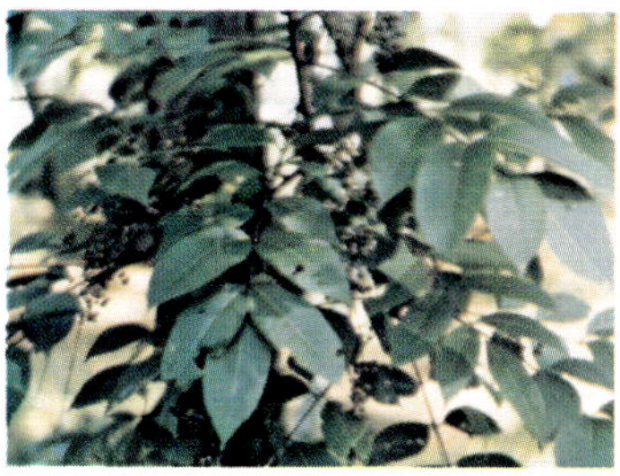

Poison Sumac

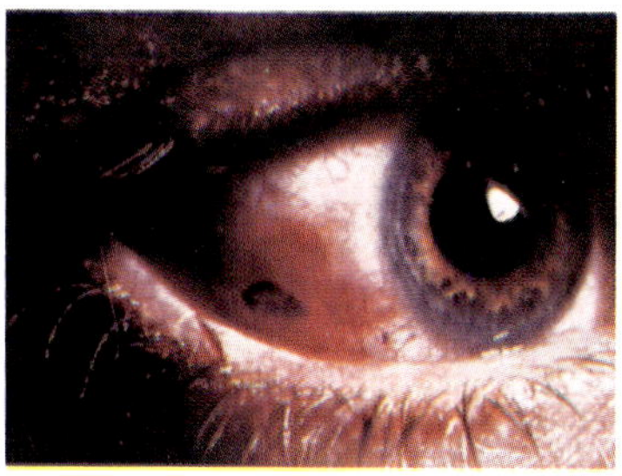

Embedded Object in Eye

SKIN COMPLAINTS

Chapter 6

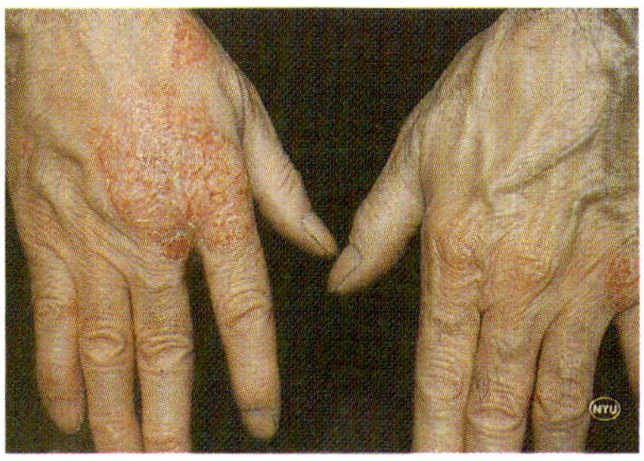

Eczema

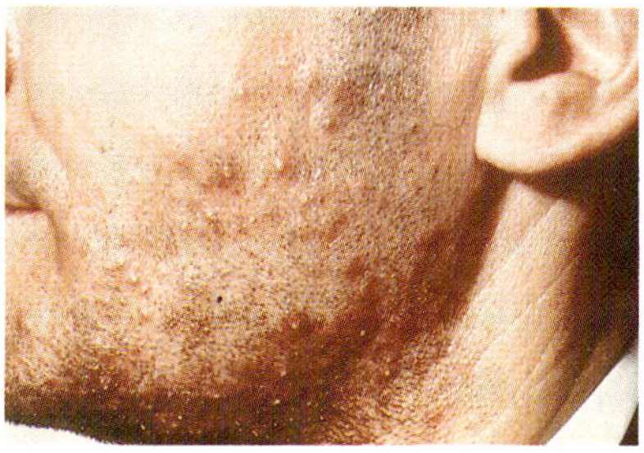

Acne

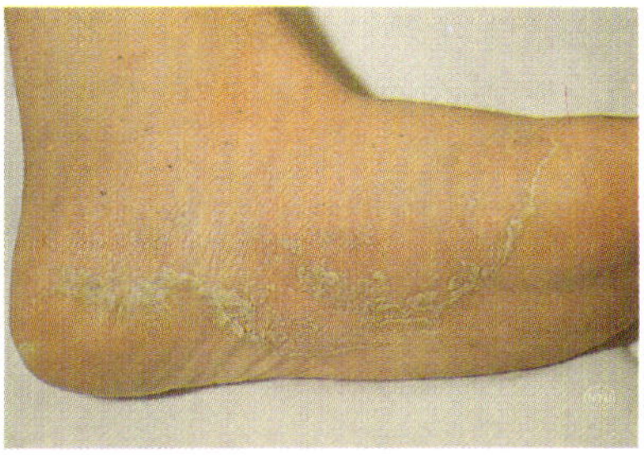

Athlete's Foot

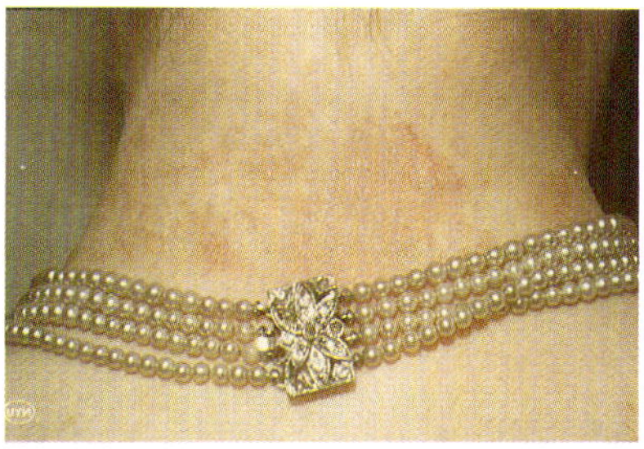

Allergic Contact Dermatitis

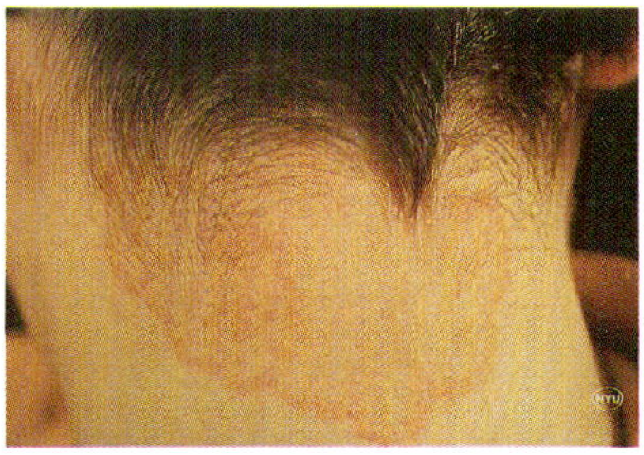

Ringworm

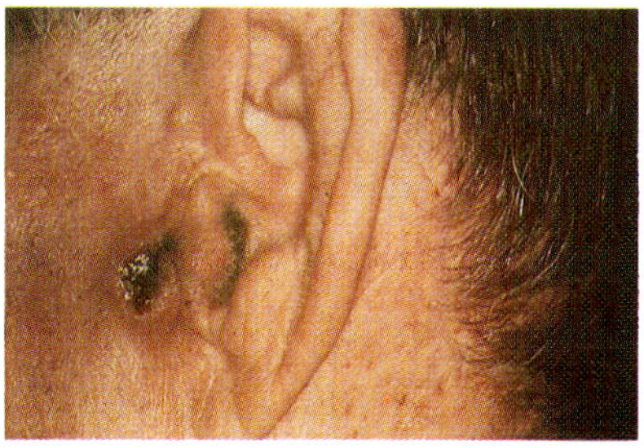

Skin Cancer

Courtesy American Academy of Dermatology and Institute For Dermatologic Communication and Education

SKIN COMPLAINTS
Chapter 6

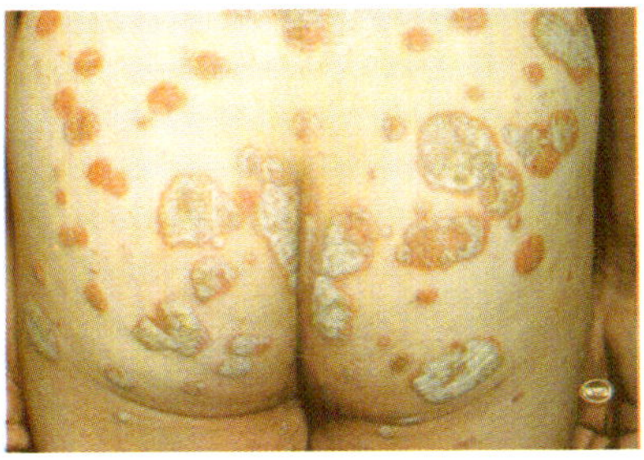
Psoriasis

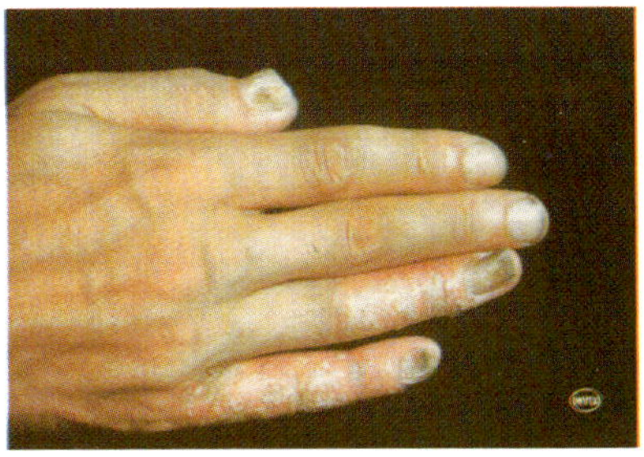
Psoriasis

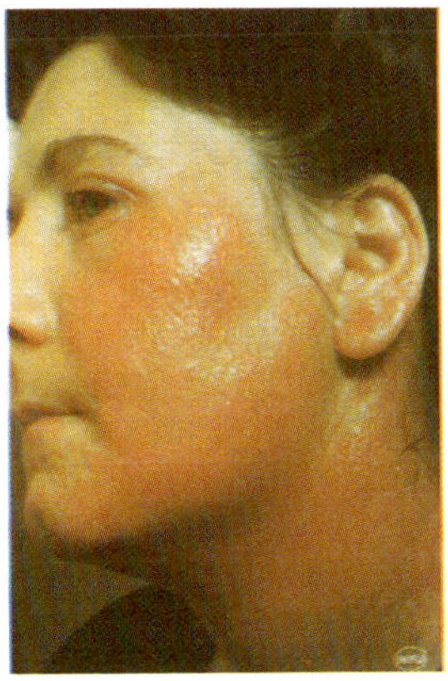
Allergic Contact Dermatitis

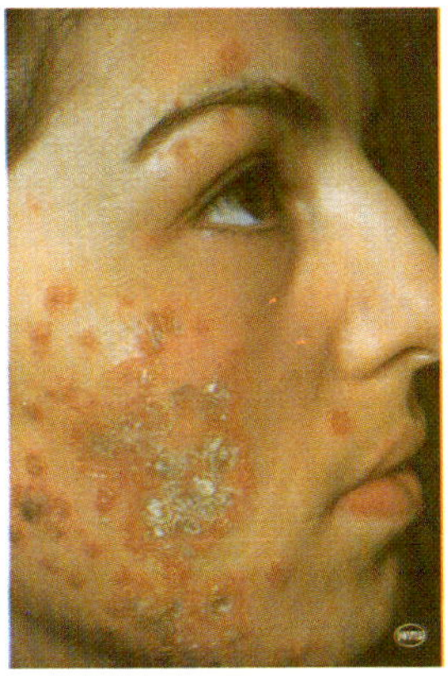
Impetigo

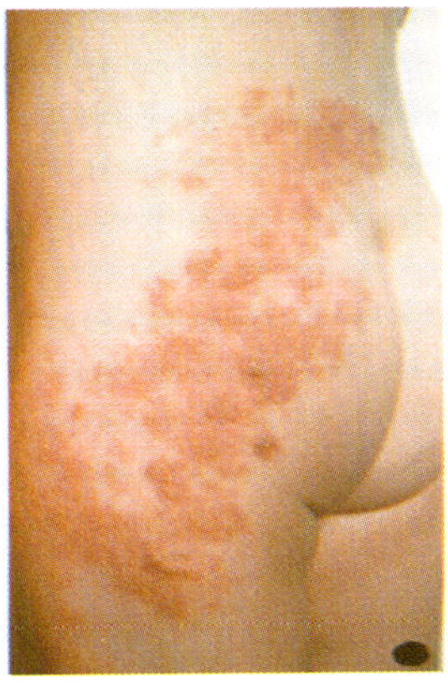
Shingles (Herpes Zoster)

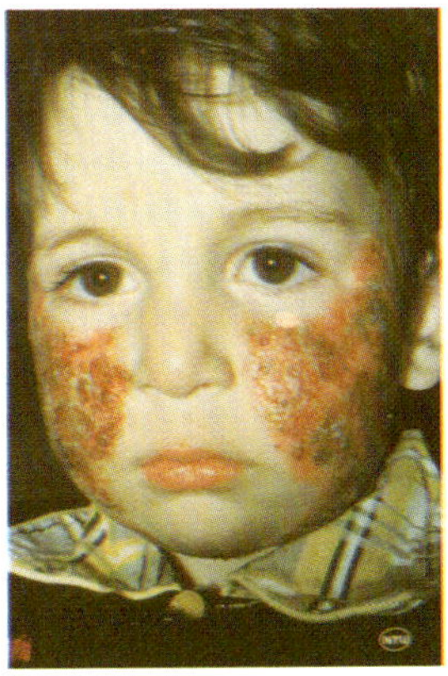
Atopic Dermatitis

Courtesy American Academy of Dermatology and
Institute For Dermatologic Communication and Education

MUSCLE, BONE AND JOINT COMPLAINTS

Chapter 7

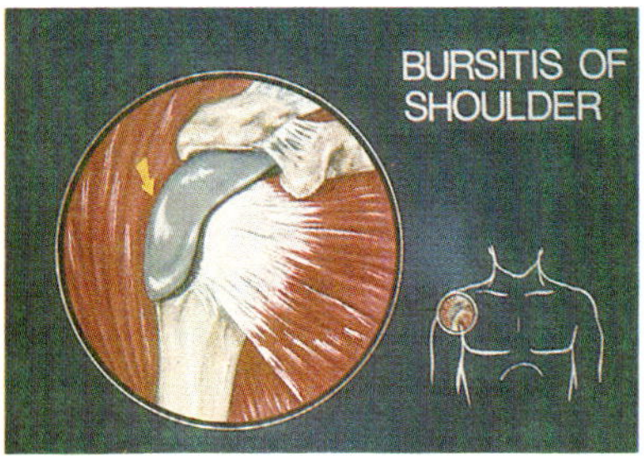

Inflammation of Sac Around Joint

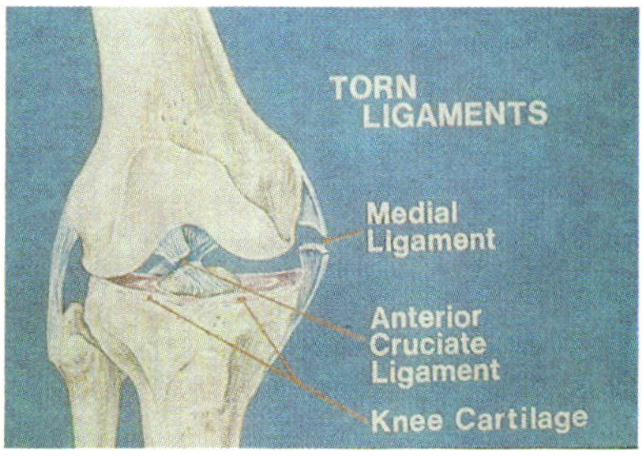

Sprain

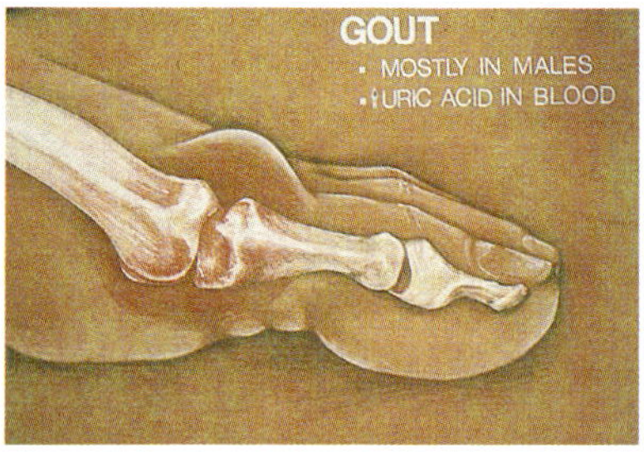

Deposits and Inflammation in Joint

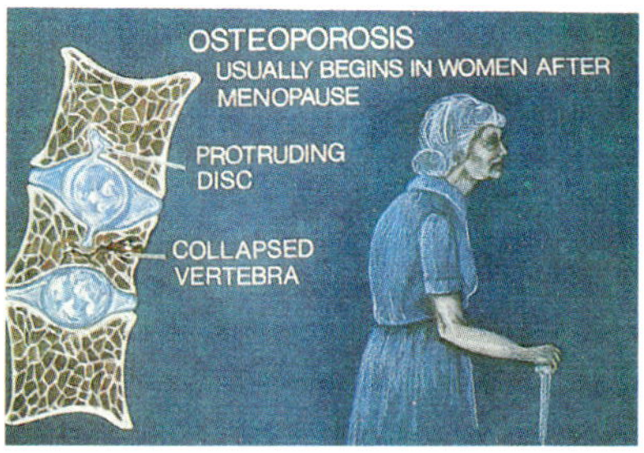

Thinning of Bones

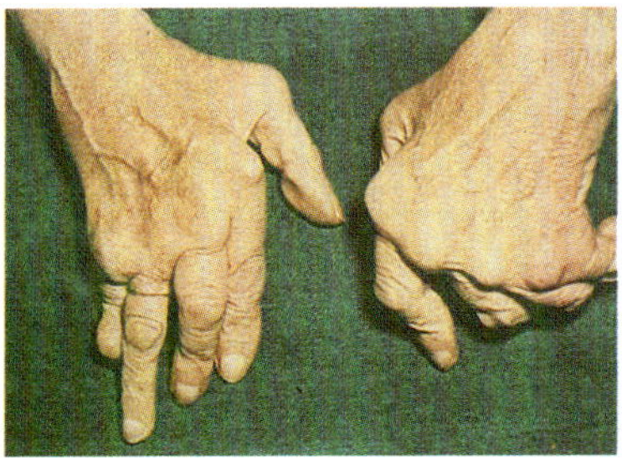

Rheumatoid Arthritis

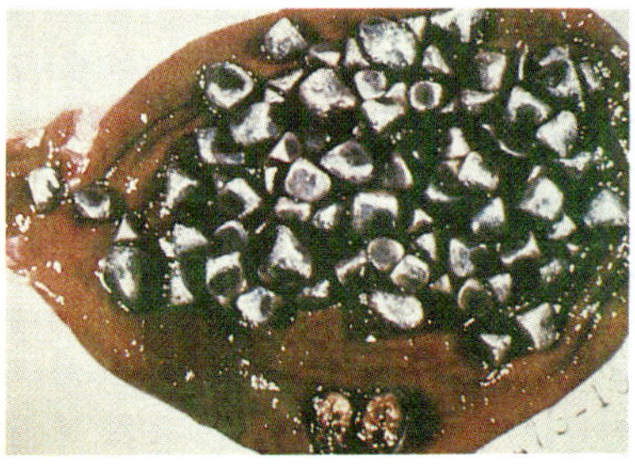

Gallstones

Courtesy Spenco Medical Corporation, Waco, Texas

EYE AND EAR COMPLAINTS

Chapter 8, 9

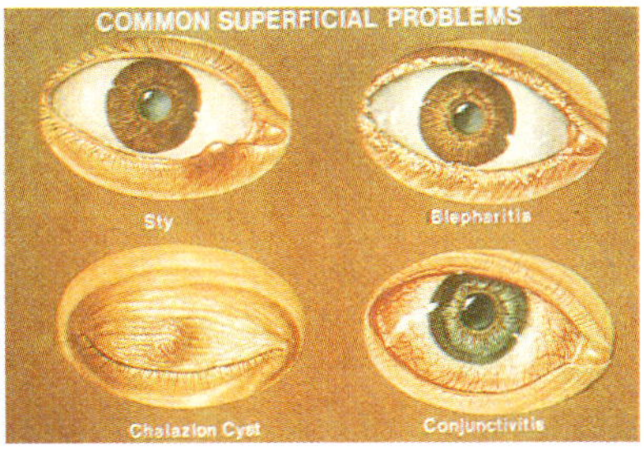

Sty-Pimple like Inflammation
Blepharitis - Inflammation of eyelid margins
Chalazion Cyst - Infection of Oil Gland
Conjunctivitis - Inflammation of Membrane Covering Eyeball & Eyelid

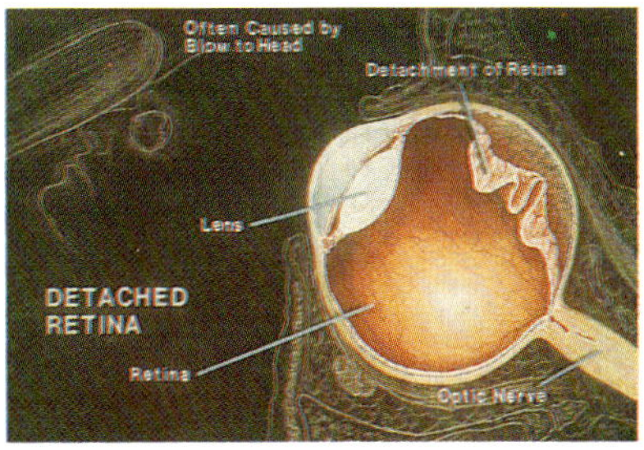

Detached Retina

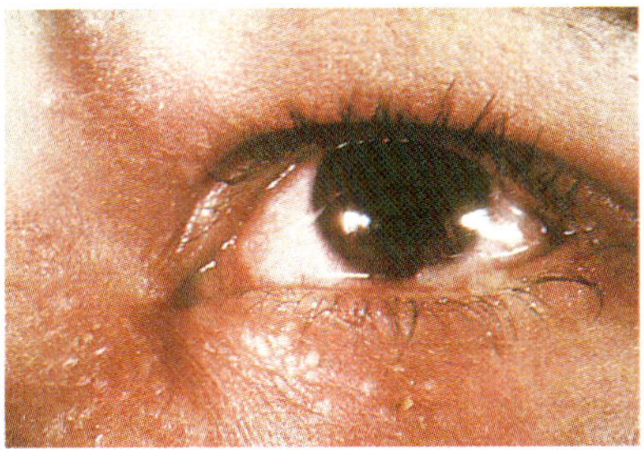

Virus Infection of Eye

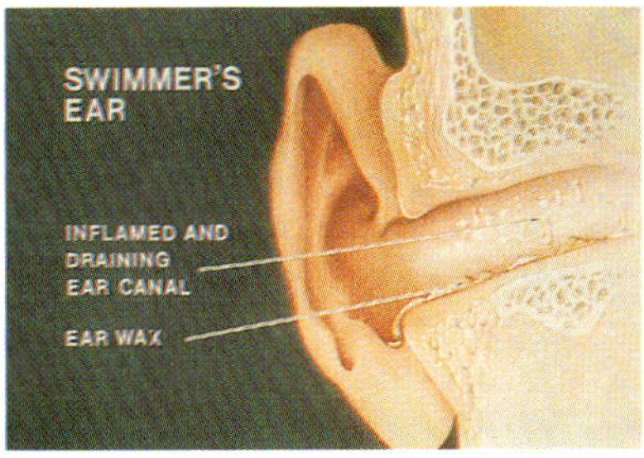

Swimmer's Ear

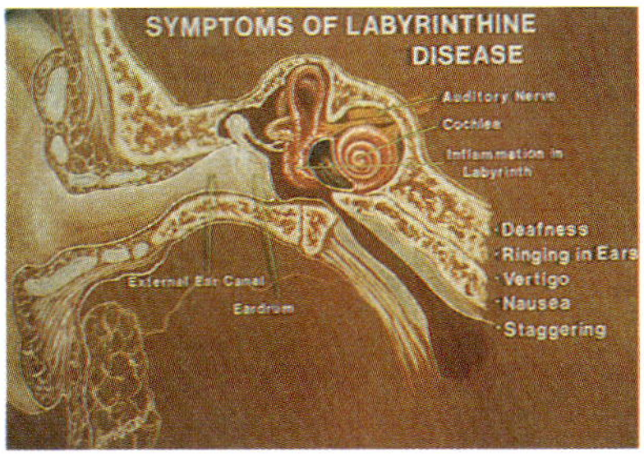

Inflammation and Disorder of Inner Ear

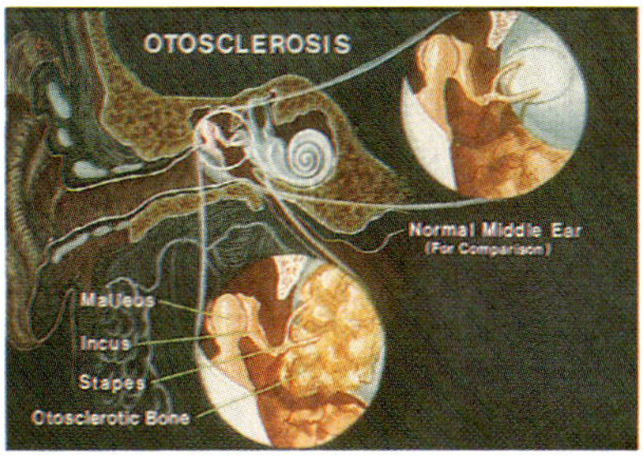

Conductive Hearing Loss

Courtesy Spenco Medical Corporation, Waco, Texas

NOSE AND THROAT COMPLAINTS
Chapter 9

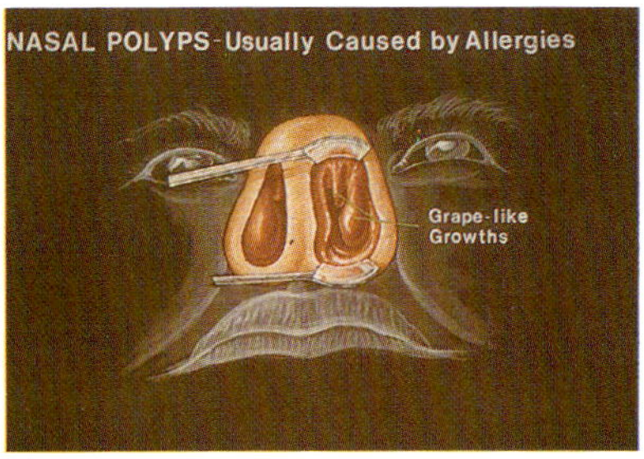

Nasal Polyps

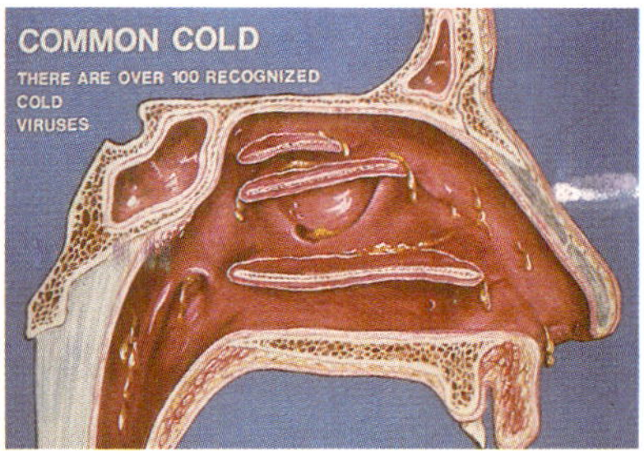

Location of Discharge from Common Cold

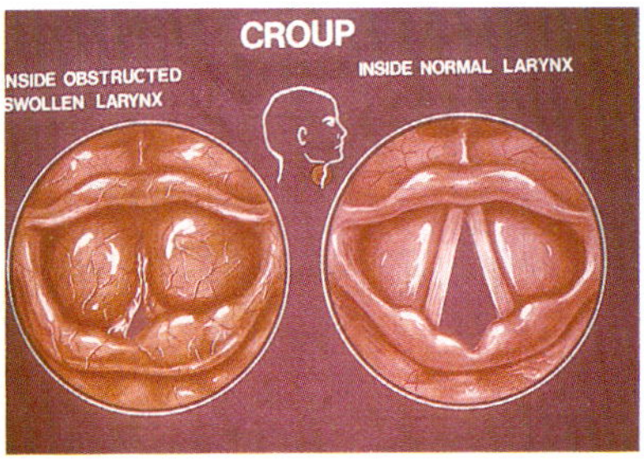

Croup - Obstruction of Larynx

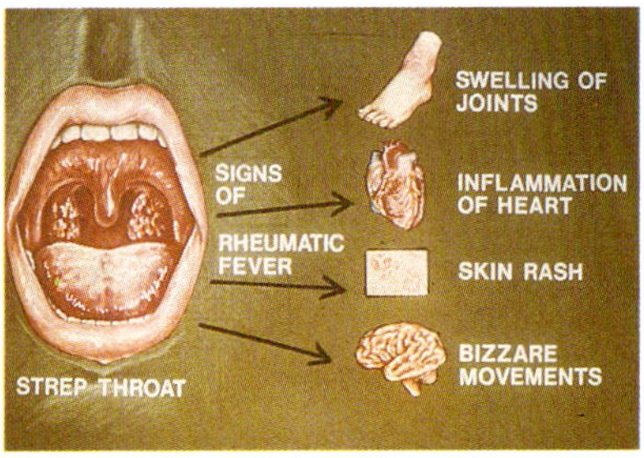

Strep Throat and Rheumatic Fever

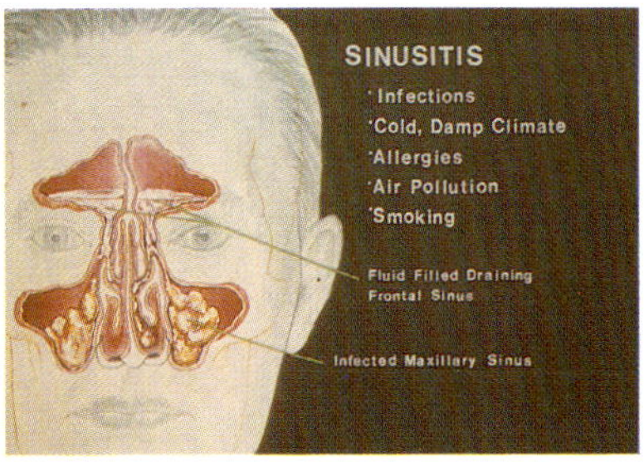

Inflammation of Sinuses

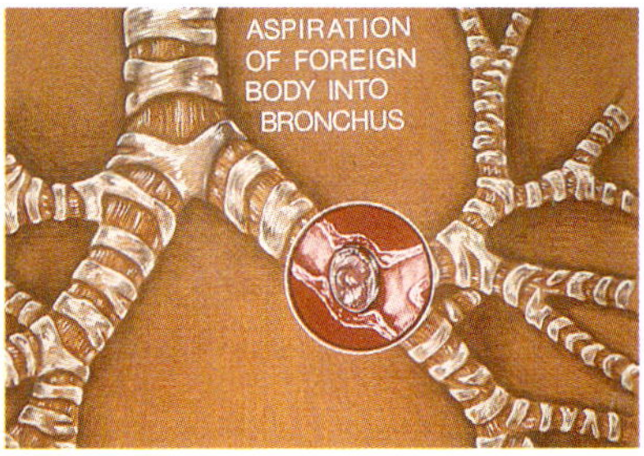

Obstruction of Air Passage

Courtesy Spenco Medical Corporation, Waco, Texas

MOUTH, TOOTH AND RESPIRATORY COMPLAINTS

Chapter 10, 11

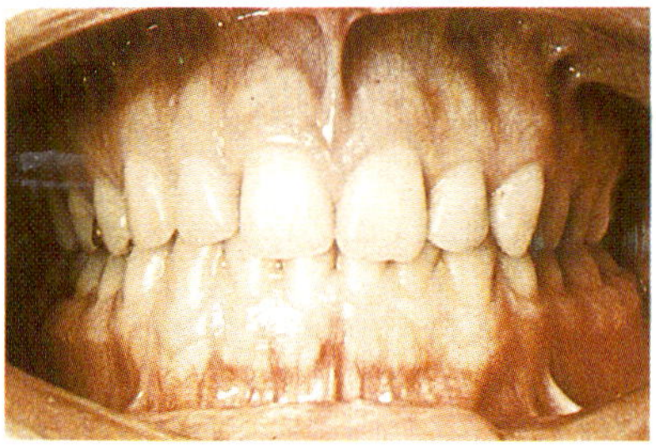

Normal Teeth and Gums

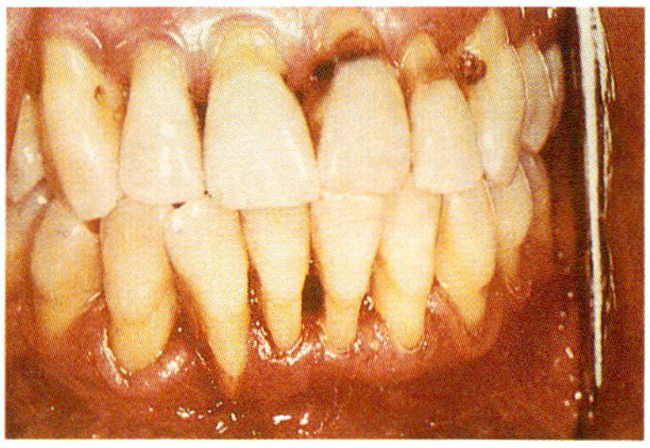

Tooth Decay and Inflammation of Gums (Gingivitis)

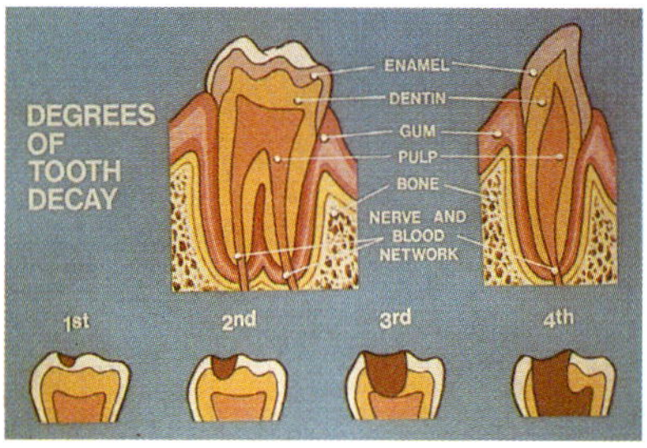

Degrees of Tooth Decay

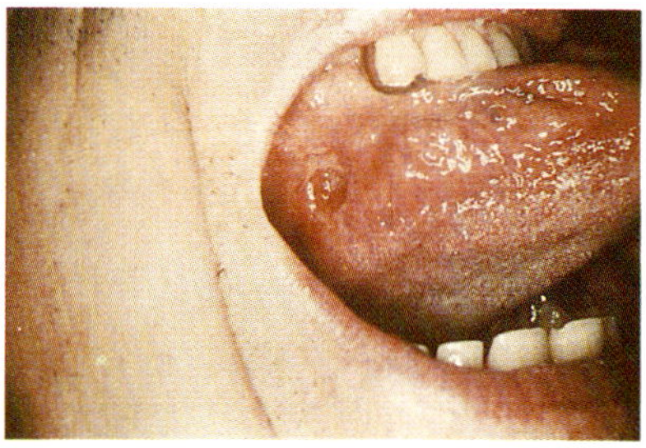

Cancer on Side of Tongue

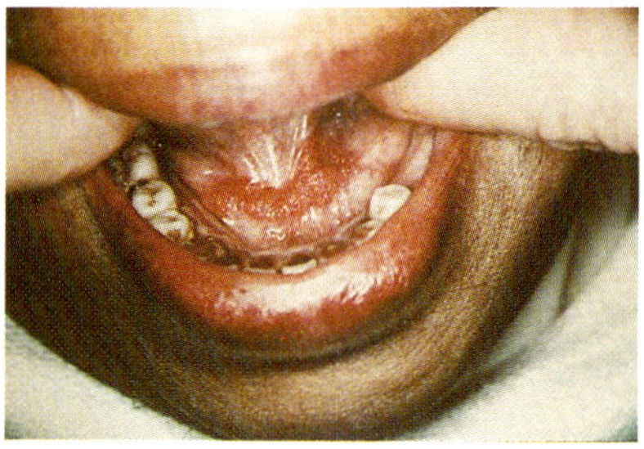

Cancer on Floor of Mouth

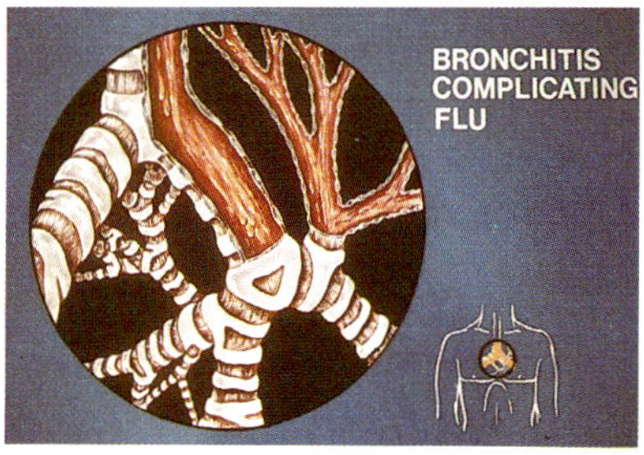

Inflammation of Air Passages

Courtesy Spenco Medical Corporation, Waco, Texas

GASTROINTESTINAL, ABDOMINAL AND REPRODUCTIVE COMPLAINTS
Chapter 12

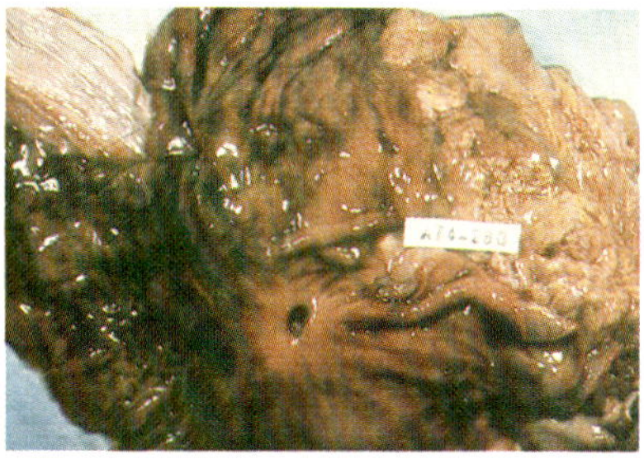

Stomach Ulcer

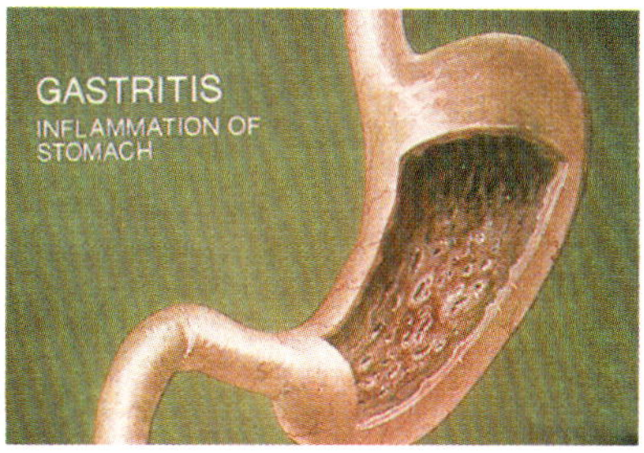

Inflammation of the Stomach

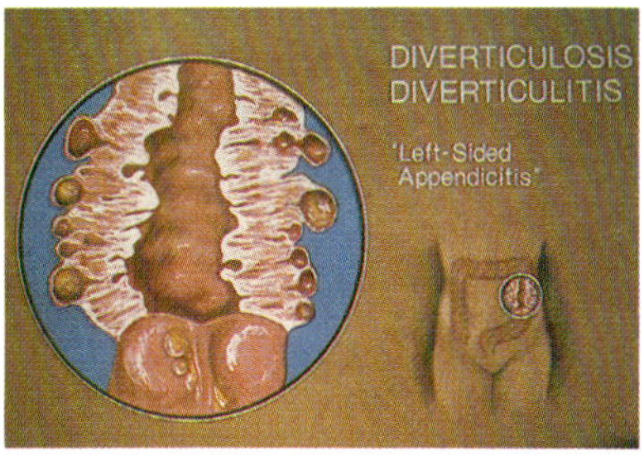

Pouches in Wall of Colon

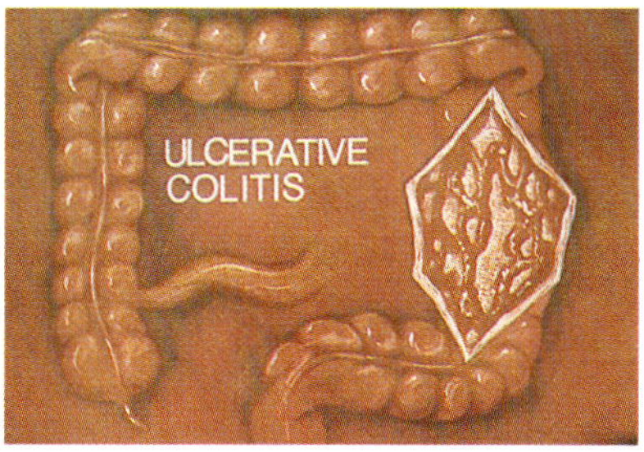

Inflammation of the Colon

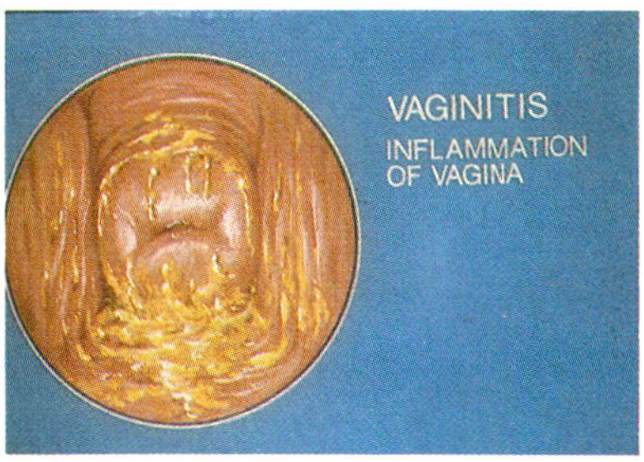

Inflammation of Vagina

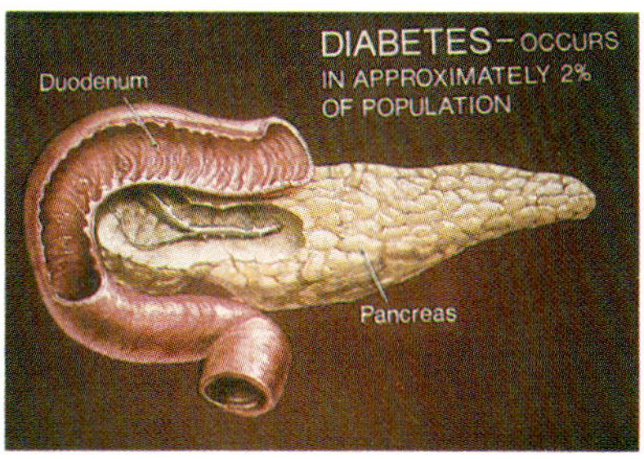

Disorder of Carbohydrate Utilization

Courtesy Spenco Medical Corporation, Waco, Texas

HEART AND CIRCULATORY COMPLAINTS

Chapter 13

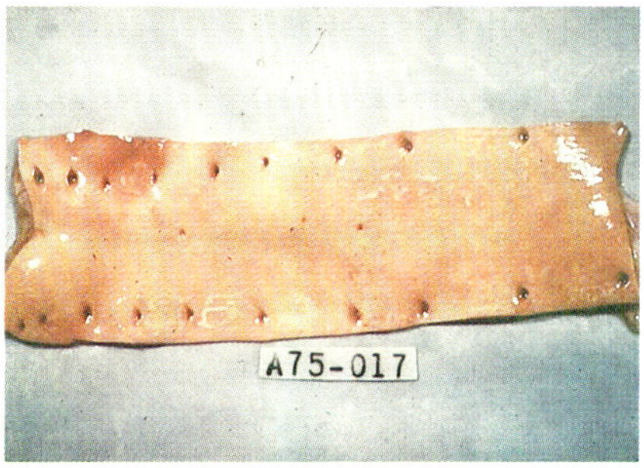

Inside Surface Normal Artery

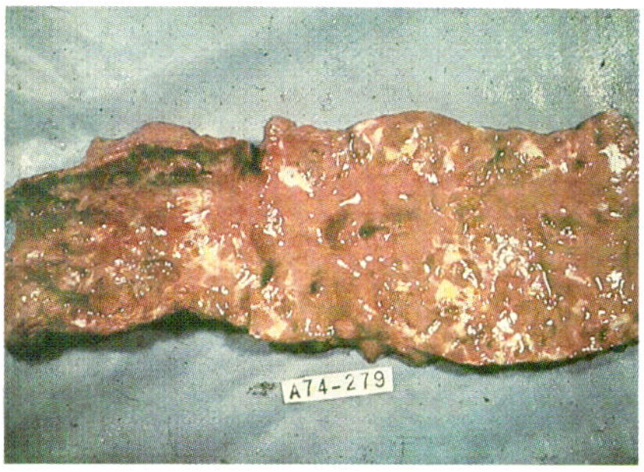

Inside Surface Severe Atherosclerosis

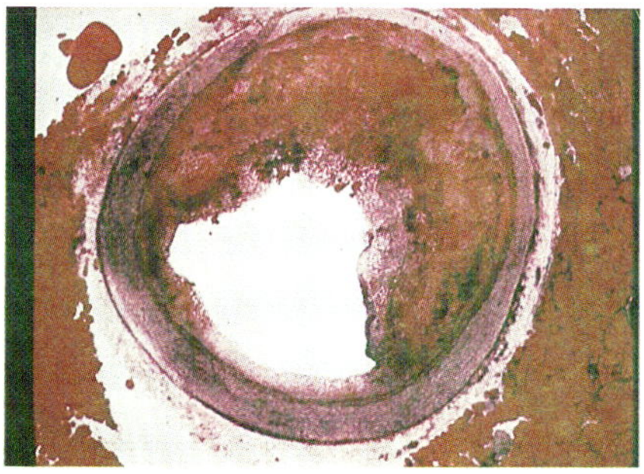

Artery Cross-Section Atherosclerosis

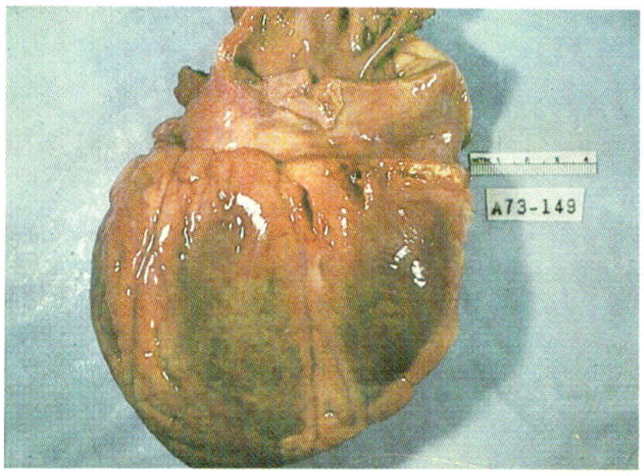

Myocardial Infarction
(Heart Attack)

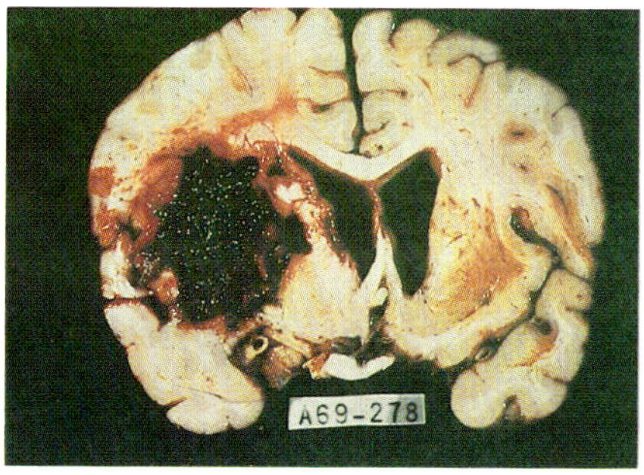

Cerebralvascular Accident (Stroke)

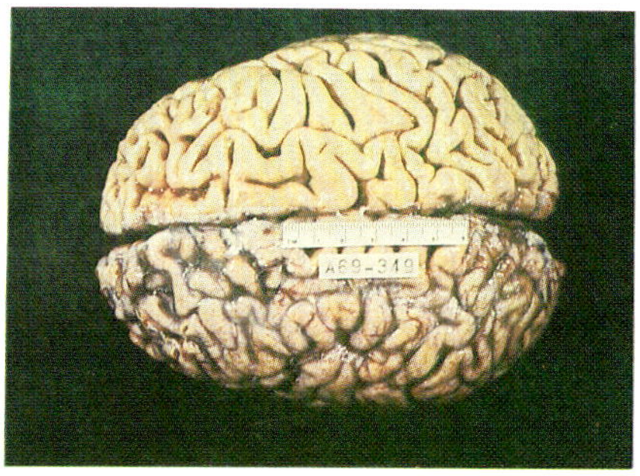

Stroke Damaged Brain

Courtesy Spenco Medical Corporation, Waco, Texas

CHILDHOOD HEALTH COMPLAINTS

Chapter 6, 14

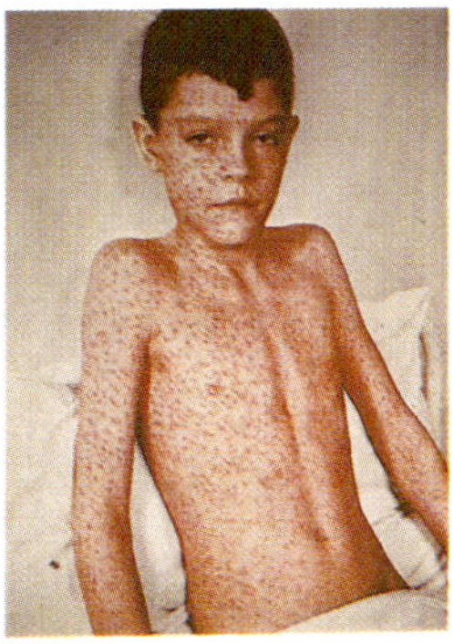

Measles

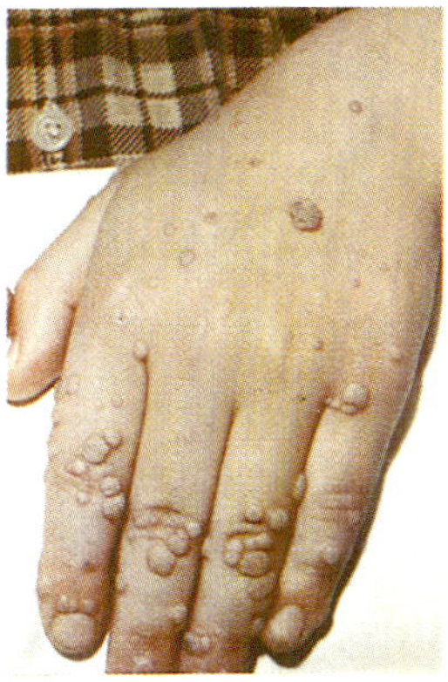

Warts

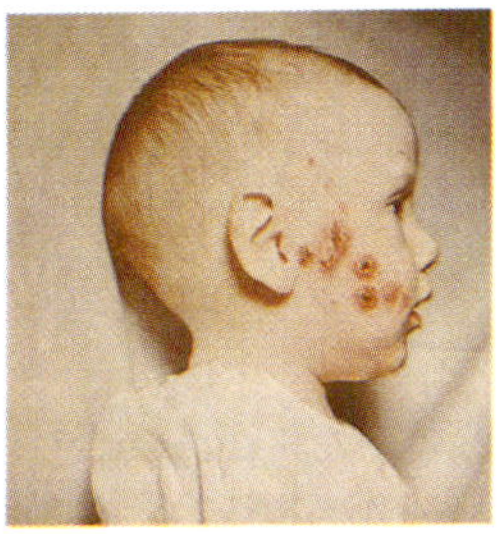

Impetigo

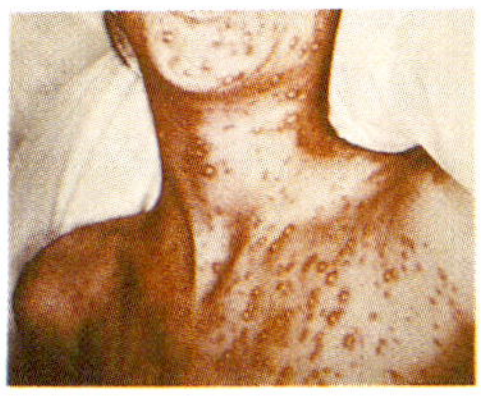

Chicken Pox

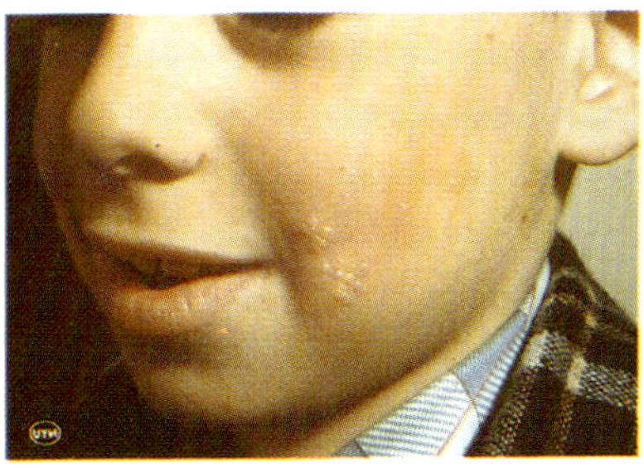

Herpes I Virus

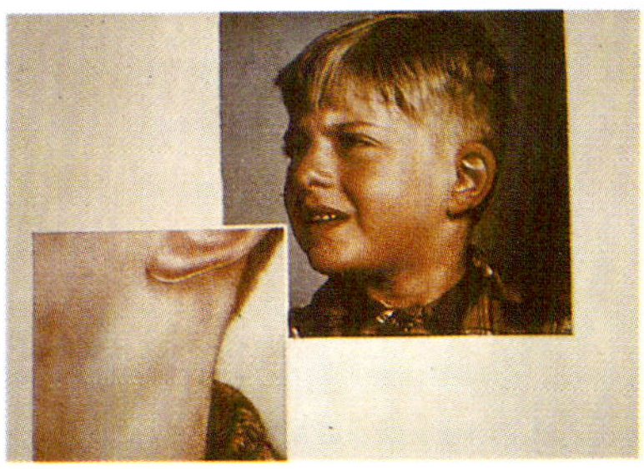

Mumps

Courtesy American Academy of Dermatology and Institute For Dermatologic Communication and Education and Metropolitan Life Insurance Co.

infection, redness in body creases, difficulty in swallowing, difficulty in breathing, or excessive drooling. You should take the child to the doctor if he or she acts extremely sick, even though none of the above symptoms have developed.

If the child is given an antibiotic prescription by a doctor, be sure that the child finishes the full course of antibiotics. Otherwise, a strep infection may still be present, and the child could develop any number of serious complications.

Caution: There has been recent concern about giving infants and children aspirin for fevers caused by some viruses because it may induce Reye's syndrome. Consult your physician.

LARYNGITIS (Hoarseness)

Acute or chronic inflammation of the larynx — the voice box — has many of the same causes and implications as sore throat. The most common cause of laryngitis is the common cold; the most important symptom is hoarseness. Other causes include sore throat, sinusitis, tonsillitis, bronchitis, flu, pneumonia, whooping cough, syphilis, measles, excessive or improper use of the voice, poor ventilation, inhalation of irritating gas, allergies, irritation from dust or smoke, hot or corrosive liquids, violent weeping, polyps in the throat, and use of alcohol or tobacco.

Signs and Symptoms

A mild case of laryngitis begins with a dry, tickling sensation of the larynx followed quickly by partial or complete loss of the voice. The patient may experience a slight fever, minor discomfort, poor appetite, rawness in the throat, heat in the throat, pain in the throat, difficulty in swallowing, and a dry cough followed by expulsion of mucous matter. Use of the voice is painful or absent. Swelling of the larynx may impair breathing and creates a constant urge to clear the throat.

Self-Care Treatment

Rest your voice completely; communicate only in sign language and whispers, and don't strain to try and use your voice. Completely avoid smoking and alcohol consumption; drink plenty of fluids, especially fruit juices.

Keep the temperature in your home even and warm; keep the air moist with a humidifier or vaporizer. To relieve pain, keep an icebag on the throat for fifteen to twenty minutes at a time four or five times a day.

When to Call the Doctor

If laryngitis persists more than a week or if you develop a fever, you should call your doctor. You should also make an appointment to see your doctor if your laryngitis becomes recurrent.

Laryngitis in Children

Laryngitis in infants is usually the result of a birth defect or is caused by excessive crying. In older children, it is usually caused by a viral infection. Make sure that the room is humid, that the child drinks plenty of fluids, and that the child rests his or her voice. You can help relieve the pain by wrapping a warm towel around the child's neck or applying warm compresses to the neck.

Any child under the age of three months who develops laryngitis should see a doctor. Also call a doctor if a child of any age develops difficulty in breathing, difficulty in swallowing, or excessive drooling, or if the laryngitis persists for longer than five days or grows worse, despite home treatment.

HALITOSIS

The most common source of halitosis — bad breath — is poor dental hygiene; anyone who does not daily clean the teeth and surrounding mouth tissues is almost certain to have bad breath or at least an unpleasant mouth odor. There are a number of other causes of bad breath, though: decayed teeth, an abscessed tooth, coated tongue, infected sinuses, infected tonsils, chronic lung disease, gastrointestinal disease, liver disease, severe dieting (resulting in acetone in the lungs), diabetes, some medicines or drugs, and a number of foods and spices that enter the bloodstream and are exhaled from the lungs — including alcohol, tobacco, coffee, garlic, onions, and a number of other spices.

Self-Care Treatment

The first key to overcoming halitosis is to practice good oral and dental hygiene. Clean your teeth after every meal with a good toothbrush and some kind of dental paste (you can use commercial toothpaste or a combination of table salt and baking soda). Floss between your teeth once a day to remove stubborn particles of food that may become lodged. Once a day, brush your tongue gently to cleanse it; brisk, rough brushing or brushing more often than once a day can stimulate the taste buds to grow long and form traps that will act as collectors and increase halitosis.

Stop smoking; tobacco is one of the primary sources of halitosis and is difficult to overcome, since it is exuded from the lungs.

Mouthwashes have some germicidal action, but they are extremely limited. Do not rely on mouthwashes to conquer halitosis; you can use them if you need to mask odor for a short period of time. A better idea is to regularly clean your teeth and rinse your mouth out with a slightly salty solution to complete the cleansing.

Avoid eating foods that you know cause bad breath.

Halitosis in Children

The most common source of a child's bad breath is a foreign object lodged in the nose; this will result in a white, yellowish, or bloody discharge from the nose. Don't give children a mouthwash. Teach them proper dental habits, and help them practice brushing their teeth and flossing.

Take your child to a doctor if you notice a white, yellowish, or bloody discharge from one nostril or if the child has sores in the mouth. He or she should see a dentist if you can see a decaying tooth.

When to Call the Doctor

If your halitosis does not respond to a treatment regime composed of improved dental hygiene and the other elements listed above, you should see your doctor or dentist so that the underlying causes of halitosis can be identified and corrected.

CHAPTER 10

COMMON MOUTH AND TOOTH COMPLAINTS

TOOTH KNOCKED OUT

Anyone can lose a tooth due to injury or a blow to the mouth, but it is most common among children because the bone structure of a child's mouth is more supple; when a child's tooth is placed under pressure, it may "pop out." The same amount of pressure exerted on an adult's tooth will usually just cause the tooth to break off.

Self-Care Treatment

If the tooth is a baby tooth, have the child rinse the mouth out with a slightly salty solution of warm water and a teaspoon of salt; have the child swish the water gently. There is usually little bleeding, but if the socket does bleed, have the child bite down on a thick piece of sterile gauze for fifteen minutes or until the bleeding is under control.

If the tooth is a permanent tooth, your first aid and speed can enable the tooth to be replanted. There are two primary keys:

1. Keep the tooth moist. Immerse the tooth completely in clean, plain warm water or in clean saltwater as soon as you find it. If you don't

have access to any water, put the tooth under your tongue, where it will be kept moist with your saliva.

2. Get to the dentist as quickly as you can. The faster you can get to the dentist, the greater the chance that the replant will work. In order to be effective, the replant procedure must be done within thirty minutes of the injury.

No replant is permanent; if the replanted tooth survives the first three to six months, it will probably last about eight years before the body eventually rejects it. The value of replanting, however, is that during the crucial period of adolescence, when the facial structure is forming and the last of the permanent teeth are coming in, the tooth enables proper formation and development. In addition, it allows an individual to be older and more mature before having to cope with a partial denture.

TOOTHACHE

Like pain in any other part of the body, a toothache is a signal that disease has attacked the tissue. The most common cause of toothache is dental caries, which begins as a small break in the outer enamel and then spreads into the center of the tooth, or the pulp. The pulp contains a rich supply of blood vessels and nerves and is extremely painful when irritated. Pulpitis—a serious infection of the pulp cavity—may result if the caries is not treated.

Toothache can also accompany ear infection, sinusitis, and other diseases, particularly those affecting the mouth and oral cavity.

Signs and Symptoms

The chief symptom, of course, is pain in a tooth. The pain may be intermittent at first but usually becomes more severe and constant. The neck of the tooth may be sensitive when touched with a fingernail or the bristles of a toothbrush, and the tooth is usually sensitive to sweets, fruit juices, and hot or cold liquids. When the victim lies down, the tooth may throb with a sharp, intermittent pain. The gums seldom swell, and there is no fever.

Self-Care Treatment

Use aspirin as a temporary method of pain relief; an ice pack on the jaw can also help relieve pain temporarily. **Any** case of toothache should be seen by a dentist as soon as possible, even if the toothache seems to go away. Avoid eating irritating foods until you can see the dentist, and rinse the mouth out every few hours with a mild, warm saline (salt) solution to relieve pain.

Regular dental checkups and improved dental hygiene can help prevent toothache.

Toothache in Children

While dental caries is the primary cause of toothache in children, a child's toothache may also be due to an ear infection, a sore throat, an injury to the jaw joint, or the mumps. You should take your child to the doctor instead of the dentist if he or she complains of earache and/or has a fever.

DENTAL ABSCESS

When infection attacks the root of a tooth, a dental abscess occurs. An abscess is a potentially serious condition, since pus from the abscess may leak into the bloodstream and cause a systemic infection that involves the entire body.

Signs and Symptoms

The most characteristic symptom of a dental abscess is acute pain at the base of a tooth; other symptoms include swollen gums, puffy eyes and lips, tender and swollen lymph glands in the neck on the side of the toothache, and spasms in the muscles of the jaw. If the spasms are severe, the victim has trouble opening the mouth.

Self-Care Treatment

Any case of an abscessed tooth should be seen by a dentist as soon as possible. Until you see the dentist, try the following to reduce pain:

1. Apply warm mouthwashes and warm compresses. In some cases, heat may increase the pain; if it increases your discomfort, use ice packs and cold mouthwashes. Swish the mouthwashes gently to avoid irritating the tooth and surrounding tissues. Apply the compresses to the jaw, outside and over the area of the toothache.
2. Take aspirin. Never apply aspirin directly to the tooth or the gums—it can cause local burns of the mucous membranes of the mouth.
3. If the gum near an aching tooth gets inflamed and reddened, swish a saline solution—one teaspoon of salt to eight ounces of warm water—gently around the gum as frequently as you can. This may cause the abscess to rupture; if it does, continue the saline rinses.
4. Avoid eating irritating foods or drinking irritating beverages.

When to Call the Doctor

See a dentist as soon as possible if any of the above symptoms occur—even if they later go away.

BLEEDING GUMS (Pyorrhea)

A direct result of untreated inflammation of the gums, pyorrhea is an acute inflammation of the gums that involves discharge of pus. Pyorrhea can also be caused by local irritation, including dental caries, tooth decay, irritation from a filling, improperly fitting dentures, or lodged food particles.

Constant swallowing of the pus can cause indigestion and results in chronic ill health.

Signs and Symptoms

In its initial stages, pyorrhea causes the gums to be painful and to bleed easily when the teeth are brushed. The gums between the teeth become infected and exude pus, which causes bad breath and indigestion. As pyorrhea advances, the gums recede, exposing the base of the tooth to hot and cold foods—causing intermittent and severe pain. Advanced pyorrhea causes loosening of the teeth, resulting in chewing difficulty, and is one of the major causes of tooth loss in the United States.

Self-Care Treatment

See a dentist promptly for any of the above symptoms—even if they are not severe. Use a saline mouthwash until you can get to the dentist.

GINGIVITIS

Gingivitis, inflammation of the gums, can be caused by accumulation of food particles between the teeth, general poor health, irregular teeth, badly fitting fillings or dentures, vitamin deficiencies, anemia, unremoved tartar, poor oral hygiene, blood disorders, mouth breathing, diabetes, allergic reactions, and pregnancy. Gingivitis can lead to more serious disorders, chief among them pyorrhea.

Signs and Symptoms

Whereas pyorrhea causes a recession of the gums, gingivitis causes an overgrowth. The gums swell in a band at the neck of the teeth and may bleed upon slight contact, but little or no pain is involved. Other signs and symptoms include swollen red or purple gums; gums that bleed at the slightest touch; gums that separate from the teeth and form pockets; growth of polyps between the teeth; formation of abscesses between the teeth; inflammation of the entire mouth; black spots on the gums and mouth; reddened and cracked lips; a scalded feeling on the tongue; a bright red and smooth tongue; and ulcerated lesions in the mouth.

Self-Care Treatment

See your dentist immediately if you experience any of the above symptoms, even if they disappear. For temporary relief until you get to the dentist, use frequent warm saline (salt) mouthwashes and brush your teeth thoroughly and frequently. Stimulate your gums with finger massage, and avoid gum irritants.

To prevent gingivitis, brush your teeth after each meal, floss once a day, and take proper care of your gums. Eat a healthy diet containing an adequate amount of nutrients, calcium, and vitamins.

TRENCH MOUTH (Vincent's Disease)

Most frequent among young adults and adolescents, trench mouth is usually caused by bacterial infection and can be caused by poor dental fillings, vitamin C deficiency, lead and bismuth poisoning, blood diseases, gastrointestinal diseases, diabetes, insufficient rest, emotional stress, a faulty dental arch, untreated cavities, heavy smoking, poor oral hygiene, and general nutritional deficiency.

Signs and Symptoms

The gums are painful, red, and spongy; they bleed easily. There is usually a bad taste in the mouth, and the mouth and throat are sore. Fever and malaise may occur; lymph nodes in the neck usually swell. A dirty gray or yellowish membrane may form on the mucosa of the mouth, and sores or ulcers may appear on the gums, the inside of the cheeks, and sometimes on the tonsils and in the throat. Swallowing and talking may be painful.

Self-Care Treatment

Rinse your mouth frequently with a solution of two teaspoons of 3 percent hydrogen peroxide in eight ounces of water. Get plenty of bed rest, and eat a diet well-balanced with nutrients and vitamins. It will be easier to get the nutrients you need if you eat a soft diet that is easier to chew.

During acute flareups, refrain from brushing your teeth. Stop smoking and drinking alcohol. Take aspirin to relieve pain and reduce fever.

When to Call the Doctor

It is essential that you see a dentist for trench mouth; professional cleaning of the teeth is critical to proper healing of trench mouth. In addition, see a doctor if your fever rises above 100° F, and if you experience prolonged sickness.

SORE TONGUE

A sore tongue is caused by the direct irritant effect of a variety of substances. Tongue inflammation accompanies anemia, scarlet fever, nutritional deficiencies, and general infections. A coated tongue may be a symptom that accompanies a number of diseases, but it does not necessarily indicate illness. A dry tongue can result from fever and dehydration. Common causes of sore tongue include smoking (especially pipes), eating extremely spicy foods, eating extremely hot food (which often affects the roof of the mouth as well as the tongue), having an allergic reaction (to toothpaste, mouthwash, or food dye), or experiencing a vitamin deficiency especially of the B vitamins).

Signs and Symptoms

Signs and symptoms of a sore tongue include reddening of the tip and edges of the tongue, painful ulcerations on the tongue, whitish patches on the tongue, smooth areas on the tongue, hair on the tongue, and burning, tenderness, or painful swelling.

Self-Care Treatment

Try to determine the underlying cause or agent that is making your tongue sore; remove it if you can. Eat a well-balanced, nutritious diet.

For relief of pain and tenderness, swish a mild alkaline solution—one alkaline aromatic solution tablet or one teaspoon of baking soda in eight ounces of warm water—through your mouth four times a day.

When to Call the Doctor

If your tongue does not heal within twenty-four to forty-eight hours with the treatment regime described above, consult your doctor.

CANKER SORES

Canker sores are recurring sores that form inside the mouth and on the lips; they are generally confined to the movable areas of the lining of the mouth. Most cases occur sporadically and involve only a few lesions. Women get canker sores twice as often as men do, and canker sores are more common among lower income groups.

The exact cause of canker sores is not known. Aggravating factors include psychosomatic stress (business problems, sexual difficulties, intense grief), physical stress, injury to the mouth or lip (often incurred in biting), menstruation, and gastrointestinal upset. Canker sores may occasionally occur on mucous membranes other than those of the mouth.

Ninety percent of the time, the tendency toward canker sores runs in families. They are not contagious, and anything that affects the lining of the mouth can aggravate the sores. If left untreated, the sores heal in ten to fourteen days.

Signs and Symptoms

Hours before the lesions appear, the mouth gets oversensitive, often with a tingling or burning sensation. The lesions appear as small, egg-shaped ulcers with yellow or white centers surrounded by a reddish halo. The ulcer, extremely painful and tender, looks like a small, punched-out hole—never a raised blister. The surrounding tissue may swell, but rarely is fever present. The diameter of the sores varies from one-third of an inch to one and a quarter inches.

The sores can appear singly or in batches. Within a week, they get covered with a yellowish opaque coat.

Self-Care Treatment

Avoid eating foods that contain acid—specifically, ketchup, lemon

Canker Sores Aren't Herpes

Many people confuse canker sores with oral herpes, but the two afflictions are unrelated. Canker sores are not contagious and almost always show up inside the lips and cheeks, on the tongue, or at the base of the gums as oval, grayish-white sores with bright red rims. The cause is unknown, but canker sores (or aphthous ulcers, as they are technically called) often appear during periods of emotional and physical stress and after eating certain foods. They tend to run in families, and women are about twice as likely to get them as men. Untreated, most canker sores go away on their own within ten to 14 days.

Diets, vitamins or special supplements usually do nothing to get at the underlying cause, with the possible exception of canker sores that appear in the 20% of the population who are deficient, for one reason or another, in iron, folic acid or vitamin B_{12}. Studies reported by Dr. David Wray of the National Institute of Dental Research show that from half to 85% of such patients appeared to get rid of their canker sores after receiving supplements to make up for the three nutrient deficiencies. However, if canker sores are not due to deficiency, taking supplements probably does no good. Tests for the condition are complex and generally not available in the offices of private physicians.

Source: *Changing Times*, October 1981, p. 42

juice, citrus fruits, tomatoes, and mustard. Increase your fluid intake. Don't take vitamin supplements; they are useless against canker sores, and retention of some fat-soluble vitamins can result in disease.

To relieve pain, take aspirin and gargle with warm saltwater (one teaspoon of salt to eight ounces of water). Apply a poultice of baking soda and water, or try a mouthwash of baking soda and water. Sucking anesthetic lozenges or cough drops can also relieve pain.

If you have obtained a prescription of tetracycline from your doctor, hold a suspension of tetracycline (antibiotic) in the mouth for several minutes, then swallow it; it soothes pain when absorbed and speeds healing to five to seven days.

When to Call the Doctor

If canker sores do not heal within fourteen days or if they continually recur, see your doctor.

LEUKOPLAKIA

Characterized by whitish growths on the mucous lining of the mouth (usually the tongue and cheeks), leukoplakia occurs mostly in men (about two-thirds of the cases occur in men) who are middle-aged or elderly. Because leukoplakia can be precancerous, the growths should be constantly monitored.

Leukoplakia can be caused by a combination of conditions in the mouth and the body in general—including badly fitting dentures, jagged teeth, nicotine (from cigarettes, pipes, or cigars), faulty dental work, hot spices, alcohol, syphilis, vitamin A or B deficiency, or a deficit of sexual hormones, or eating extremely hot food.

Signs and Symptoms

Leukoplakia features white or yellowish-white patches on the floor of the mouth, the tongue, and the inside of the cheeks. The patches are thickened and leathery and sometimes become fissured or ulcerated. Unfortunately, pain does not occur until late in the disease and sometimes does not occur until the disease has become cancerous. The lesions on the floor of the mouth are particularly likely to develop into cancer.

Self-Care Treatment

Keep your mouth scrupulously clean, and avoid all irritants (such as nicotine, spicy foods, hot foods, alcohol, and irritating dentures). Suck a vitamin A tablet (as recommended by your pharmacist) two to three times a day.

When to Call the Doctor

See a doctor immediately if you begin to develop any of the symptoms of leukoplakia. Because it can develop into cancer, it is a serious condition that requires medical treatment and close monitoring. In severe cases, the patches may need to be surgically removed.

CARE OF THE TEETH AND MOUTH

Cleaning teeth and gums is the key to preventing all major gum diseases and the **only** way to prevent dental decay. Proper and effective cleaning includes the use of flossing techniques, and the correct brushing procedure.

Flossing

There are many places in your mouth that your toothbrush can't reach: spaces in between your teeth, areas along your gum line, and the rear surfaces of your back molars. These places still need to be cleaned—they're major sites of plaque buildup and frequent sites of oral and dental disease. Flossing will enable you to clean the areas your toothbrush can't reach or can't properly clean.

Follow these easy steps:

1. Hold the floss between your thumbs and forefingers. There should be about an inch of floss between your two hands; use your thumbs and forefingers to guide the floss as you proceed.
2. Insert the floss between two teeth with a gentle sawing motion. Never snap the floss down into the gums—you'll cut or bruise them. As the floss approaches the gum line, curve it tightly in a C-shape against the tooth and gently slide it into the space between your gum and your tooth; continue sliding it gently until you feel a slight resistance.
3. Keep the floss held tightly against the tooth; scrape the side of the tooth as you move the floss away from the gum and back toward the chewing surface of the tooth.

Don't get discouraged at first; as you break up the plaque deposits and as you remove the bacteria, your gums will get sore and might bleed. This tenderness will probably continue for the first five or six days, or until you have succeeded in removing the stubborn deposits. As the plaque is removed, your gums will heal and will stop bleeding. If you discontinue flossing, your gums may swell up and start to bleed again due to fresh plaque and bacteria deposits.

If the bleeding from flossing doesn't stop after a week, consult your dentist. It's important to floss every day to keep the plaque from building back up.

Basic Brushing

The key to good toothbrushing, of course, begins with a good toothbrush. Yours won't do the job properly if it's worn down or missing bristles—you need to replace your toothbrush often. A soft bristle brush is best.

It's best if you brush your teeth after each meal, but you should make sure that you brush them at least once a day. Your toothbrush can be either manual or electric: both kinds are effective. You may find that an electric toothbrush makes brushing easier if you are handicapped or have arthritis; in addition, children may be delighted by the novelty of an electric toothbrush and may brush more often.

While oral irrigators—devices that shoot a high-powered stream of water that can be directed along the gum line and between teeth are **not** substitutes for regular brushing or flossing (oral irrigators can't remove plaque by themselves); they are useful in helping remove food particles, in stimulating the gums, and in aiding cleaning for those who wear orthodontic braces. Make sure you adjust the water pressure to a safe level—water that's too strong can damage the delicate tissues of the gums.

Your choice of toothpaste depends on personal taste, but you should choose a toothpaste that contains fluoride to give you the maximum protection against dental decay. Read the labels on different brands of toothpaste; some fluoride toothpastes are effective in preventing up to 30 percent of the cavities in children.

Correct brushing procedure includes the following steps:

1. Angle your toothbrush so that it rests with the bristles along the gum line—an area where many cavities are prone to start and where plaque buildups can be particularly stubborn.
2. Move the brush back and forth with short strokes; you should use a gentle scrubbing motion. Concentrate on only a few teeth at a time—don't try to clean the whole side of your mouth at once. The toothbrush is designed to clean only a few teeth at a time, so change position frequently and concentrate on only one or two teeth.
3. When you have finished cleaning the inner and outer surfaces, thoroughly scrub the chewing surface.
4. To slightly freshen your breath, brush the surface of your tongue gently. Don't exert too much pressure: brushing vigorously can cause the papilla-like taste buds to lengthen, creating tiny traps for bacteria and food particles.

CHAPTER 11

COMMON RESPIRATORY COMPLAINTS

COUGHING

A cough is a reflex mechanism that acts as a defense to clear the breathing passages of mucus; even when voluntary, a cough is caused by a reflex action and is desirable if it acts to clear matter from the breathing tubes.

Coughing develops with a number of conditions, including chronic upper respiratory infections, asthma, heart failure, foreign bodies in the throat, diphtheria, tuberculosis, influenza, the common cold, inhalation of irritants, blood clots in the lungs, a sudden or extreme change in temperature, smoking, and a number of illnesses and infections.

Normal lungs form about half a cup of mucus every day. The tiny, fine hairs that line the respiratory passages—the cilia—sweep the mucus up to the back of the throat, where it can be expelled or swallowed. Coughing aids in that process.

Signs and Symptoms

A productive cough is one that is accompanied by copious amounts of sputum—it can be yellow, green, or brown material and may be streaked with blood, depending on the cause of the cough. A dry (or nonproductive) cough usually is a hacking cough that brings up no sputum; it is characteristic of bronchitis, pneumonia, the early stages of tuberculosis and follows inhalation of a foreign body.

Self-Care Treatment

In general, administer aspirin to reduce fever (do not administer aspirin if there is no fever, since aspirin does not act in any way on the cough), and increase the humidity in your home with a vaporizer, humidifier, or steamy shower.

If you have postnasal drip that is irritating your throat, take a decongestant every four hours; an over-the-counter cough syrup may help contain the cough and should be taken every four hours. Don't take antihistamines, because they dry out the lining of the throat and bronchial passages.

If your throat is irritated, gargle with warm salt water (one teaspoon of salt to eight ounces of warm water), or suck on throat lozenges or hard candy if your throat is dry and tickly. Increase your fluid intake—especially important if you have a fever.

Completely stop smoking. Don't rest too much—lying in bed can actually cause you to cough more.

If someone in your family starts to cough up frothy blood, have the person lie on his or her back with the head elevated. Apply ice packs to the neck and chest, and give nothing by mouth. Get the person to a doctor as soon as possible.

When to Call the Doctor

Contact a doctor immediately if you cough up blood; if your cough produces large amounts of thick, foul-smelling, yellowish or greenish sputum; if you have a fever of more than 102° F.; if you have a fever of over 100° F. that lasts longer than three days; if your cough lasts longer than ten days; if your cough worsens after twenty-four hours of treatment; if you have pain other than a mild headache; if you have a sore throat or suffer from excessive weakness for longer than a week; or if you have to maintain treatment longer than a week.

Cough in Children

You should take a child to the doctor immediately if he or she develops a violent, sudden cough without a cold; if the child is under three months of age; if he or she is breathing rapidly; if he or she has difficulty in breathing; if the child is wheezing; if the child runs a fever for longer than four days; if the cough continues for longer than ten days; if the cough wakes the child from sleep; if the child has significant changes in breathing patterns; if the child has a cold and is under three years of age; and if the child develops a sudden fever.

If Your Child is Coughing, Call the Doctor . . .

1. When a severe cough and fever are present for more than 24 hours.
2. When a severe cough alone is present for more than 72 hours and not improving.
3. When the child's activity is greatly decreased.
4. When there are several signs of severe breathing distress—come in immediately:
   - Fast breathing rate (consistently greater than 40 breaths per minute—one breath in plus one breath out equals one breath).
   - Blueness of the lips or elsewhere (not due to cold skin).
   - Nose enlarging with each breath.
   - Skin caving in below ribs, between ribs, or above breastbone with each breath.
   - Trouble breathing out.
   - Difficult, raspy breathing.
   - Grunting.
5. When frequent, severe, barklike coughs are present—the child should be seen as soon as possible.
6. When severe nasal congestion or runny nose lasts more than 3 days in a child less than 12 months old.
7. When child complains of earache, or pulls, digs at, or rubs one or both ears.
8. When child with very frequent ear infections has a severe cold for more than 4 days.
9. When a sore throat is present—come in for a throat culture.
10. When there is any uncertainty about any of the above.

HICCUPS

Hiccups, a simple body reflex, have no protective function; they may be minor and may occur only infrequently, or they may last so long and become so severe that they completely sap the victim's strength. In severe cases, they can lead to depression or death.

Normal hiccuping can be set off in several ways: gulping hot or cold liquids, overeating, overdrinking, smoking excessively, being fatigued, laughing after a big meal, having indigestion, being nervous, exercising after a meal, swallowing food in the wrong way, having a hiatal hernia or pleurisy, being pregnant, or having a brain disorder. Serious cases of hiccups can occur with mental or emotional shock, prolonged mental strain, drug addiction, postpartum depression, and cardiospasm.

Normally, in signalling the diaphragm to contract on schedule, the phrenic nerves act in harmony; sometimes, however, a message carried from one of the abdominal organs by way of sensory nerves to the brain causes a disruptive reflex action in the phrenic nerves and interrupts the rhythm. In turn, the diaphragm "goes berserk," resulting in spasms that cause the victim to inhale with each contraction. The end result is hiccups.

Signs and Symptoms

In normal cases, hiccups taper off and go away without too much trouble; a simple disruption of the spasm effect of the diaphragm causes hiccups to stop.

Hiccups lasting more than two days can cause discomfort, fatigue, exhaustion, and interference with sleeping, eating, and resting. Those suffering from syphilis, pneumonia, pleurisy, meningitis, encephalitis, and brain or spinal cord tumors are much more likely than usual to suffer prolonged attacks of hiccups.

Self-Care Treatment

Treatment of hiccups is aimed at shocking the phrenic nerves back into normal harmonic activity. Try any (or all) of the following:

- Hold a paper bag over your nose and mouth, and breathe in it for several minutes

- Take a deep breath, hold it, and blow it out slowly
- Drink a large glass of water in one draft, without taking a breath
- Apply slight pressure on the eyeballs with the eyes closed
- Swallow crushed ice
- Place an icebag on your diaphragm (located just beneath your rib cage)

Don't restrain a baby who has the hiccups; gently pat him or her on the back between the shoulder blades, and the hiccups will gradually resolve themselves. A baby who has the hiccups for longer than a day should receive medical attention.

BRONCHITIS

Bronchitis results when cells in the mucous lining of the bronchial air passages are irritated and damaged by bacteria, virus, or irritants (such as cigarette smoke), and when the cells secrete a sticky mucus to trap and help move out the irritant. Unfortunately, the mucus is so sticky that it is difficult for the body to move it out of the bronchial passages, and it serves as an ideal breeding ground for bacteria.

The cough associated with bronchitis is the body's attempt to move the sticky mucus out of the bronchial air passages. Because the mucus is sticky, the cough is usually severe.

Signs and Symptoms

A cough that produces clear white or clear yellow sputum is common with bronchitis; the stickiness of the mucus causes a wheezing sound that accompanies the cough. Adults often experience chest pain with bronchitis, but it is not a common symptom in children. The chest pain is intermittent and varies in intensity (steady chest pain is indicative of other, more serious conditions). Prolonged, severe coughing can result in muscle aches at certain points between the ribs. Bronchitis is highly contagious. Fever is generally present.

Self-Care Treatment

1. Avoid breathing in irritating substances—such as cigarette smoke or

heavy air pollution—until all of your symptoms have disappeared.

2. If your bronchitis is severe, stay in bed; if it is mild to moderate, strictly limit your activities. Keep your sleeping room humid and warm.
3. Take a cough medicine (an over-the-counter preparation will work well) at night to help you get to sleep. Increase your fluid intake—you should drink about one gallon of fluid a day to help thin the sticky mucus.
4. Have another family member massage your chest and back; you can have the person rub in a mentholatum preparation if it helps you feel better. The massage stimulates blood circulation to the area and helps speed healing.
5. Twice a day, lie on your stomach with a pillow under your abdomen and your head lowered; stay in the position for about five minutes, coughing gently and expelling sputum. Using the pillow to elevate your hips, turn first to your left side, then to your right side, and finally on your back; hold each position for five minutes, and cough gently while you expel sputum.

When to Call the Doctor

Call a doctor if you experience pain on one side of the chest, blood in the sputum, a fever over 101° F., shortness of breath when not coughing, or wheezing. See a doctor if you are over sixty years of age, if the cough persists for longer than ten days, if you have diabetes, if you smoke more than a pack of cigarettes a day, if you have frequent bronchitis, or if your bronchitis worsens instead of improves after three to four days. See a doctor if you have bronchitis more often than once a year.

SHORTNESS OF BREATH (Dyspnea)

Shortness of breath following heavy exertion or exercise is normal, but shortness of breath that is not preceded by heavy exertion is abnormal and is usually due to some form of oxygen shortage, such as inadequate ventilation, respiratory problems that prevent adequate circulation of oxygen in the blood, cardiac and circulatory problems, or emotional difficulty. Any disease that keeps normal oxygen from getting into the blood or any injury that prevents its circulation through the body can cause shortness of breath.

Signs and Symptoms

A victim may experience shortness of breath while at rest or after slight exertion; he or she may wake up in the morning out of breath and may need to sleep propped up in order to breathe. There may be hyperventilation, and tingling of the fingers may result.

Self-Care Treatment

Rest in bed until you can catch your breath. Sitting may be easier. See a doctor as soon as possible.

When to Call the Doctor

Make an appointment to see a doctor if you have any of the symptoms of dyspnea—a doctor will need to determine and correct the underlying causes. See a doctor immediately if you experience shock, chest pain, arm pain, neck pain, abnormal pulse, or cyanosis (bluish coloring of the skin and nails).

A child who has dyspnea symptoms should be taken to a doctor immediately if he or she develops fever, drooling, hoarseness, difficulty in inhaling, wheezing, tingling in the fingers, dizziness, or if he or she begins breathing with the chin jutting out and the mouth open.

HYPERVENTILATION

Caused by stress, alcohol consumption, sudden and dramatic illness, and severe pain (usually in the abdomen), hyperventilation means an abnormally rapid breathing rate. There is usually an increase in both the rate and depth of breathing, and there is a constant diminution of carbon dioxide. More common among women, it occurs almost exclusively among young adults. While in some cases the individual is not aware that he or she is breathing too fast, some victims become extremely concerned with the rapid breathing.

Signs and Symptoms

Hyperventilation is characterized by a feeling in the top of the head that is hard to describe; dizziness or lightheadedness; blurring of vision; dryness or bitterness in the mouth; tingling of the hands or tingling around the mouth; tightness or a "lump" in the throat; pounding of the heart; shortness of breath; a feeling of great fatigue or weakness; a feeling of being in a dream; fainting; and panic.

Other symptoms include numbness of the hands, fingers, and other body parts; prickling of the skin; trembling; cramping of the muscles; and curling of the fingers and toes.

Self-Care Treatment

Have the victim rest in a quiet place for a few minutes; reassure the person that nothing is wrong physically and that he or she is breathing too fast because he or she is frightened or anxious. Assure the victim that once the anxiety passes, breathing will return to normal.

Put a poncho or a paper bag (never a plastic bag) over the person's mouth and nose to trap the exhaled carbon dioxide; force him or her to rebreathe it. Leave the cover in place for six respirations, then remove it for six. Continue the cycle until the breathing slows.

When to Call the Doctor

If hyperventilation becomes a recurrent problem, make an appointment to see your doctor.

WHEEZING

Wheezing is an audible, high-pitched whistling sound that occurs during exhalation due to a narrowing of the air passages in the lungs; as the air is forced out, it makes a whistling sound as it passes through the narrow tubes. Wheezing can result from asthma, bronchitis, respiratory infections, and heart conditions.

Signs and Symptoms

A wheezing attack is characterized by a sense of tightness in the chest, shortness of breath, and an audible wheezing sound during exhalation. The wheezing sound may or may not be associated with cough or sputum. Wheezing associated with congestive heart failure causes difficulty in breathing and enlargement of the neck veins; cyanosis (bluish coloring of the skin, lips, and fingernails) results.

Self-Care Treatment

Sit in a bed or chair to make it easier to breathe. Drink plenty of fluids, and stop smoking.

When to Call the Doctor

Anytime wheezing occurs, you should see the doctor so that the underlying cause can be identified and treated.

INFLUENZA

Influenza is a respiratory disease produced by three groups of viruses: A, B, and C. The B and C strains are generally more mild; the A strains become mutant and are responsible for the new strains of flu that are most resistant to treatment. The incubation period (from time of exposure to onset of symptoms) for influenza is only twenty-four to forty-eight hours; the disease is highly contagious and is spread the same way as the common cold.

Signs and Symptoms

The following are symptoms of the flu: listlessness, headache, muscular aches, backache, moderate fever (usually 101° F. to 103° F.), chills, sore throat, watering eyes, nasal discharge, cough, nausea, vomiting, headache, limb soreness, fatigue, weakness, loss of appetite, anxiety, and mild distress beneath the breastbone. While the fever generally lasts only a few days, the weakness and listlessness may persist for several weeks. Secondary infections are common and are signalled by cough with sputum production and fever above 103° F.

Self-Care Treatment

Stay in bed while your symptoms persist; keep warm, and keep the air moist in your sleeping room with a humidifier or vaporizer. Increase your fluid intake; drink at least eight ounces of fluid every two hours.

Take aspirin to reduce fever and relieve body aches; make sure that you take aspirin with milk or food to prevent stomach upset.

To decrease your chances of getting the flu, stop smoking, eat well-balanced meals, keep the air in your home moist, and avoid crowded areas during the flu season (late fall and winter).

See the aspirin caution mentioned elsewhere in this text.

When to Call the Doctor

Call your doctor if the flu does not clear up after twelve days, if a serious sore throat is your major symptom, if your fever goes above 103° F., and if you begin to cough up sputum.

PNEUMONIA

Usually bacterial, pneumonia can sometimes be viral; the viral form of pneumonia usually develops from the flu and is sometimes fatal. An inflammation of the air sacs in the lungs and the small bronchioles leading to them, pneumonia is the most common acute infectious disease of the lungs next to bronchitis.

The incubation period (from time of exposure to onset of symptoms) for pneumonia is one to seven days; the disease is airborne and is spread by droplets in the air. The bacterial presence in the air sacs causes them to fill with fluid, and the moist environment encourages further bacterial growth.

Pneumonia can occur on its own or can occur in combination with other diseases, most often the common cold, bronchitis, a serious injury, or surgery. Pneumonia is critical in infants and the elderly.

Signs and Symptoms

Pneumonia usually begins with or is preceded by a common cold; the secretions are unusually heavy, and the cold grows more intense. Typical signs and symptoms of pneumonia include sudden shaking chills, fever between 102° and 104° F., cough (that produces yellow, green, or rusty sputum that may be streaked with blood), rapid pulse, fast respiration, cyanosis (bluish coloring), and difficulty in breathing. The chills of pneumonia are often so violent that the victim's teeth chatter and the bed shakes.

Viral pneumonia is somewhat different; it has a gradual onset, the temperature is lower and more variable, and the cough is seldom productive. The chest is more achy, and the pulse and respiration are slower.

Bacterial infection that leads to pneumonia can in some cases cause a flushed face, sweat on the forehead and face, and hot, moist skin.

Self-Care Treatment

In all cases of pneumonia, you should notify a doctor immediately. While you are waiting to see the doctor, you can alleviate symptoms by following these guidelines:

1. Get in bed; stay isolated from others.
2. Dispose of your tissues and handkerchiefs where they cannot contaminate others.
3. Take aspirin to reduce fever and relieve pain.
4. Drink as much fluid as you can; keep your mouth moist so that your lips don't dry out and crack from fever.
5. Eat a soft, bland diet high in proteins and salt (unless you have congestive heart failure).
6. If you experience severe chest pain, wrap your chest tightly with an elastic or cloth bandage. Lie on your side during coughing spells to alleviate chest pain.

Continue with this treatment once your doctor has diagnosed you; follow his or her suggestions and treatment regime strictly. Make a gradual return to recovery, and get as much rest as you need.

PLEURISY

Inflammation of the pleura—the double membrane that covers the lung—results in pleurisy, a condition that results from any disease that also inflames the lung (such as pneumonia, tuberculosis, or a tumor). Pleurisy can also accompany the common cold, influenza, bronchitis, kidney disease, rheumatic fever, and rheumatism. Sometimes it appears without apparent cause and can be either dry or wet.

Signs and Symptoms

In dry pleurisy, the dry surfaces of the double membrane rub against each other, producing sharp, knifelike pain that is always made worse by breathing or coughing. The pain can sometimes be felt in the neck, shoulder, or abdomen. There is usually shortness of breath.

If dry pleurisy is not treated, tissue fluid gets in between the membranes and causes wet pleurisy. Symptoms include rapid and shallow breathing, pain on bending or twisting, shortness of breath, cough, painful breathing, and fever of about 101° F.

Self-Care Treatment

Stay in bed, whether or not you have a fever. If possible, get fresh air and sunshine in your room; don't exert yourself at all until your symptoms have disappeared.

If coughing is painful, lie on the painful side during coughing spells. Practice deep, careful breathing. Take aspirin for pain, and eat a diet rich in protein and vitamins.

When to Call the Doctor

Call your doctor whenever you develop symptoms of pleurisy, because pleurisy is a forerunner of tuberculosis, lung cancer, and other lung diseases. Occasionally, fluid that accumulates in cases of wet pleurisy will have to be removed by a physician.

ASTHMA

Asthma—a spasm of the bronchial tubes and swelling of the mucous membranes in the breathing passages—is a chronic, recurrent, allergic condition that is caused by sensitivity to an agent such as pollen; in some cases, it is caused by severe respiratory infection. Approximately 2 to 3 percent of the American population suffers from asthma; half of the victims are children under the age of ten. The condition often runs in families.

One-third of those who develop asthma also develop a life-threatening allergic reaction to aspirin—especially so if they developed the asthma after they were ten years old. Emotional problems can cause the asthma to lead to emphysema and other disorders of the lungs. Asthma is a dramatic disease, and the severity and duration of the asthma attack depends on the victim's general health.

In asthma, the spasms of the muscles of the respiratory system and the swelling of the mucous membrane make it difficult to breathe, and the victim has to force the air out of the lungs. Asthma attacks can be precipitated by things such as dust, pollen, infection, smoke, food, medication, exertion, cold and damp weather, emotional upsets, or fatigue.

Signs and Symptoms

While most people suffer asthma attacks in response to the presence of allergens, some people suffer asthma in a chronic state, and any exertion can bring on the symptoms of an attack. Those symptoms include shortness of breath, coughing spells, wheezing respiration, tightness of the chest, sweating, flushing of the face, or paleness and bluish coloration of the skin. By the end of the attack, the cough is usually producing thick, sticky sputum. After the attack is over, the lower chest muscles ache due to the coughing and strain on the lungs. Most asthma sufferers are symptom-free between attacks.

Self-Care Treatment

Much of the treatment of asthma is based on prevention. Don't lie on a carpet unless you are separated from it by a clean, lint-free blanket or a plastic sheet. Keep the windows in your car and house closed; don't smoke. Avoid nasal irritants, such as dust, wet paint, or air pollution. Exercise mildly to increase your strength, and keep in good general health. Reduce anxiety and tension as much as you can, and try to avoid getting a common cold.

During an asthma attack, sit up; don't lie down, because it will be harder to breathe. Humidify the air with a vaporizer, humidifier, or steamy shower, and stay warm. Drink a glass of warm liquid every hour, and take an over-the-counter cough syrup if it helps you breathe. Stay away from sources of emotional excitement during an asthma attack.

When to Call the Doctor

Asthma should be under the general treatment of a doctor at all times. Call a doctor immediately if you experience fever; if you can't talk or eat; if you experience too much pain to lie flat or to sleep; if it hurts to breathe; if your sputum changes color; and if you vomit more than twice in a period of twenty-four hours.

Asthma in Children

One of the most important elements of treatment for asthmatic children is to keep them away from other children who are ill. Keep the child's environment as free from allergens as possible—especially feather pillows and comforters, rubber pillows (they can get moldy), pets, house dust, and cigarette smoke. Encourage the child to drink plenty of fluids, and use a vaporizer in the sleeping room at night to keep the air moist. Encourage the child to exercise frequently to increase strength and endurance; swimming is an excellent exercise for both.

CHEST PAIN

Chest pain can originate in the heart, chest walls, or abdominal organs; it can be caused by exertion, strong emotion, a heavy meal, sudden exposure to extreme cold, infection, injury, cancer, or psychological factors.

Signs and Symptoms

Chest pain can be in the center of the chest (beneath the sternum) and can be described as dull, stabbing, or cutting. It may be a shooting pain that lasts for only a few seconds; such a pain is common and normal, especially among adolescents. Chest pain may be aggravated by deep breathing, coughing, or sneezing. Associated signs and symptoms include fever, cough, sputum, shortness of breath, ashen face, cold sweat, and increase in pulse rate.

Self-Care Treatment

Take aspirin to reduce the fever and relieve the pain. Increase your fluid intake, and eat light meals. To further reduce pain, apply heat, use topical ointments (such as *Ben-Gay* or *Vicks*), and wrap adhesive strips around the chest to prevent spasm.

When to Call the Doctor

Because chest pain can be a symptom of any of a number of serious disorders, consult a physician if you experience any kind of chest pain other than the common and normal shooting pain that lasts only a few seconds. Contact a physician immediately if you experience shortness of breath, irregular pulse, dizziness, severe pain, or profuse sweating.

Chest Pain in Children

Most chest pain in children is a result of severe and prolonged coughing that weakens and fatigues the chest muscles. As with adolescents and adults, a brief shooting pain is normal.

The child should see the doctor immediately if he or she experiences shortness of breath, rapid breathing, rapid pulse, severe pain, or irregular pulse; a doctor should see the child if the chest pain lasts longer than a week or if it is accompanied by dizziness or tingling in the fingers.

CHAPTER 12

COMMON GASTROINTESTINAL, ABDOMINAL, AND REPRODUCTIVE TRACT COMPLAINTS

INDIGESTION

Heartburn, indigestion, or acid stomach can stem from any of a number of causes, including organic disease in the gastrointestinal tract, overeating, eating too rapidly, inadequate chewing, eating unusual food, eating improperly cooked food, consuming too much fat in the diet, being constipated, eating during emotional upsets, experiencing severe emotional strain, swallowing large amounts of air, or smoking excessively.

Symptoms begin an hour or two after eating and are made worse by coffee, cola drinks, alcohol, or spicy foods (such as tomato paste, onions, garlic, or pepper). Indigestion symptoms are relieved by consuming milk, simple antacids, and bland foods (such as cereal, bread, potatoes, dairy products, and ice cream).

Signs and Symptoms

Signs and symptoms of indigestion include nausea, heartburn, upper abdominal pain, a sense of fullness or abdominal distention (bloating), stuffiness, headache, cramps, disagreeable taste in the mouth, chest pain, gaseousness, belching, diarrhea, and vomiting. If it is caused by indigestion, vomiting brings its own relief.

Self-Care Treatment

Once indigestion has occurred, try to belch; if you can't, try to pass gas from the colon. One way to pass gas from the colon is to get down on your hands and knees, lower yourself onto your elbows, raise your buttocks into the air, and bear down slightly.

To relieve the indigestion, take an over-the-counter antacid or a mixture of half a teaspoon of baking soda to four ounces of water. Take

Guidelines For Using Antacids

- Don't use *any* antacid longer than two weeks unless your doctor has given you the go-ahead.
- Use antacid containing sodium bicarbonate or calcium carbonate (such as *Alka-Seltzer*) only occasionally; if you need to take an antacid more than twice, switch to one that doesn't contain either of these ingredients, preferably one with calcium carbonate.
- If you are on a sodium-restricted diet, stick to an antacid that is low in sodium; *Di-Gel, Gelusil, Maalox, Mylanta, Pepto-Bismol,* and *Phillips' Milk of Magnesia* are all low in sodium content fall below 9 milligrams). If you're unsure, ask your doctor or pharmacist for a recommendation.
- For the greatest effectiveness, use a liquid whenever it is possible and convenient. If you do use a tablet, chew it thoroughly.
- If a certain food or beverage consistently causes you stomach upset or indigestion, cutting out the offending item makes much more sense than constantly trying to mask its effects with medicine. If you can't identify the culprit, call your doctor.
- If you are pregnant, steer clear of antacids containing aspirin or a lot of sodium. You should check with your doctor before taking any antacid.
- If your indigestion lasts longer than two weeks, or if it gets worse as a result of your self-medication efforts, immediately stop taking the antacid and call a doctor.
- When asking your doctor or pharmacist about which antacid to use, tell him or her about any other medications you are taking.
- If you change antacids, notify your pharmacist or doctor.
- Remember that no antacid is entirely free of side effects.

sips of water or milk, but avoid food for several hours; don't drink coffee, tea, or alcohol.

If all other methods fail, touch the back of your throat with your finger to induce vomiting.

To prevent indigestion in the first place, avoid tension and argument while you eat; don't eat standing up, and don't smoke during, before, or after your meal. Don't drink water with your meals—drink it either before or after your meal. Eat at a leisurely pace, and don't bolt or gulp your food. A bland diet can help prevent indigestion if you can't tolerate spicy foods.

To correct constipation: drink at least a quart of water daily, and eat cooked fruit twice a day. Exercise for thirty minutes a day—including taking a long, brisk walk, running, bicycling, swimming, hiking, or digging a hole. This can help prevent constipation and indigestion.

When to Call the Doctor

See a doctor if indigestion does not respond to treatment or if it becomes a recurrent, persistent problem. A doctor should also check you if your indigestion is accompanied by other gastrointestinal symptoms.

GASTRITIS

Acute gastritis involves inflammation of the lining of the stomach, and it is usually sudden, violent, and of brief duration. It can be caused by too much alcohol, the excessive use of drugs (including aspirin), spicy foods, intake of poisons or alkalies, influenza, diphtheria, pneumonia, scarlet fever, or any intestinal fever.

Signs and Symptoms

Gastritis usually begins eight to twenty-four hours after ingestion of the offending substance. Symptoms include a severe burning pain at the pit of the stomach, loss of appetite, malaise, nausea, vomiting, and a coated tongue. Headache and dizziness occasionally occur. If the gastritis is from foods or alcohol, symptoms usually disappear within two days.

If the gastritis is from ingestion of a poison or corrosive agent, symptoms include severe stomach pain, collapse, rapid pulse, cyanosis, difficulty in swallowing, excessive thirst, vomiting of blood, blood in the stools, cold moist skin, and rigid, tender stomach muscles.

If the gastritis is caused by infection (such as the flu), symptoms include loss of appetite, vomiting, and a feeling of fullness and pressure in the stomach.

Self-Care Treatment

If the gastritis is caused by food or alcohol ingestion or by infection, stay in bed and avoid eating solid foods for several days. When you begin eating, start out with bland foods.

When to Call the Doctor

If you ingest a corrosive agent or a poison, call a doctor or poison control center immediately. The physician will have to empty the contents of your stomach, and you will need to be under constant medical supervision until the poison is out of your system.

If your gastritis does not subside after two to three days, or if you vomit more than twice during a twenty-four-hour period, you should call a doctor.

GASEOUSNESS

Gas and its associated abdominal bloating is one of the most common complaints of the human race; about one-tenth of all people have symptoms of gas. Gas can be caused by too much swallowed air, ingestion of gas-producing foods, intolerance of some foods (most commonly milk), disease of the pancreas, gallbladder disease, spastic colon, diverticulitis, stress, and a diet high in refined foods.

Everyone produces gas as a natural byproduct of the fermentation of food in the intestinal tract; normally, the gas passes from the colon and rectum without notice. When the gas gets trapped in the intestine, however, pressure builds up and results in pain.

Signs and Symptoms

The characteristic sign of gaseousness is severe, cramping pain in the abdomen; strong spasms and severe bloating may accompany the cramping pain. There is a sensation of fullness and pressure in the abdomen, and the victim is unable to voluntarily pass gas from the rectum. When gas is passed, it is often explosive, passing in strong spurts.

Self-Care Treatment

To reduce gaseousness, avoid eating foods that produce gas—including milk, cheese, buttermilk, puddings, ice cream, cream pies, milk gravies, beans, broccoli, cabbage, cauliflower, brussels sprouts, turnips, cucumbers, radishes, applesauce, and onions.

Eat a diet high in bulk and fiber to keep the intestinal tract healthy and moving smoothly. Eliminate sources of stress and nervous tension as much as you can. Take measures to eliminate constipation; when you feel the urge to have a bowel movement, do not suppress it.

Improve your eating habits. Eat slowly, with your mouth closed; never gulp liquids. Keep talking to a minimum while you are eating, and don't gulp your food. Avoid coffee, alcohol, tobacco, chewing gum, and carbonated drinks—all of them lead to increased gas formation.

In some cases, antacids help relieve spasms and allow for less trapping of gas.

BELCHING

Belching occurs when the stomach is distended with excess food or gas from swallowing air while eating, chewing gum, smoking, or drinking fluids. It is also caused by excessive stretching of the stomach due to overeating or overindulgence in alcohol.

Self-Care Treatment

Eat and drink in moderation. Chew small bites of food carefully, and drink slowly and carefully, taking care not to swallow too much air. Avoid foods that produce gas—especially beans, cabbage, corned beef, and cucumbers.

HEARTBURN

Heartburn is irritation of the stomach and esophagus that results from smoking, drinking alcohol or coffee, taking aspirin, experiencing stress, having ulcers, and eating food that produces excess acid.

Signs and Symptoms

The characteristic symptom of heartburn is a burning pain located just below the breastbone or ribs. It is aggravated by coffee, tea, or alcohol and is relieved by milk or bland food.

Self-Care Treatment

Many of the treatment tips for indigestion also apply to heartburn. Avoid any substances that aggravate the problem—especially spicy foods, alcohol, coffee, tea, and aspirin.

You can relieve the burning pain by taking a nonabsorbable antacid (such as *Maalox* or *Mylanta*) every one to two hours. While sodium bicarbonate may provide quick relief, you should not use it frequently or repeatedly.

Eliminate stress as much as you can, and stop smoking.

If the pain is worse when you lie down, it is probably because acids flow into the esophagus. To prevent such a backflow, avoid lying down right after eating; elevate the head of your bed about six inches with blocks under the legs. Avoid eating for two to three hours before you go to sleep.

When to Call the Doctor

Call the doctor immediately if you have pain that goes through to the back or if you vomit bloody or black material or pass tarlike black stools.

NAUSEA AND VOMITING

Common with viral infections, nausea and vomiting can be caused by the flu, stomach upset, food poisoning, communicable disease, excess food or alcohol, emotional stress, appendicitis, radiation sickness, pregnancy, severe shock or fright, or exposure to unpleasant odors.

Nausea results when irritated nerve endings in the stomach and other parts of the body send messages to the brain center controlling the vomiting reflex. When the nerve irritation becomes intense enough, vomiting results. Intense pain in almost any part of the body can cause nausea; nausea in the first twelve weeks of pregnancy is common and normal, but after that it is cause for concern.

Signs and Symptoms

Nausea is accompanied by faintness, weakness, dizziness, headache, and sweating. The force and frequency of nausea and vomiting help determine the cause. For example, forceful vomiting without nausea suggests increased pressure within the skull, perhaps due to brain injury. Vomiting accompanied by fever and headache suggests the onset of the flue or a communicable disease. Nausea and vomiting in young women of childbearing age suggests the possibility of pregnancy.

Too much vomiting can result in dehydration, signalled by dryness of the mouth and tongue, extreme thirst, and scanty urine.

Self-Care Treatment

Try to determine the cause of upset, and treat the underlying cause first. Do the following:

1. Lie down as much as you can. Don't eat or drink anything until you stop vomiting; then begin with liquids, add bouillon and jello, soups, and applesauce, and gradually work up to a solid diet.
2. To begin taking food and drink again, gradually drink a solution of one teaspoon of salt and a half teaspoon of baking soda in a quart of water. Follow it with fruit juices; sip clear liquids, such as ginger ale, *Seven-up,* clear soup, and water.
3. If the vomiting is caused by a contagious disease, keep your eating dishes and utensils separate from those of other family members. Wash your hands frequently, and dispose of tissues where they will not spread contamination.

When to Call the Doctor

Call a doctor promptly if you experience persistent nausea and vomiting accompanied by headache, eye pain, dizziness, postnasal drip, fever, history of skull injury, black or bloody vomit, or the inability to retain any fluids or food after twelve hours. Contact a doctor if you vomit and you are diabetic, if you may be pregnant, or if you are taking medication of any kind.

Vomiting in Children

Vomiting in children is usually caused by illness (most often the flu, pneumonia, ear infection, tonsillitis, meningitis, urinary tract infection, or appendicitis), intussusception (a condition where a segment of the bowel is pushed into a segment that is ahead of it), croup, head injury, nerves, ingestion of poison, extreme excitement, or allergic reaction to food or medication. Spitting up small amounts of food or milk is common and normal among infants.

To treat a child who is vomiting, give no fluids or solids for two to four hours. Then give the child *Coca-cola* syrup every fifteen minutes; repeat the dosage six times. If you don't have *Coca-cola* syrup, give one teaspoon of ginger ale or *Seven-up* every ten minutes. If the child does not vomit, give him or her one ounce of ginger ale every twenty to thirty minutes. Tea with sugar can also be given to settle the stomach.

Don't give the child any solid food or milk for twenty-four hours after the vomiting has stopped, but make sure that the child drinks plenty of clear fluids to prevent dehydration. Start progressing the diet after vomiting has stopped for twenty-four hours; jello, applesauce, popsicles, and other mild, bland foods are good for starters.

Call a doctor immediately if the child continues vomiting for several hours, has a headache, has a stomachache, has swollen glands in the neck, experiences severe abdominal pain, ingests a poison or medication, has diarrhea, or shows signs of dehydration (dry skin, sunken eyes, thirst, scanty urine). Call a doctor if a child under the age of three months vomits forcefully, or if a child cannot walk, straighten up, or sit straight without severe pain. Always call a doctor if the child's vomit is black or bloody. Consult your doctor if there is no improvement in the child after twenty-four hours.

DIARRHEA

Diarrhea—frequent, watery, loose stools—can result from the rapid movement of fecal matter through the intestines, resulting in poor absorption of the water and nutrients usually absorbed from the feces. Diarrhea can be caused by infectious disease, irritation of the intestinal tract, emotional stress or disorder, food intolerance, and reaction to some medication. Dehydration is the greatest danger with diarrhea and is more likely if there is also vomiting. Watery stools can number up to twenty in a day, depending on the cause and severity of the problem.

Signs and Symptoms

The signs and symptoms of diarrhea are the repeated passage of unformed watery stools accompanied by gas and abdominal cramps; the number may range from five to twenty-five in a single day. The amount of material excreted from the bowels each time is usually small and consists largely of water, mucus, and sometimes blood. The urge to defecate is strong, and there is a feeling of fullness in the abdomen.

Self-Care Treatment

Discontinue food for a period of twenty-four hours; drink plenty of water to prevent dehydration, and drink a solution of one and a half tablespoons of sugar and a quarter of a teaspoon of salt in a quart of water.

Keep your environment calm and restful. Avoid situations or people that cause emotional stress.

After each bowel movement, carefully cleanse the anal region with soap and water to prevent irritation of the skin surrounding the anus.

It may be best to give the intestines a rest when diarrhea is present. These guidelines may be helpful:

1. Do not eat solid foods or milk products until diarrhea has stopped. Clear, cool, or lukewarm liquids are in order, but avoid liquids that are ice-cold or extremely hot. Some liquids that are suggested are water, flat cola or ginger ale, liquid gelatin, or *Gatorade.*

Over-The-Counter Diarrhea Medication

There are three main elements in the over-the-counter diarrhea medication.

Kaolin and Pectin. Kaolin, a gelling agent, is usually combined with pectin in diarrhea medication. The gelatin in kaolin helps you produce more solidly formed stools.

Kaolin and pectin medications are generally mild, and they are not effective against severe bouts of diarrhea. Because of its mildness, kaolin/pectin medicine is particularly good for children, when the doctor authorizes it.

Take about two to four tablespoons each time you have a loose bowel; medications containing a kaolin/pectin combination include *Kaopectate, Kalpec, Kao-Con,* and *Donnagel.*

Because of their mildness, you should start treating diarrhea with kaolin/pectin mixtures. If they do not control your diarrhea in 24 hours, you should call your pharmacist and reassess the situation with him or her. A pharmacist is likely to suggest something a little stronger. You should take the stronger drug for another 24 hours, and, if your diarrhea is still not under control, you should call your doctor.

Paregoric. Paregoric, a mild narcotic preparation available in most states without a prescription, stops the propulsive, wavelike motion of the intestines.

Since paregoric is stronger than kaolin/pectin, you might try one to two tablespoons after each loose bowel movement for a couple of days. You should not use paregoric more often than four times a day without your doctor's permission. Paregoric can be taken in combination with medicines that contain kaolin and pectin; there is no side effect from either medication when the proper dose is taken.

Bulk-Forming Compounds. Diarrhea medicine that contains bulk-formers serves to increase the mass of the stools and to reduce the watery quality of the stools. Most of the medicines containing bulk-formers rely on psyllium; *Metamucil* is a common one. Psyllium is generally not very effective when used alone, so it's a good idea to use it in conjunction with some other medication or to find a medication that combines ingredients. There are no side effects when the medication is taken in the usual dose.

---

2. As the condition improves, eat a bland diet that includes plenty of liquids. Suggested easily digested foods are bananas, rice, baked potato (without butter), applesauce, fresh fruits, vegetables, bran, and whole wheat bread.
3. Resume a normal diet pattern slowly and avoid milk products, alcohol, and spicy or fatty foods for several days after normal bowel movements occur.

When to Call the Doctor

Consult a physician if your diarrhea does not improve with treatment in three days, if your stools get black or bloody, if you have severe abdominal pain, if you have frequent or painful urination, if you are diabetic, or if you are taking medication of any kind.

Diarrhea in Children

Diarrhea is common to small children; it is usually caused by ingestion of poison, nervousness, bacterial infection, viral infection (most common), appendicitis, or food poisoning. It's common for infants to have watery stools, but they are **not** considered diarrhea; an infant that has greenish, mucus-covered, watery stools for a period of a week is considered to have diarrhea.

Give a child nothing by mouth for two to four hours; then give him or her a little ginger ale until the diarrhea stops. If necessary, keep the child on a liquid diet for a few days. When you start feeding the child again, avoid milk and fats (eliminate butter, fatty meats, peanut butter, and fruits), and give the child applesauce, rice, bananas, and toast. Don't give a child an over-the-counter diarrhea medicine.

If diarrhea occurs in an infant, omit one or two feedings, or give the infant smaller amounts at each feeding. If you are nursing, let the baby nurse as long as he or she wants to, and then give him or her as much boiled water as he or she will take after the feeding. If the baby is bottle fed, dilute the milk mixture with an equal amount of cool, boiled water.

If the diarrhea persists, give the baby a mixture of sugar, salt, and water (one and a half tablespoons of sugar and a quarter of a teaspoon of salt to one quart of water). As the diarrhea improves, return the infant to the regular formula.

Consult a doctor if the child has diarrhea for more than forty-eight

If Your Child Has Diarrhea, Call the Doctor . . .

1. When diarrhea persists in a child less than 8 weeks old. If severe, frequent diarrhea persists in a child this age, he or she should be seen quickly. If you are unable to reach the pediatrician within an hour, go to the hospital.

2. When the child is still having more than five large, watery stools per day after 24 hours of clear fluids only.

3. When the child shows any of the following signs of dehydration:
   - Dry, parched lips (unexposed portion).
   - Decrease in frequency or amount of urine, dark yellow.
   - Greatly decreased activity.
   - Obvious weight loss.

4. When the child shows any of the following signs of dehydration—call immediately. If you are unable to reach a pediatrician within an hour, go to the hospital.
   - No urination for 6 hours (4 hours in children 6 months or less). Sometimes this is difficult to determine due to frequency of watery stool.
   - Sunken "soft spot" (while lying down).
   - No tears when cyring.
   - Hard to arouse.
   - Sunken eyes.

5. When the child has loose bowel movements for more than a week.

6. When the child normally has frequent, large, soft, smelly, fatty stools.

hours, has a fever, vomits three or more times, has mucus in the stools, has grayish skin, has frequent or painful urination, has scanty or absent urination, or has severe abdominal pain.

CONSTIPATION

Constipation, a condition in which the waste matter is too hard to pass easily or in which the bowel movements are infrequent or uncomfortable, can be caused by not intaking enough fluids and fiber, habitually ignoring the urge to defecate, overusing laxatives, overusing enemas, or being afraid to pass a bowel movement because of an anal fissure or hemorrhoid that will cause pain. Constipation affects the elderly, invalid, and bedridden and those who have a lack of physical activity.

Constipation/Using Laxatives

Constipation sometimes refers to an incomplete evacuation of the bowels or a feeling that bowel movements should be more frequent. It is not necessarily "normal" to have a bowel movement once a day; it is normal to have as many as three bowel movements a day or as few as three a week. Bowel movements can also remain normal and change in color, bulk, and texture.

Food that fails to move smoothly or quickly enough through the intestine is slowed, and excess moisture is absorbed; the fecal matter is dry and hard.

Over-The-Counter Laxatives

Most laxatives work in one of two ways: Either they soften the stool, or they increase peristalsis (the wavelike motion of the colon). The basic types of laxatives follow.

Stimulants. Chemical stimulants act directly on the colon, causing it to contract and eliminate the bowel movement. The waste products are simply pushed along by the increased wavelike movement of the colon.

Saline. Saline laxatives, containing magnesium and sodium salts, work by retaining water in the intestines, eventually causing a mechanical stimulus that triggers the urge to expel bowel matter.

Bulk-Formers. Bulk-formers expand and swell when they come into contact with water. When they encounter the moisture present in the digestive tract, they form a large mass that, in turn, stimulates the wavelike motions of the colon.

Lubricant-Softeners. Lubricant-softeners aren't actually laxatives, because they don't really stimulate a bowel movement: They simply help the body form softer, moister stools that are easier to pass. This kind of laxative is good for those who need to avoid straining during bowel movements—those with hernias, hemorrhoids, heart disease, or other medical conditions that may be aggravated by straining to eliminate hard stools.

Castor Oil. Although castor oil has been used as a laxative for years, its exact mechanism of action is unknown. However it is known that it does have an overall irritant effect which increases peristalsis (the wave-like movements that move fecal material along the intestinal tract). Castor oil is not generally recommended for laxative use because prolonged use may cause excess fluid loss, which can lead to dehydration.

Suppositories. These work much as the enema does—in the lower colon only—but they are much more convenient to use. There are three different kinds: stimulant, lubricant—softener, and saline/lubricant-softener.

CAUTION: Read the labels carefully—some people should not use certain kinds of laxatives. Over dependence on laxatives can be habit forming and cause undesirable side effects.

Signs and Symptoms

Symptoms of constipation include a chronic feeling of fullness associated with a vague urge to evacuate the bowels. Blood is not present in the stools unless the anus is fissured slightly during evacuation; then the blood is on the outside of the stool in tiny streaks, not mixed in with the feces. Nausea, headache, or a dull and aching distress in the rectal area may persist until the stool is passed.

Self-Care Treatment

Eat naturally laxative foods—fruits, vegetables, and prune juice are excellent choices. Drink at least eight glasses of water a day, and defecate when you feel the urge.

Inactivity and bed rest promote constipation. Get some exercise every day; if you are confined to bed, make some adjustments in your diet to prevent constipation. Vegetables, fruits, whole wheat bread, celery, and cereals are all good foods that help prevent constipation.

Avoid unnecessary tension and worry. Try to forget about your bowel elimination. If nothing else works, occasionally take bulk-forming laxatives that do not irritate the bowel (such as *Metamucil*).

When to Call the Doctor

Call your doctor if you have constipation with thin, pencil-like stools; if you have severe abdominal pain and bloating; if you have unexplained weight loss; if your constipation alternates with diarrhea; if other gastro-intestinal symptoms are present; or if your constipation represents a trend that could be classified as a change in bowel habits.

Constipation in Children

Hardness of the feces, not frequency of bowel movements, is the factor to consider in children. A child may have six bowel movements in one day, but if they are hard and dry, the child is constipated. It is normal for a child to have a bowel movement only once every three or four days.

About 95 percent of all constipation in children is **not** due to a physical abnormality. Some is due to emotional tension—especially true at toilet training time. Infants with diaper rash may hold back to keep from irritating the rash (treatment, then, should center on the rash, not the constipation).

When fecal matter is hard enough to form a plug, liquid seeps around the plug and escapes, a condition known as "soiling." Soiling should always be treated by a physician.

Diet change should be sufficient treatment for most children. Eliminate rice from the diet, and give the child prune juice every day. Give infants one tablespoon of *Karo Syrup* in four ounces of water or milk. Mineral oil can be given to older children but never to infants. Avoid giving enemas.

Call your doctor immediately if the child has pain with a bowel movement, has blood on the stool, has no bowel movement for four to five days, has a crack or fissure on the rectum, is constipated for a period of four weeks, has soiling, has bouts of constipation more than three times when unaccompanied by illness, and when the problem interferes with school or social activities.

ULCERS

An ulcer—an ulcerated sore in the mucous lining of the stomach or the small intestine—can be caused by too much stress, production of excess acid in the stomach, and a host of psychological problems. If an ulcer goes untreated, it can bleed and eventually hemorrhage; in some cases, it may ulcerate completely through the wall of the stomach, leaving a hole and spilling stomach contents into the sterile abdominal cavity.

Signs and Symptoms

The most common symptom is steady, rather than intermittent, pain in the abdomen. The pain is usually absent in the morning before breakfast but often appears at night (between one and three in the morning). The pain is usually boring and burning and can cause a constant cramp in the abdomen between the end of the breastbone and the navel. Eating, taking antacids, and resting almost always relieve the pain.

Other symptoms include vomiting, bright red or black blood in the stools, and black or bloody vomit.

Self-Care Treatment

It takes an average of forty days for an ulcer to heal, but it can heal as quickly as thirteen days, or it may take as long as a year; you must continue treatment until you are completely symptom-free. Do the following:

1. Eat small, frequent meals so that there is food in the stomach most of the time; eat bland foods, and avoid very hot foods, very cold foods, and very fibrous vegetables. Don't drink alcohol, coffee, or tea, and avoid heavily spiced foods.
2. Avoid taking aspirin.
3. Eat your food slowly, and chew it thoroughly. Don't rush your meals. Never go for more than three hours without eating.
4. Take good care of yourself, and do what you can to prevent catching the common cold. Stop smoking.
5. Take antacids for pain. You may also want to try drinking milk to relieve the pain.

When to Call the Doctor

Call a doctor immediately if you are not able to gain relief from the pain, or if your vomit or stools are black or bloody. Call the doctor if you lose your appetite, feel full without eating much food, or if you suspect that you have an ulcer.

Ulcers in Children

Ulcers are fairly uncommon among children; when they do occur, it is among children who are intense, highly motivated, and competitive and who have family conflicts. Ulcers in children may also accompany extensive burns, diseases of the brain, or severe infections (such as meningitis or blood poisoning).

IRRITABLE COLON

Irritable colon is responsible for more than half of all the disorders of the digestive system; almost everyone suffers from it at one time or another. It can be caused by severe anxiety or tension, emotional flareup, hasty gobbling of food, overuse of laxatives, overuse of enemas, and failure to have a bowel movement when needed.

Signs and Symptoms

The most characteristic symptom of irritable colon is that it flares up in connection with emotional upsets. There is chronic constipation, consisting of small, hard, dry stools covered with mucus. Diarrhea is often interspersed with the constipation, consisting of several watery stools in the morning and no stools for the rest of the day. Pain is usually moderate to severe in the upper left side of the abdomen; manual pressure, passage of feces, or passage of gas relieves the pain. Other symptoms include bloating, headache, vomiting, insomnia, loss of appetite, fatigue, and anemia.

Self-Care Treatment

Treatment centers on resolving and avoiding emotional stress and tension. You can reduce pain in the abdomen by applying heat (with a heating pad or moist heat) at regular intervals—not during times of stress. Eat a midly bland diet consisting of some fruit and some roughage. Take time to move your bowels daily. Avoid the use of laxatives and enemas.

When to Call the Doctor

If you are unable to control the condition with home treatment, contact your doctor for possible treatment using sedatives or tranquilizers and some psychiatric treatment.

DIVERTICULITIS

When walls of the colon begin to thicken (usually around the age of sixty, but sometimes as young as thirty), increased pressure within the colon results in the formation of small pockets (called diverticula) at weak spots in the muscular wall of the colon.

Signs and Symptoms

Diverticulitis goes unnoticed in many, but symptoms may include abdominal pain, gas, constipation, diarrhea, and fever. In some cases, fecal matter may become lodged in one or more of the pockets, causing inflammation and fever.

Figure 12-1
Diverticulitis occurs when the muscles in the wall of the colon thicken, causing increased pressure in the colon and leading to the development of diverticula.

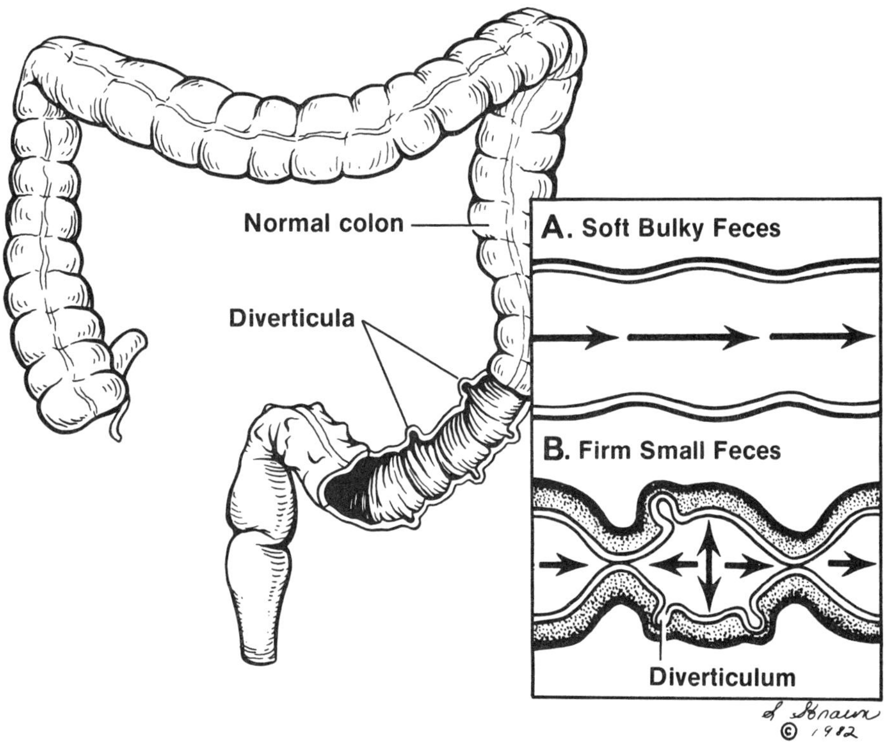

Self-Care Treatment

Eat a bland diet consisting of apples, peaches, bananas, pears, oranges, seedless grapes, seedless raisins, prunes, carrots, lettuce, turnips, bran cereals, whole wheat breads, and miller's bran. Avoid eating fruits or prepared foods that contain small, hard seeds that may become lodged in the diverticula. Avoid eating nuts, popcorn, corn, raw celery, tomatoes, cucumbers, grapes, figs, strawberries, raspberries, or other fruits with seeds or any breads that contain seeds—including poppy, sesame, or caraway seeds.

When to Call the Doctor

You should be under a doctor's general care if you have diverticulitis, since the doctor can prescribe medication to combat infection, relieve pain, and regulate your bowel function.

Call your doctor immediately if you are unable to move your bowels for a period of two days or if you develop an unexplained fever.

ABDOMINAL PAIN

Disease of almost any origin in the abdomen can produce abdominal pain.

Signs and Symptoms

Pain in the upper part of the abdomen is often due to gastritis or simple indigestion; cramping in the lower part of the abdomen can be due to viral infections and diarrhea. Lower abdominal pain on the right side may be due to appendicitis, muscular strain, or a stone in the right kidney. Pain at the midline or across the entire lower abdomen can be due to bowel obstruction. Upper abdominal pain is usually due to conditions of the esophagus, stomach, upper small intestine, pancreas, or bile ducts. Lower abdominal pain is usually due to the female organs, rectum, gallbladder, kidneys, spleen, liver, or colon.

Pain from hollow organs is usually intermittent.

Self-Care Treatment

Don't take aspirin or other painkillers. Avoid solid food, and sip clear liquids. Try to have a bowel movement, pass wind from the rectum, or belch. Soak in a warm tub, go to bed, and apply heat to the painful area.

When to Call the Doctor

Call your doctor immediately if you have sharp pain when you release a gentle compression of the abdominal wall, if the pain was caused by injury, if the pain remains the same or gets worse over several hours, if the pain is severe, or if the pain is accompanied by fever, vomiting, rectal bleeding, or diarrhea.

Abdominal Pain in Children

The causes of abdominal pain in children change with the age of the child. Common ones include colic, constipation, vomiting, stomach flu, viral infections, obstruction of the intestines, bacterial infection, sore

If Your Child Has Abdominal Pain, Call the Doctor . . .

1. When abdominal pain is present and not followed by diarrhea or vomiting soon thereafter.
2. When there is persistent abdominal pain after an injury.
3. When abdominal pain is associated with urinary symptoms (painful urination, frequent urination, or bloody or pink urine).
4. When there is pain associated with a rash from the waist down.
5. When severe constant abdominal pain lasts several hours.
6. When any abdominal pain persists beyond 2 days.
7. When worms are passed.
8. When there is persistent fever higher than 103 degrees.
9. When there is any uncertainty about any of the above.

throat, ear infections, excessive coughing, pneumonia, hepatitis, urinary tract infection, or appendicitis. Appendicitis is the least common cause of abdominal pain in children.

Give the child nothing by mouth but ginger ale; let him or her soak in a warm tub bath. Give the child small amounts of clear fluid, and don't give aspirin.

Call your doctor immediately if the child is under four years of age and has no symptoms of infection, has urinary difficulty, was injured, has severe pain in the abdomen, has black or bloody stools, vomits without having a bowel movement, vomits with intermittent pain, has pain in only one part of the abdomen, or has yellowing skin, sore throat, rapid breathing, swollen glands, rash, or joint pain. Call a poison control center if you think that your child might have ingested poison.

PINWORMS

A distant relative of the earthworm, the pinworm lives only in humans and higher apes; the adult pinworm is white, about as thick as a sewing thread, and measures about one-quarter of an inch long. Moving with a caterpillarlike motion, the pinworm lives in the large intestine, comes out at night to lay microscopic eggs around the skin of the anus, and crawls back into the intestine. The eggs are transmitted to the mouth by the hands, toys, or food, are swallowed, and hatch in the intestines — and the process begins all over again.

Signs and Symptoms

A child who has pinworms will complain of itching or burning around the anal and genital area, especially at night. You can see pinworms around the anus if you turn on a light suddenly and search quickly; sometimes a pinworm may be mistaken for a piece of lint. Occasionally, you can see pinworms in the bowel movements.

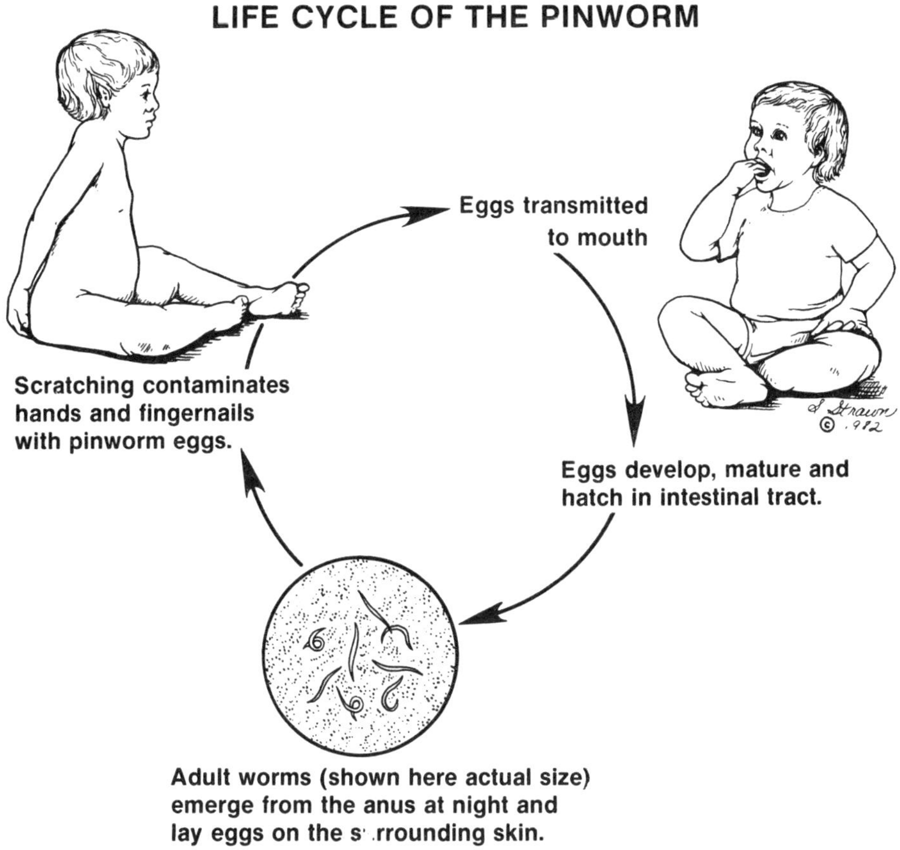

Figure 12-2

Self-Care Treatment

A child with pinworms must be treated with a vermifuge to kill the worms, and the medication is available only by prescription. Your doctor may recommend that all members of the household be treated at the same time to prevent the spread of infestation.

Cut and scrub the child's fingernails to remove eggs; launder the clothing, bedding, and towels frequently to destroy the worms. You need to exercise great caution to prevent other family members from picking up the worms.

HEMORRHOIDS

The most common of all digestive disorders, hemorrhoids are varicose veins of the anus or rectum. There is a familial tendency to develop hemorrhoids; they can result from the constant straining that accompanies chronic constipation, pregnancy, rectal disease, and diarrhea. They can also result from pressure on the veins due to liver or heart disease. Hard, impacted fecal matter can tear the hemorrhoids and cause them to bleed.

Signs and Symptoms

Hemorrhoids are the most common cause of rectal bleeding; the blood is bright red and is streaked only on the outside of the bowel movement and on the toilet paper. Hemorrhoid blood is never mixed in the feces. Other symptoms include rectal irritation, itching, burning, mucus leakage from the anus, and pain, although some hemorrhoids do not cause pain.

Hemorrhoids are subject to irritation by constipation, diarrhea, or vigorous wiping.

Over-The-Counter Hemorrhoid Medicines

You can get hemorrhoid medicine in three forms.

Ointments. Ointments are the most effective, because they allow for direct application of active ingredients to the sites of external itch, inflammation, and pain. You should use an ointment if the cause of your discomfort is from external, not internal, hemorrhoids. *Never* insert the ointment applicator into your rectum in an attempt to soothe internal hemorrhoid symptoms.

Suppositories. These are best if you are suffering from internal hemorrhoids; inserted into the anus, they coat the rectal wall with medication. Suppositories are ineffective in treating pain and itch of external hemorrhoids, because the medication from a suppository never comes into contact with the external hemorrhoid.

Aerosols. Designed to treat external hemorrhoids, aerosols are generally ineffective because the delivery of active ingredients to the site is usually erratic. The only advantage of aerosols is that they keep fastidious persons from having to touch themselves.

Self-Care Treatment

Self-treatment is dangerous; you should have a physician check all cases of hemorrhoids. For temporary pain relief, apply cold compresses to the anus if bleeding does not stop spontaneously; take sitz baths of water and baking soda or water and vinegar solutions. Apply analgesic ointments to the hemorrhoid if you have your doctor's approval.

Keep your rectal area clean; when you can, shower instead of using toilet paper following a bowel movement. After gently drying the rectal area, apply a zinc oxide solution on the hemorrhoids.

Avoid straining by taking measures to avoid constipation; keep your stools soft by eating fresh fruits, bran, and whole wheat bread and by drinking prune juice. Drink plenty of fluids, and get some exercise every day.

Contact your doctor if your hemorrhoid bleeds for a period longer than one week.

Hemorrhoids in Children

Give a child a diet to soften the stools. Good foods include fruits, vegetables, prune juice, bran, and whole wheat bread. Make sure that the child drinks plenty of fluids. Call your doctor if there is blood in the stool of a newborn, if a child complains of itching or pain that is most intense at night, if hemorrhoids seem to be a problem for longer than five days, or if the blood is **in** the stool instead of just streaked on the outside or on the toilet paper.

HERNIA (Rupture)

A hernia is the protrusion of a portion of the abdominal contents, usually a section of intestine, into a weak place in the wall of the abdomen. Rupture can be in any area of the abdominal wall, but it is most frequent in the groin area and is most often the result of severe muscular strain from lifting, pushing, or jumping. Strenuous activities increase the pressure within the abdomen and force out a section of the abdominal contents through an existing weak spot in some cases.

Signs and Symptoms

A sharp pain is felt at the moment of protrusion, accompanied by a feeling of something "giving way" at the site of the hernia. Nausea or vomiting may occur. Herniation may occur with little or no pain or discomfort, and swelling at the site may be the first indication. The swelling is tender to touch and may range in size from a marble to a fist.

Self-Care Treatment

1. Never push a hernia back into place with the fingers. This can cause internal damage.
2. Keep the victim quiet and still. Have him or her avoid sudden movements or lifting, even of moderate weights.
3. Most hernias are reduceable. Have the victim lie flat on the back with the knees drawn up over the chest for several minutes. In this position, the section of the abdominal contents is likely to return to the abdomen and reduce the hernia. If this is unsuccessful, have the victim turn over on the abdomen (unless it is a navel hernia) and bring the knees up under the chest so that the buttocks are raised.
4. If the hernia is reduced, improvise a truss out of a block of wood, metal, or any similar material that is about an inch thick. Cover the block with a thick layer of cotton, and place it directly over the protruding part. Apply a gauze bandage to hold it firmly in place. When a rupture cannot be reduced, protruding intestines may become compressed by adhesions or swelling to such a degree that the blood supply is shut off. In these cases, the symptoms are similar to those of bowel obstruction.

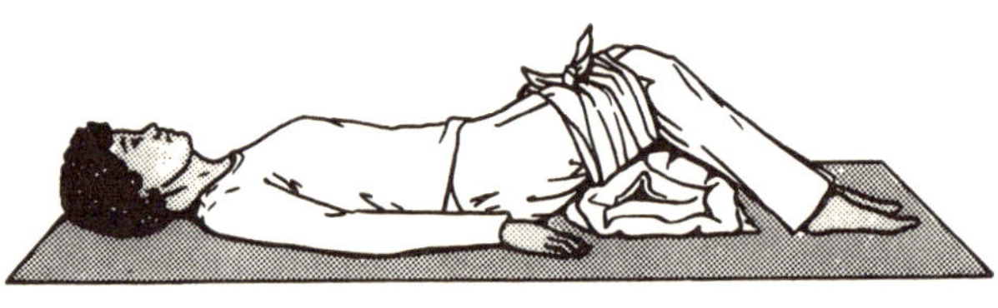

Figure 12-3
Treatment for a rupture or hernia.

5. Whether the hernia is reduced or not, apply cold compresses at the site.
6. Give soft foods and ample fluids.
7. Give aspirin for pain.
8. Do not give laxatives or cathartics unless prescribed by a physician.
9. Contact a physician as soon as possible.

APPENDICITIS

Appendicitis is an inflammation of the appendix, which is a small hollow "thumb" hanging off the colon in the lower right side of the abdomen. Appendicitis is a serious disease, usually requiring surgery to prevent rupture, spillage of contents into the sterile abdominal cavity, and resulting peritonitis.

Signs and Symptoms

When the appendix becomes blocked or plugged (usually by a small piece of fecal matter) and cannot drain properly, the muscles of the appendix cramp to try to unblock the opening. Resulting symptoms include pain, first under the belly button and then moving to the lower right side of the abdomen; nausea, vomiting, or loss of appetite; local tenderness in the lower right quarter of the abdomen; and fever of 100° F. to 102° F. — in that order. It isn't likely to be appendicitis if there is no fever, if a high fever is present, or if a fever appears before pain.

Additional symptoms include diarrhea, firm muscles in the abdomen that remain rigid, and pain during walking. If the problem is not appendicitis, pain will disappear within six to eight hours; the pain from appendicitis grows worse.

Self-Care Treatment

Notify a physician immediately. While you are waiting for the doctor, keep the victim in bed with the head and shoulders elevated; keep an icebag over the lower right quarter of the abdomen. If you can't get ice, use cold water compresses.

Don't give the victim anything by mouth, and never give laxatives or apply heat to the abdomen — both speed rupture of the appendix. If the patient cannot see the doctor for some time, give small amounts of clear fluids every half hour to maintain fluid balance.

PREMENSTRUAL TENSION

While the cause is not understood, some women experience premenstrual tension that begins a week to ten days before the menstrual period and ends a few hours after the menstrual flow begins.

Signs and Symptoms

Signs of premenstrual tension include mild to severe headaches, irritability, nervousness, emotional changes, pain in the breasts, general body puffiness, and a tendency to retain water.

Self-Care Treatment

If there are no debilitating symptoms, you are best to ignore premenstrual tension; if you experience headache or pain in the breasts or abdomen, take aspirin.

If you tend to retain water prior to your menstrual flow, exclude salt from your diet for three days prior to your menstrual flow.

When to Call the Doctor

Call your doctor immediately if premenstrual tension is accompanied by vaginal bleeding between menstrual periods.

VAGINAL DISCHARGE

While a certain amount of discharge from the vagina is common and normal, increased or abnormal discharge is generally due to fungus or bacterial infections of the vagina, generally lowered resistance, lack of sleep, poor diet, and insufficient liquid intake.

Signs and Symptoms

Vaginal discharge associated with bacterial or fungal infection can result in thin, foamy discharge that is yellowish-green or gray in color, or a cottage cheese-like discharge that has a strong, offensive odor. Both discharges result in severe itching at the vaginal opening and irritation to the tissue of the genital region.

Common Sexually Transmitted Diseases in the United States

Disease	Pathogen	Incubation Period	Symptoms	Possible Complications	Treatment	Immunity
Genital Herpes	Virus: Herpesviris (Herpes type II)	2 to 10 days after sexual contact	Blister-like sores usually on and inside the genital organs that reoccur often with genital pain and fever; can occur on body at virus contact points	Cannot be cured; can cause miscarriage, death to infected newborns, brain damage to newborns, and increased cervical cancer	No effective cure at present; symptomatic treatment only	None No vaccine
Gonorrhea	Bacterium: Neisseria gonorrhea (gonococcus)	2 to 9 days after sexual contact	Pus discharge from penis and vagina; painful urination in males (women often show no symptoms)	Pelvic inflammation in women; infection causes plugging of fallopian tubes in women and vas deferens in males resulting in sterility; Newborns develop eye infections	Penicillin, tetracycline, ampicillin (injections required)	None No vaccine
N.G.U. (non-gonococcal urethritis)	Bacterium: Chlamydia trachomatis	5 to 21 days after sexual contact	Men often have painful urination with pus discharge from penis. Women seldom exhibit outward symptoms	Males: Epididymitis and prostatitis resulting in infertility; Females: inflammation of the cervix and fallopian tubes resulting in infertility; Newborns: eye infections	Erythromycin, tetracycline (injections required)	None No vaccine
Syphilis	Bacterium: Treponema pallidum	10 to 90 days after sexual contact	Primary stage: chancre sores on or inside the genital organs or on body at infection contact. Secondary stage: body rash, fever, tiredness, loss of hair, mouth lesions	Organ disease and death; Unborns: congenital defects, brain damage, miscarriage	Penicillin, erythromycin, cephaloridine, tetracycline (injections required)	None No vaccine

Self-Care Treatment

Contact your doctor to get medication that will effectively treat bacterial and fungal infections. While you are on medication, refrain from sexual intercourse until your medication has been used and you are symptom-free. Don't stop using the medication when your symptoms clear up—keep using it until it is gone.

Wear cotton underwear, and avoid wearing pantyhose, tight nylon or synthetic body suits, or tight pants that discourage air circulation and absorption of perspiration. Clean the bathtub out carefully after bathing so that you won't spread the infection to others.

If your doctor approves, vinegar douches can help relieve itching. Don't scratch or rub the area, because the genital tissues can get irritated and can fall prey to a secondary infection.

Since oral antibiotics often cause yeast infection due to a disruption of the normal balance of yeast and bacteria in the vagina, eat one cup of yogurt three times a day while you are taking an antibiotic.

When to Call the Doctor

Call your doctor if you are still having vaginal discharge after you have finished using the medication or if you experience bleeding between your menstrual periods.

Vaginal Discharge in Children

A mucous discharge from the vagina is normal during the first two weeks of a girl's life and during the one to two years preceding the onset of menstruation. Vaginal discharge at that time can be quite thick, but it has no odor and is not irritating to the skin.

Abnormal vaginal discharge in children is usually due to insertion of a foreign body (such as a pebble or marble) into the vagina, use of irritating chemicals in the bath (often found in children's bubble baths), wearing panties made from synthetic materials, improper wiping of fecal material following a bowel movement (pushing fecal matter into the vagina), having pinworms or a urinary tract infection, lack of cleanliness, or masturbating. Occasionally, a child will get a bacterial or fungal infection, although these are not commonly the cause of vaginal discharge in children.

Vaginal discharge that is puslike, irritating, foul-smelling, or bloody is abnormal. Instruct your child to wipe herself from front to back after using the toilet, and inspect her for signs of pinworms. Avoid using bubble baths, and don't let her use feminine hygiene deodorant sprays. Avoid letting her wear synthetic underwear; she should use cotton. To soothe irritation, have the child sit in a tub of warm water to which a cup of vinegar has been added; apply a soothing jelly (such as *Vaseline, A and D,* or *Desitin*) to the genital and vaginal area following the bath.

Your child should see a doctor if you took DES (diethylstilbesterol) while you were pregnant with her; she should also see a doctor if you cannot control or stop the vaginal discharge with home treatment.

MENSTRUAL CRAMPS

Dysmenorrhea—menstrual cramping—affects half of the female population under the age of twenty-five and occurs just before and during the menstrual period. Dysmenorrhea is caused by congestion of the pelvic tissues, by inflammation of the pelvic tissues, or by obstruction of the menstrual flow. This can be due to infection, long-standing anxiety, sex pressures, a sedentary life-style, constipation, or general lack of exercise, but in many cases the cause is unknown. Menstrual cramps are no longer a problem after a woman gives birth once, possibly due to dilation of the cervix and stretching of the uterine muscles.

Cramps that are continuous but that worsen during the menstrual period may be due to infection of the cervix, gonorrhea, or other diseases that should be treated by a physician.

Signs and Symptoms

Signs and symptoms include mild to severe pain in the lower abdomen with headache, irritability, mental depression, malaise, fatigue, mild nausea, or occasional vomiting. Bowel function is normal, and there is usually no fever. Pain sometimes runs down the legs and thighs and can result in a low backache. The victim may be pale and sweating; the menstrual flow may be either copious or scant. Cramps last about twelve hours from onset to resolution.

Table 10-1
PROBLEMS ASSOCIATED WITH MENSTRUATION

Problem	Symptoms	Cause	What to Do
Toxic Shock	Vomiting, diarrhea, fever, rash on palms and soles of feet.	Extended retention of tampons; prevents normal removal of staphylococcal toxin by menstrual flow.	1. Avoid highly absorbent tampons. 2. Change every 3-4 hrs. 3. Alternate tampons with sanitary pads. 4. Remove tampons and see a physician if symptoms appear.
Premenstrual Syndrome	Most common in middle-aged adults. Breast tenderness, bloated feeling, headache, tension, irritability, fatigue and depression. Flaring of other chronic problems.	Salt and fluid accumulation in all body tissues.	1. Decrease salt & fluid intake. 2. Mild analgesics aspirin. 3. If symptoms remain, see your doctor.
Dysmenorrhea	Cramping in lower abdomen during menstruation occassionally with nausea and vomiting, headache, pain in back and thighs.	*Simple* — poor posture, sedentary life style, fatigue. *Complex* — hormonal, cysts, tumors, pelvic inflammatory disease.	Usually treated with analgesics, heat to the abdomen, rest and exercise. Hormones, drugs or surgery if cause is more complex.
Endometriosis	Pelvic pain 2-7 days before menstruation until cessation of flow, abnormal uterine bleeding, painful intercourse and/or defecation, sterility.	Retrograde menstruation through fallopian tubes into abdominal cavity. Endometrial tissue outside of uterus.	Become pregnant if condition has just begun; hormone therapy, and/or surgery.

Self-Care Treatment

Get adequate rest, and avoid constipation. Exercise daily, and pay special attention to stretching the abdominal muscles. Avoid situations that bring on nervous tension. Take aspirin for pain, and apply hot compresses to the abdomen; remove restrictive clothing. A hot water bottle usually works well. Avoid getting fatigued.

When to Call the Doctor

If pain is repeatedly more severe with each menstrual period and if you are debilitated and unable to control the pain, call your doctor.

MENOPAUSE

Menopause, the cessation of menstruation and the discontinuation of secretions of certain hormones that regulate menstruation, after the woman has menstruated for about thirty-five years, usually occurs at about the age of forty-five to fifty. Although menopause may not actually take place until the age of fifty, the woman may start feeling symptoms as early as thirty-five years of age—or ten to fifteen years before the menstrual flow actually stops.

Signs and Symptoms

The most characteristic sign of menopause is cessation of menstruation. Menstruation may stop abruptly (no more periods after the end of a regular period), gradually (the periods slowly diminish in amount of flow and length of flow until they stop completely), or irregularly (by far the most common, marked by irregular menstrual cycles and flows until the periods stop).

Other symptoms of menopause include hot flashes, loss of skin elasticity, dry skin, dry hair, hair loss, constipation, backache, pain in the joints and bones, headaches, bloating, general body swelling, muscle aches, and depression.

Self-Care Treatment

Because symptoms of the menopause may continue for several years or more, treatment becomes a basic way of life and is aimed at making the adjustment comfortable. You will need to add moisturizers to your hair and skin, take measures to avoid constipation, lose excess weight to avoid bloating, and take measures to relieve low back pain, headache, and joint pain.

One of the most baffling symptoms of menopause is the hot flash. When you feel a hot flash coming on, don't panic—sit down in a quiet place and make yourself comfortable while you wait for the hot flash to pass. If you can take off your shoes, go ahead; loosen any tight clothing (especially belts and collars), and take elastic bands and hairpins out of your hair. Take a few deep breaths, and exhale slowly. Most hot flashes last only a few seconds; few last longer than a minute.

When to Call the Doctor

If any of the symptoms of menopause become debilitating and

interfere with your daily activities, you should get medical help. A few women require extensive medical help for deep depression that can accompany menopause.

URINARY TRACT INFECTION

Urinary tract infections result from bacterial invasion of the urinary bladder tract; they are generally caused from improper wiping (forcing fecal matter into the urethra), kidney stones, an undeveloped kidney, or a bladder hernia.

Urinary tract infections are not contagious, even through sexual intercourse. Sexual intercourse may, however, force bacteria into the urethra and speed the appearance of urinary tract infection symptoms.

Common Reproductive Tract Infections

Problem	Symptoms	Treatment
Vaginitis — Bacterial infection, spread by sexual contact	Yellow or grey-green vaginal discharge, vaginal itching	Antibiotics, medicated douche
Trichomoniasis — protozoan; spread by sexual contact or contaminated objects	Itching; thick greyish-white discharge; foul odor. Painful and frequent urination	Medication, douche. Treatment somewhat difficult; risky during pregnancy
Manilia Candida — Yeast infection	Itching and redness of Labia. "Cottage cheese" discharge	Antibiotic vaginal cream, vinegar douching (1 Tbsp./quart of water) may prevent reinfection
Pubic Lice (crabs) Sexual or other close contact	Mild to intense itching	Shampoo, cream, or lotion, called *Kwell,* applied after thorough cleansing
Venereal Warts Virus	Warts on the genitals	Various medications, surgical removal, freezing cauterization

Signs and Symptoms

Signs and symptoms of urinary tract infections include a burning sensation during urination, a need to urinate often coupled with scanty urination, cloudy urine (due to pus), bloody urine, low back pain (due to infection in the kidneys), fever, and chills. Some people lack well-defined symptoms but feel tired and weak.

Self-Care Treatment

It is essential that all urinary tract infections be treated with antibiotics, so you should see your doctor immediately if you devlop any of the above symptoms. To aid in your recovery, try the following:

1. Avoid drinking alcohol, tea, coffee, or carbonated beverages.
2. Drink lots of water or fruit juice — at least eight glasses a day — to flush out your entire urinary system. Cranberry juice inhibits the growth of bacteria and is an excellent choice.
3. Empty your bladder completely whenever you urinate.
4. Don't hold your urine for prolonged periods; if you can, urinate every time you feel the urge.
5. Avoid fatigue.

When to Call the Doctor

If you follow the above-listed home treatment tips and take the antibiotic prescribed by your doctor, your infection should clear up rapidly; call your doctor if your symptoms have not eased up considerably within five days.

Preventing Urinary Infection

To prevent urinary tract infection, wash your genitals throroughly every time you bathe — preferably every day. Wipe toward the rear after having a bowel movement to avoid pushing fecal matter into the urethra. If you frequently get urinary tract infections following intercourse, try to urinate within one hour of intercourse, and cleanse the area around the urethra with warm, soapy water.

CHAPTER 13

HEART AND CIRCULATORY COMPLAINTS

FAINTING

Fainting is a sudden loss of consciousness due to an insufficient supply of blood to the brain. Fear, hunger, an unpleasant sight, bad news, standing too long, pain, the sight of blood, the taking of a blood sample, exhaustion, weakness, heat, lack of air, or any emotional or physical shock can trigger fainting. Fainting becomes more frequent with increasing age.

Signs and Symptoms

A person may collapse suddenly without any obvious warning, but the usual signs and symptoms include weakness, dizziness, extreme paleness, sweating, coldness of the skin, black spots appearing before the eyes, forehead covered with perspiration, numbness and tingling of the hands and feet, nausea, disturbance in vision, shallow breathing, and a feeling of lightheadedness with yawning. The pulse may be rapid and weak.

Self-Care Treatment

If the person is about to faint, have him or her lie down with the legs somewhat elevated, or lower the head between the knees for about five minutes.

If the person has lost consciousness, keep him or her lying down with the feet and legs slightly elevated. Cover the individual to maintain body heat, but do not overheat. Loosen any tight clothing. Keep the victim lying down for a reasonable period of time after consciousness returns.

If the victim vomits, turn him or her on the side so that the vomitus can escape from the mouth. Wipe out the victim's mouth with your fingers wrapped in a cloth. Bathe the face with cool water, but do not pour water over the face.

Do not give the victim any liquids until he or she is revived. Examine the victim to see if he or she has suffered from any falling injury.

Prolonged loss of consciousness indicates that the condition is more serious than simple fainting. Consult a physician if the victim does not revive quickly.

Fainting in Children

Children usually faint because they are holding their breath—a common ploy to attract attention. If a child feels faint, have him or her sit with the head between the knees. If that position is not possible or comfortable, have the child lie down flat on the back; elevate the legs. Open a window to provide some fresh air, and avoid sudden changes of position. Keep the child down for five to ten minutes, or until feelings of faintness pass.

Call a doctor if the child has a fever, loses consciousness, experiences nausea and/or vomiting, senses tingling in the fingers, gets blue dicoloration of the skin and lips, or if the fainting spells begin to interfere with school and other daily activities.

HIGH BLOOD PRESSURE

About twenty to twenty-five million people—5 to 6 percent of the total population—in America suffer from high blood pressure, now recognized as the most serious common problem in the nation. While some cases of high blood pressure are caused by kidney disease, adrenal tumors, or certain other hormonal disorders, about 85 percent of all cases originate from unknown causes.

Signs and Symptoms

High blood pressure has been called the "silent killer"—it can exist for years without manifesting any signs or symptoms at all. When symptoms do occur, they usually include headache, weakness, insomnia, dizziness, nervousness, and fatigue.

Self-Care Treatment

1. Stop smoking. Spasms of the blood vessels that result from tobacco contribute to high blood pressure.
2. Avoid drinking coffee, tea, and cola drinks—including diet colas—because all of them contain caffeine, which acts to stimulate the circulatory system and increase blood pressure.
3. Lose weight. Even twenty extra pounds can create a hazard for the circulatory system.
4. Avoid stress and tension as much as possible.
5. Maintain your physical fitness. Regular daily exercise—such as walking, running, biking, hiking, or swimming—has been shown to reduce blood pressure.
6. Rest and relax when you can. Avoid the temptation to pack your weekends full of activity and chores that can't be done during the week—use the time to relax.
7. Avoid high-fat and salty foods—both increase blood pressure.
8. Take any medication that your doctor prescribes.

When to Call the Doctor

Call the doctor immediately if you notice unexplained numbness in your face, arms, or legs; if you experience change in vision, including blind spots or loss of vision; if you either gain or lose weight without explanation; if you experience a rapid heartbeat or if you skip a heartbeat; or if you react in an unusual way to your medication (experiencing weakness, sleepiness, dizziness, depression, blurred vision, constipation, fatigue, or other symptoms). Anyone with high blood pressure should be under the care of a doctor.

HEART ATTACK

The heart is a muscle supplied with arteries. When an artery becomes blocked, because of a blood clot or narrowing of the coronary arteries, the part of the muscle that it serves dies rapidly and the individual has what is known as a heart attack. A heart attack is called a coronary thrombosis, coronary occlusion, myocardial infarction, or simply a coronary.

After a heart attack, the rest of the heart usually continues to pump. But if too much muscle is lost, the heart is unable to pump enough blood, and shock and death result.

Heart attack risk may be increased appreciably if a person is obese, smokes cigarettes, has high blood pressure, is inactive, has a diet high in cholesterol, and is under undue stress.

Signs and Symptoms

Signs and symptoms vary greatly depending upon the basic cause. But typical signs of a heart attack are weak, rapid, irregular pulse, appearance of severe illness, crushing chest pain that moves from the left arm to the neck to the left side of the chest or that remains in the upper abdomen or back of the chest, apprehension, acute fear, anxiety, perspiration, fainting,

Figure 13-1
Causes of heart pain and heart attack.

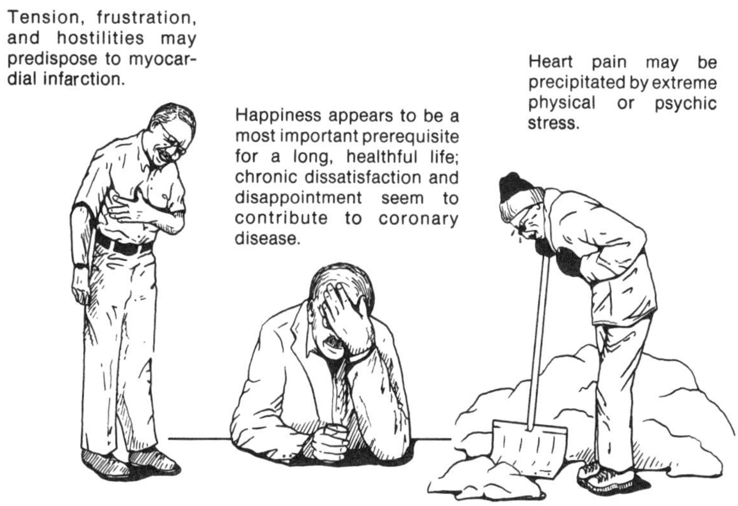

Figure 13-2

EARLY SIGNALS OF A HEART ATTACK

PAIN, in one form or another, almost always accompanies a heart attack. Ranges from a mild ache to one of unbearable severity. When severe, pain is often felt as constricting, like vise on chest. Pain also often includes the burning and bloated sensations that usually accompany indigestion. Pain may be continuous and then might subside — but don't ignore if it does. Could be in any one or combination of locations shown below.

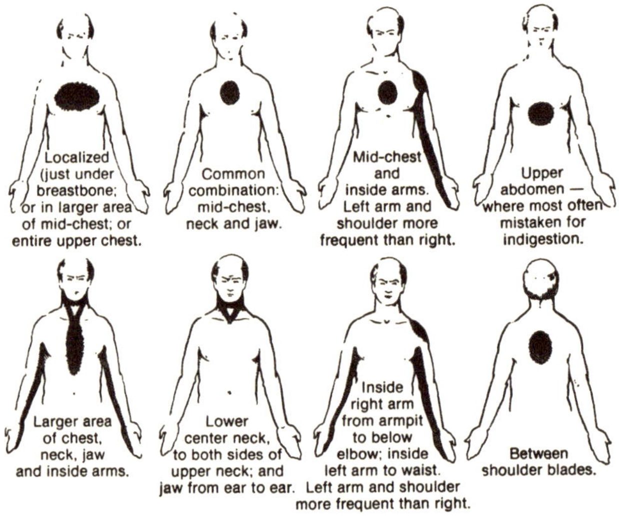

Courtesy Metropolitan Life Insurance Company ©

Figure 13-3

Checklist of Other Heart Attack Early Signals

None of the symptoms below is conclusive proof of a heart attack. But the more of them present, the more likely it is that the patient *is* undergoing a heart attack.

DIFFICULTY BREATHING	COLD SWEAT
PALPITATIONS	PALENESS
NAUSEA	WEAKNESS
VOMITING	ANXIETY

How to Help a Possible Heart Attack Victim.

You can best help — possibly save a life — if you know in advance: 1) The nearest hospital equipped to handle heart attack emergencies. 2) How to do Cardiopulmonary Resuscitation (CPR).* 3) How quickly to call a doctor, the hospital and/or an ambulance. 4) The fastest route to the hospital. Knowing these things, you should:

1 Help victim to least painful position — usually sitting with legs up and bent at knees. Loosen clothing around neck and midriff. Be calm, reassuring.

2 Quickly call ambulance to get victim to hospital via local rescue squad, police, fire or other available service. Once the ambulance is on the way, notify family physician, if you have one.

3 If ambulance is coming, comfort victim while waiting. Otherwise, help victim to car, trying to keep victim's exertion to minimum. If possible, take another CPR-trained person with you. Victim should sit up.

4 Drive cautiously to hospital. Watch victim closely (or have other passenger do so). If he or she loses consciousness, check for breathing, and feel for neck pulse under side angle of lower jaw to check for circulation. If no pulse, start CPR. Continue CPR until trained help arrives to take over.

5 If victim retains consciousness to hospital, make sure he or she is carried, not walked, to emergency room.

*Get in touch with local Heart Association or Red Cross.

Courtesy Metropolitan Life Insurance Company ©

shortness of breath and other breathing difficulty, nausea, vomiting, and possible unconsciousness.

The pain accompanying heart attack builds in intensity over the first few minutes and lasts from a half hour to several hours. It is described as a pressure or squeezing sensation and not intermittent or pulsating. The pain is not relieved by changes in body position nor affected appreciably by breathing. Pain is not always present in a heart attack.

Figure 13-4
Risk factors in coronary heart disease.

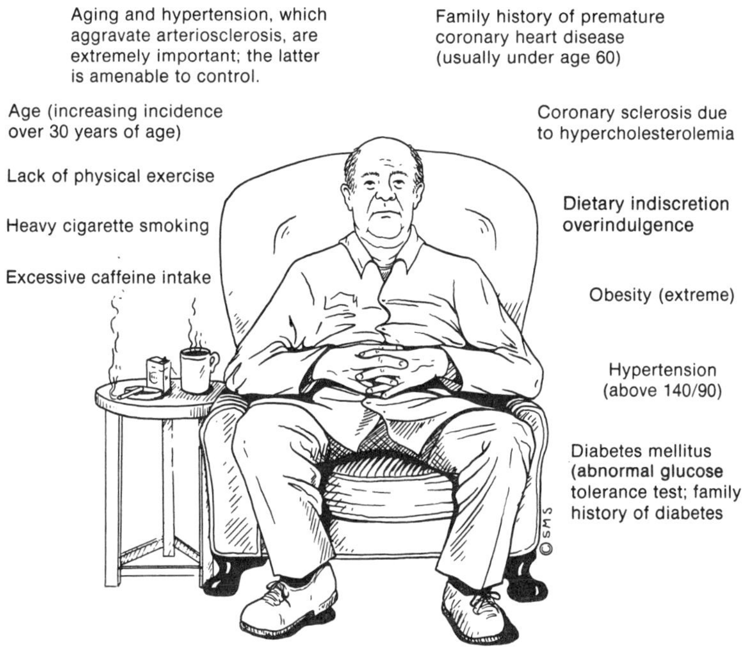

Self-Care Treatment

1. Place the victim in sitting position, and keep him or her quiet. If the victim does not have breathing difficulty, keep him or her lying down. Do not let the victim move about. Loosen any clothing.
2. Keep the victim warm, but do not overheat.
3. Administer oxygen if available. Oxygen may help some of the damaged heart muscle to survive.

4. Comfort and reassure the individual. Anxiety is likely to be intense and may worsen the victim's condition.
5. If the person carries medicine prescribed for such attacks and is conscious, help the victim take it.
6. Get medical help at once.
7. If the victim is not breathing, begin artificial respiration. If necessary, give cardiopulmonary resuscitation.

ANGINA (Chest Pain)

Angina means chest pain that is usually due to a narrowing of an artery in the heart. It occurs when the blood flow to the heart is temporarily inadequate to meet its oxygen needs. It is usually brought on by stress or unusual effort. The decreased blood flow causes a periodic, recurring pain similar to the pain of a heart attack. Angina is a warning that the heart is under undue stress and needs relief before permanent damage occurs.

Signs and Symptoms

The major symptom of angina is a sharp pain in the chest that appears during exertion and is relieved by rest and relaxation. The pain is felt first beneath the breastbone in the center of the chest. It radiates in some patients to the throat, jaw, teeth, and left or right arm. In some persons the pain is not sharp, but rather is a burning feeling (similar to heartburn) or a dull ache, and is often described as a pressured or squeezing sensation. Others describe only an "uncomfortable" feeling. The most common complaint is a sharp pain that radiates to the left side of the chest and down the left arm.

Self-Care Treatment

1. Patients are usually aware of their condition and have been given medication (nitroglycerine) by their doctor to relieve the pain. Help the person to take any prescribed medication.
2. Care for this patient the same way that you would care for a person having a heart attack.

3. The pain is usually relieved by rest and lasts three to eight minutes and rarely longer than ten minutes. Even though angina is painful, it does not lead to death. However, it *is* a warning sign that a person who has angina is more **prone** to **develop** a heart attack.

IRREGULARITIES IN HEART RATE

Irregularity in heart rate may appear without apparent cause, although smoking, coffee, alcohol, digestive disturbances, overeating, and anxiety may bring it on. Skipped beats, palpitation, fluttering, and premature beats (extrasystoles) are common and usually are no more significant than the discomfort or anxiety that they may cause when they appear. Irregularity is a momentary skip, followed by an extra strong beat, and can be detected in a pulse at the wrist. Everyone who knows that he or she has any irregularity of the heart deserves a cardiac evaluation by a physician.

Signs and Symptoms

Symptoms include a feeling that something is "turning over" in the chest, fluttering sensations, dizziness, feeling of faintness, or actual fainting.

Self-Care Treatment

1. Make the victim comfortable and reassure him or her. The condition should subside without much further treatment.
2. Have the victim drink cold water.
3. Have the victim hold his or her breath and bend forward.
4. Keep the victim quiet to lessen the load on the heart.

STROKE

Stroke, also called apoplexy and cerebrovascular accident, results

Figure 13-5

WHAT YOU SHOULD KNOW
ABOUT HEART ATTACK AND STROKE

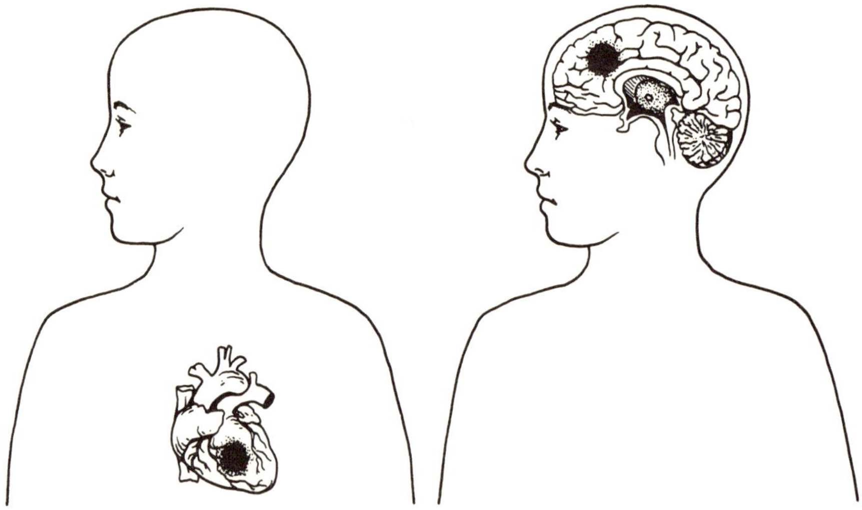

Heart Attack: An estimated 3,990,000 have coronary heart disease. More than 684,000 die of heart attack each year — 350,000 before they reach the hospital. Many thousands of these might have been saved if the victims had heeded the warning signs.
Stroke: An estimated 1,700,000 persons are afflicted by stroke. More than 214,000 suffer fatal strokes annually. Many fatal strokes could be prevented if hypertension (high blood pressure), a leading cause of stroke, is diagnosed and controlled.
The warning signs of heart attack: Prolonged, oppressive pain or unusual discomfort in *center* of chest; Pain may radiate to shoulder, arm, neck, or jaw; Sweating may accompany pain or discomfort; Nausea, vomiting, and shortness of breath may also occur.
The warning signs of stroke: Sudden, temporary weakness or numbness of face, arm, or leg; Temporary loss of speech or trouble in speaking or understanding speech; Temporary dimness or loss of vision, particularly in one eye; An episode of double vision; Unexplained dizziness or unsteadiness; Change in personality, mental ability, or the pattern of headaches.
Act immediately. Sometimes these symptoms subside, then return. When you experience one or more warning signs, call your doctor and describe these symptoms in detail. If he's not immediately available, get to a hospital emergency room at once. Be prepared to act. Instruct others to act if you cannot. Keep a list of numbers — doctor, hospital, ambulance or other emergency services, and police — next to your telephone, and in a prominent place in your pocket, wallet, or purse. Adapted from American Heart Association.

from brain damage due to a blood clot, a tumor, a blow to the head, or rupture of an artery in the brain. Actually, a stroke is just like a heart attack—except that it happens in the brain. Extensive damage causes death. The most common causes of stroke are arteriosclerosis (hardening of the arteries) or hypertension (high blood pressure). A stroke associated with total or partial paralysis on one side of the body is caused by bleeding into the brain from a damaged blood vessel, or by the blockage of the vessel—either by a clot inside the vessel (thrombosis) or by a traveling clot in the bloodstream (embolus). Stroke is most common in persons over forty years of age, and usually has a sudden onset.

Signs and Symptoms

Signs and symptoms include unconsciousness, paralysis or weakness on one side of the body, mouth drawn to one side, face usually flushed (but may be pale), slow but strong pulse, pupils unequal in size, numbness leading to difficulty in speaking and swallowing, diminished consciousness, convulsions, and sometimes loss of bladder and bowel control. Headaches are common before and after a stroke. They most often occur in the back of the head or at the base of the skull.

Self-Care Treatment

1. Handle the victim carefully. Be particularly careful with paralyzed parts. Keep the victim lying on the back, head and shoulders slightly raised.
2. When breathing is difficult, turn the victim's face to one side so that secretions may drain from the mouth.
3. Remove any loose dental bridges or false teeth.
4. Keep the victim warm, but do not overheat.
5. Do not move the victim unless it is absolutely necessary.
6. Do not use stimulants (smelling salts, etc.).
7. Keep the victim absolutely quiet. Remember, the victim may appear unconscious but may be able to hear what is being said. Be careful what you say in front of such a person.
8. Give nothing by mouth, as the throat may be paralyzed.
9. Get medical help at once.

VARICOSE VEINS

Varicose veins are abnormally dilated veins that occur most often in the legs and that most often affect women. They are sometimes caused by lack of exercise, prolonged sitting without movement, or sitting with the legs crossed. When blood accumulates in the bottom of the legs and pressure prevents its effective circulation, the valves of the veins no longer work properly, and the veins become varicose.

Varicose veins are also common in pregnancy.

Signs and Symptoms

Varicose veins appear as prominent, bluish, enlarged, twisted, lumpy veins or darkened, tortuous, raised blood vessels. Soreness, leg fatigue, occasional swelling, occasional discoloration, muscular cramps, and a feeling of heaviness in the legs accompany varicose veins. The pain is intensified by prolonged standing and is worse during hot weather or in high altitudes.

Self-Care Treatment

Essential to the effective treatment of varicose veins is weight loss that brings the weight to within a normal range. Bathe the legs in warm water to help stimulate the blood flow, and take rest periods several times during the day to elevate the legs. Change your daily routine to provide more exercise and movement for your legs. Wear stockings lightly reinforced with elastic, or an elastic bandage, to provide support. Avoid long periods of standing or sitting; wear loose clothing that does not restrict blood flow to the legs. If swelling of the leg or foot develops, rest in bed with the leg elevated.

When to Call the Doctor

If varicose veins get more serious, or if they become so painful that they interfere with daily activities, you should see a doctor.

CHAPTER 14

COMMON INFANT AND CHILDHOOD COMPLAINTS

As a parent, much of your medical treatment program will center around the telephone—how you use it to signal for help, to receive instructions, and to reaffirm that you are completing treatment. Wise use of the telephone can help you gain the most from your child's doctor and can make the telephone one of your most important treatment tools.

CALLING THE DOCTOR

Should You Call the Doctor?

Deciding whether or not to call the child's doctor can be a difficult decision; use your good judgment, refer to the information contained here, and call the doctor in most cases if your child appears to be really sick. Most doctors would rather that you call in the morning than at night—there is more help in the office, the drugstores are open, and the child can be observed during the day. If there is a real emergency, of course, you can call the doctor at night at home, but don't call at night with routine questions ("When should I get Brett's polio shots?") or mild symptoms ("Oh, I don't know, he's kind of stuffy"). Usually, a call can wait until the next morning; in only the most severe emergencies does a doctor need to be summoned at night. The doctor will be more pleasant and more willing to help if you call during the day and if you have prepared before you call.

Before You Call the Doctor

Make sure that you're ready and that you have done your homework so that you don't waste the doctor's time or your own. Have a piece of paper and a pencil by the telephone so that you are ready to jot down the doctor's instructions. On another piece of paper, have your pertinent information ready: the name and phone number of the local pharmacy where you would want a prescription phoned, a list of symptoms that you wanted to discuss with the doctor (in precise terms—not "burning up" or "feverish," but "a rectal temperature of 105° F."), a list of questions that you wanted to ask the doctor in relation to the child's illness, and a summary of the problem (the main reason why you are calling, why you are calling at this particular time, when the illness started, and how sick **you** think the child is).

How to Describe Signs/Symptoms

Pay attention to colors (is the nasal discharge white or is it yellow?), to textures (is the sputum thin and watery, or is it thick and sticky?), to sounds (is a cough barky or rattling?), and to distinct appearances (learn to describe a rash so that the doctor can visualize it: like red sandpaper across the abdomen, like little raised blisters all over the body).

Be prepared to give the doctor the child's temperature—it's critical to diagnosis—and specify whether it is oral or rectal.

DIAPER RASH

Rashes in an infant's diaper area can be caused by the chemicals used in washing the diapers (including soap, bleach, water softener, or whitener), the chemicals used in manufacturing disposable diapers, or a number of other factors. An infant's skin is sensitive and particularly prone to develop rash if irritation and wetness are both present in the interaction between urine and skin. Continuously wearing wet diapers, plastic pants, or disposable diapers (which have a plastic cover) promote wetness and lead to aggravation of diaper rash.

Signs and Symptoms

The appearance of diaper rash depends on what caused it and on the factors present. Diaper rash caused by ammonia in the urine is usually worse after the child has been asleep for a while. You can smell the odor of ammonia when changing the child's diaper. During the first weeks of life and after the child has been on antibiotics, he or she may develop a yeast rash, characterized by countless red, scaly spots, each several pinheads in size, that run together into a solid red rash that represents a colony of yeast. There are often lesions in the mouth when the child has a yeast rash.

If the diaper rash is a result of food or drug allergy, the child's cheeks usually have a rash at the same time. An infectious rash is similar to impetigo and is identified by blisters about the size of a matchhead that contain pus. Seborrhea, caused by overactive secretions of the oil glands, can appear in the diaper area at the same time that it appears on other areas of the body (and is usually a companion to cradle cap). The rash from a number of contagious diseases—such as measles, chicken pox, and scarlet fever—usually shows up in the diaper area one to two days before it shows up on the rest of the body.

Self-Care Treatment

1. Change the brand of soap that you use to wash your baby's diapers, and change your method of washing; make sure that the wash water is hot enough to kill bacteria that breed in the diapers.
2. Apply a soothing cream that will offer protection against the wetness; zinc oxide (such as *Desitin*), petroleum jelly, and others work well. Make sure to completely cover the diaper area, even if the rash is not that extensive.
3. Avoid airtight outer clothing over diapers. Some children will do better if they do not wear plastic pants to bed.
4. If the rash is an infectious one, wash the area completely with soap and warm water after every diaper change, and apply antibiotic cream (such as *Neosporin* or *Bacitracin*) frequently.
5. If the rash seems to be from an allergic reaction, stop all foods that were introduced within one month of the time the rash appeared. After the rash clears up, reintroduce the foods one at a time until you determine which one was causing the rash. List all the medications that the baby started taking within one week of the rash's appearance, and consult your doctor for advice.

When to Call the Doctor

Call your doctor if the diaper rash spreads and worsens instead of getting better; call whenever there are blisters, fever, or loss of appetite. If any other symptoms accompany diaper rash than the simple skin irritation common with the rash, you should consult your doctor.

CRADLE CAP

When a baby's system reacts to hormones that it receives from the mother, the oil glands become excessively productive and result in a condition similar to adult dandruff: cradle cap.

Signs and Symptoms

There may be a thick, adherent, oily, yellowish, crusty patch (or patches) on the scalp accompanied by oiliness and scaling of the scalp. There may be white flakes that resemble dandruff on the scalp, on the eyebrows, behind the ears, and in the diaper area. Some redness appears with cradle cap and may spread to the diaper area.

Self-Care Treatment

If the cradle cap is thick, use a scrub brush to remove it. Rub warm baby oil into the baby's scalp, cover the scalp with a warm towel, and let it soak for fifteen minutes. Remove the scales and flakes with a scrub brush and a fine-tooth comb. Wash the baby's hair and scalp with a shampoo that contains selenium sulfide; follow the package directions carefully, and make sure that you don't get any soap in the baby's eyes. Discontinue treatment if irritation and redness result.

When to Call the Doctor

Some redness is normal, but you should call your doctor if there is very much redness with cradle cap.

COLIC

A problem for 10 to 20 percent of all American babies, colic is any cramplike, intermittent abdominal pain; its causes are many, and it is extremely common during the first three months of life.

Signs and Symptoms

A baby who is suffering from colic will cry excessively, sometimes for hours at a time; he or she will often scream, clench the fists, pull the legs up, and turn red. The baby may stop crying briefly to take a bottle or nurse but will begin crying again within a few minutes. Rocking and cuddling usually stop the crying for only a few minutes; the baby is normal in other respects, with normal bowel movements and no more spitting up than usual.

A slight variation is the baby who wakes up frequently (usually about every two hours), screams fretfully, takes one to two ounces of milk, and falls back into a fitful sleep; the baby continues waking up throughout the night. Colic is usually worst in the late afternoon and the evening and may reach a peak during the middle of the night.

Self-Care Treatment

Check for obvious sources of discomfort other than colic that could be making the baby cry. Check for loose diaper pins, a trapped arm or leg, whether the baby is too hot or too cold, severe diaper rash, diarrhea or constipation, or signs of illness (including sores on the body, vomiting, cough, fever, and nasal discharge).

Your baby may simply be hungry—offer a bottle or nurse the baby; if the baby eats and falls to sleep peacefully, he or she was hungry, not colicky. If you can cuddle and rock your baby and he or she remains content, the baby was simply lonely or frightened.

Once you have ruled out other causes or conditions, assume that the baby has colic. If you are nursing, take care of your nipples; check to make sure that they aren't bleeding, because swallowed blood causes cramps for the baby. Keep the baby sitting partially upright in an infant carrier between feedings so that he or she won't swallow regurgitated food.

Apply gentle heat to the abdomen. If the colic continues, induce a bowel movement by inserting a glycerin suppository, small soap stick, or lubricated thermometer into the baby's rectum.

If you are bottle feeding, make sure that you prepare the formula properly; make sure that the nipple holes are large enough to prevent straining during feeding, and keep the nipple full of formula during the feeding to cut down on the amount of air the baby swallows. If the nipple hole is big enough and the baby is not swallowing air, he or she should get enough formula within twenty minutes.

Following any feeding, burp the baby until you can get a good burp. Try burping in several different positions if you don't get success at first; if gentle patting between the shoulder blades does not yield success, try lying the baby across your knees on his or her stomach and gently but rhythmically stroking the baby from the buttocks to the nape of the neck.

When to Call the Doctor

If the baby's colic continues for a period of more than two days, and if you are unable to calm and quiet the baby, call your doctor.

CROUP

A common, contagious illness among children, croup is an acute obstruction of the airway that is caused by allergy, a foreign body, or infection. Croup is highly contagious and is spread by droplets in the air.

There are two general kinds of croup. Spasmodic croup is due to virus infection and is similar to laryngitis. Epiglottitis is a bacterial infection that is severe, rapidly progressing, and life-threatening.

The croup occurs most frequently in infants and children and is most common during the winter months. It usually follows a mild common cold, and the onset is sudden. The membranes of the larynx, trachea, and lungs become severely inflamed and swollen, producing a heavy, sticky, choking mucus.

Signs and Symptoms

Spasmodic croup is characterized by an absent or low-grade fever (up to 101° F. orally) and by hoarseness—a spasmodic cough that sounds like the child is barking, and a croaking sound when the child inhales.

Epiglottitis is characterized by sudden and rising fever (usually 103° to 105° F. orally), difficulty in breathing, difficulty in swallowing, choking, convulsions, and a swollen bright red epiglottis. The child usually prefers to sit with the head forward, chin jutting out, and the mouth open.

Self-Care Treatment

Spasmodic croup usually responds to home treatment that consists of keeping the air warm and moist (use a vaporizer or humidifier, or sit the child in a bathroom with the door closed and run a hot shower), keeping the air cool and moist if the child is running a low-grade fever, keeping the child dry and comfortable, preventing chilling, remaining calm and relaxed when dealing with the child, reassuring the child that he or she will be all right, and giving the child lozenges or hard candy to suck on.

When to Call the Doctor

Epiglottitis does not respond to home treatment and can be fatal if not treated. Call your doctor immediately if your child develops the symptoms of epiglottitis; also call the doctor if the croup gets worse instead of getting better and if it persists for more than one week. If the child is an infant, call the doctor immediately.

BEDWETTING

Many children can't remain dry through the night until they reach the age of four or five; about 10 percent of all children over the age of five continue to wet the bed. Even children who do not usually wet the bed can do so if they are overtired or ill.

True bedwetting (enuresis) can be due to a physical disease or abnormality, infection of the urinary tract, diabetes, or a neurological disorder. Heredity, emotional upset (especially centered around toilet training), taking children out of night diapers too soon, and severe family problems (especially divorce) can cause or aggravate bedwetting. The cause of many cases of bedwetting is unknown.

Self-Care Treatment

Before you attempt to treat the child at home, he or she should be seen by a doctor to rule out the possibility of infection or physical deformity and abnormality (a cause in only about 10 percent of all cases). If there is no physical reason for the bedwetting, try some of these suggestions:

1. Don't take the child out of night diapers until he or she stays dry throughout the night consistently. Don't make a fuss out of the fact that the child has to wear diapers to bed, and don't act as if you resent the child for it or that there is anything wrong. Act as if the night diaper is a regular, routine part of life.
2. Don't make a big fuss out of toilet training. A child who is ready to be trained will generally cooperate. If you try to force the child before he or she is ready or if you make a major production out of it—offering the child candy every time he or she avoids having an accident, for example—you will contribute to the tendency to bedwet.
3. Don't try to shame the child out of wetting the bed or reward him or her if he doesn't—these tactics rarely work. Don't punish the child for wetting the bed. Avoid forms of punishment that the child may interpret as being related to the bedwetting—not allowing him or her to drink in the afternoon or evening, for instance.
4. If the child wakes up with a wet bed, allow him or her to stay in the room with you while you change the sheets and find dry bedclothes. Behave in a relaxed, calm manner; talk to the child in a soothing tone of voice about other things—what he or she did the day before, plans for the morning, what he or she is making at school, and other things. Don't confront the issue of the bedwetting. Don't act angrily. Gather up the soiled bedding and nightclothes in a calm way, and carry them quietly from the room. If it is the middle of the night, return to the room and spend some time with the child—singing to the child, telling a story, holding the child, or just sitting by the bedside until he or she falls asleep.
5. Never allow siblings to tease or taunt a bedwetter about the problem.
6. Use rubber sheets, draw sheets, and soakers to protect your mattress until the bedwetting stops.

COMMON COMMUNICABLE (Infectious) DISEASES

Due to a number of myths—that childhood diseases have been wiped out in this country, that immunization isn't necessary until a child reaches school age, that vaccinations are only required for children, or that a single vaccination will offer lifetime protection—there has been an alarming decline in the number of children who are immunized against polio, measles, rubella, pertussis, and diphtheria. National surveys indicate that over one-third of the one- to four-year-old children in America are unprotected. Epidemics are still possible, because all but smallpox are still thriving in this country. Those children who are unprotected get ill and carry and spread the disease to others who are unprotected.

See Tables 14-1 and 14-2 for more detailed information regarding some of the major childhood diseases.

Figure 14-1
Sites on the body where rashes appear in chicken pox, measles, rubella, and scarlet fever.

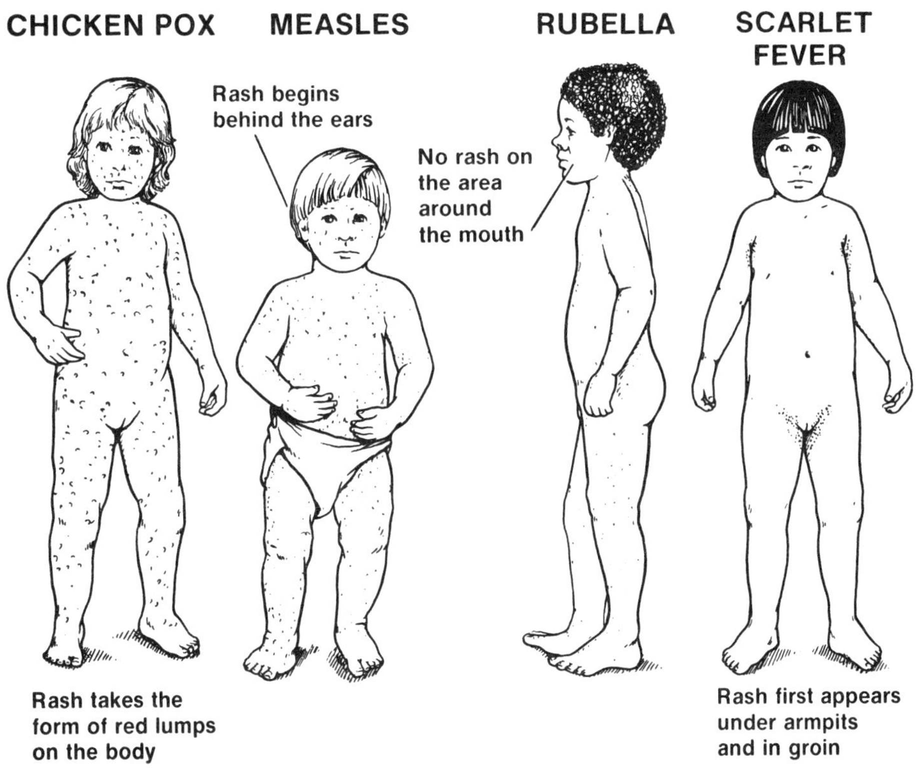

Table 14-1

Every Child Needs Protection Against These Seven Serious Childhood Diseases

<table>
<tr><th>Disease</th><th>Dangers</th><th>Prevention</th></tr>
<tr><td>Polio</td><td>Polio often cripples and sometimes kills. Little can be done if a child gets polio. Early protection is necessary.</td><td>Polio can be prevented. The vaccine must be given in a series of 4 doses.
Start when a child is 2 months old.</td></tr>
<tr><td>Diphtheria</td><td>Diphtheria can make a child choke so badly that all breathing stops. Sometimes it causes heart failure or pneumonia.</td><td rowspan="3">These three diseases can all be prevented by one 3-in-1 vaccine known as DPT. DPT is given in a series of 5 shots.
Start when a child is 2 months old.</td></tr>
<tr><td>Whooping Cough</td><td>Whooping cough can cause convulsions and brain damage. It is very dangerous for very young children.</td></tr>
<tr><td>Tetanus</td><td>Tetanus (lockjaw) is very painful and can kill. It may develop when something sharp like a nail pokes through the skin.</td></tr>
<tr><td>Measles</td><td>Measles can cause pneumonia, blindness, deafness, and brain damage.</td><td rowspan="3">These three diseases can all be prevented by just one dose of a 3-in-1 vaccine.
Get this shot at 15 months.</td></tr>
<tr><td>German Measles</td><td>German measles is dangerous because it can have serious effects on a pregnant woman who may catch it from a child. It can cause a miscarriage or lead to birth defects in the baby.</td></tr>
<tr><td>Mumps</td><td>Mumps can cause deafness, diabetes, and brain damage. It can make boys sterile.</td></tr>
</table>

THE DANGER IS GREATEST DURING THE PRESCHOOL YEARS.
START IMMUNIZATIONS EARLY — BE SURE YOUR CHILD GETS THEM ALL.
KEEP A RECORD FOR EACH CHILD.

Table 14-2

Table of Childhood Diseases

DISEASE	INCUBATION PERIOD	COMMON SYMPTOMS	ISOLATION PERIOD OF INFECTED CHILD	ISOLATION PERIOD OF EXPOSED CHILD	PREVENTIVE MEASURES
CHICKEN POX	14 to 21 days.	Mild fever, upset stomach, headache, blisterlike rash that appears suddenly. Blisters become crusted in 1 to 3 days.	Isolate for 6 days after rash first appears.	None.	None. One attack usually gives immunity.
DIPHTHERIA	1 to 10 days (average, 2 to 6 days).	Severe sore throat, fever, yellowish-gray patches on tonsils, throat, or palate. Breathing may become difficult.	Isolate until doctor has taken 3 consecutive bacteria-free cultures, one every 24 hours.	Quarantine 7 days and until 2 consecutive bacteria-free cultures have been taken, with a 24-hour timespan between them.	Shots of diphtheria toxoid (usually begun as part of 3-in-1, DPT shots in infancy). One attack usually gives immunity.
GERMAN MEASLES (Rubella)	About 14 21 days (average, 17 days).	Sore throat and headache. Rash on face and head, spreading to neck and trunk. Slight fever during rash. Rash lasts 2 or 3 days. Glands at back of head and neck and behind ears become enlarged.	Isolate from first symptoms to 5 days after rash.	None.	Vaccination. One attack usually gives immunity.

(Continued)

Table 14-2 (continued)

Table of Childhood Diseases

DISEASE	INCUBATION PERIOD	COMMON SYMPTOMS	ISOLATION PERIOD OF INFECTED CHILD	ISOLATION PERIOD OF EXPOSED CHILD	PREVENTIVE MEASURES
MEASLES (Rubeola)	Fever, 10 days after exposure. Rash, 14 days after exposure.	Resembles cold. Fever, runny nose, watery eyes, cough, White spots on inside of cheeks. Rash begins on forehead, spreads downward.	Isolate from first symptoms to 5 days after rash.	Quarantine 7 to 14 days under some conditions, but quarantine of no value during epidemic.	Vaccination of all susceptible children. Gamma globulin in special cases for temporary immunity. One attack usually gives immunity.
MUMPS (Infectious parotitis)	About 14 to 21 days (average, 18 days).	Swelling and pain in one or more salivary glands. Difficulty in swallowing.	Isolate until swelling subsides, 7 to 10 days.	None.	Mumps vaccine. One attack involving one or both sides usually gives immunity.
POLIO-MYELITIS (Infantile Paralysis)	7 to 21 days (usually 10 to 12 days).	Fever, sore throat, dull pain on bending neck, headache, muscle spasms, stiff back. Symptoms may begin suddenly or gradually.	Isolate for 7 days from onset, or for duration of fever.	None usually, except to avoid exertion.	Oral polio vaccine should be given beginning in infancy.
SCARLET FEVER	2 to 5 days.	Begins very suddenly with headache, chills, fever, sore throat, vomiting. Neck glands enlarged and tender. Tongue coated and pitted-looking at first, then becomes red and rough. Rash appears about 3 days after first symptom.	Isolate about 7 days, or longer if doctor advises.	None. But should have throat culture.	None. One attack usually gives immunity.

(Continued)

Table 14-2 (continued)

Table of Childhood Diseases

DISEASE	INCUBATION PERIOD	COMMON SYMPTOMS	ISOLATION PERIOD OF INFECTED CHILD	ISOLATION PERIOD OF EXPOSED CHILD	PREVENTIVE MEASURES
WHOOPING COUGH (Pertussis)	5 to 21 days (average, 10 days).	Increased nose and throat secretions. Spells of coughing, which are worse at night. Slight fever. Whooping develops in 2 weeks. Coughing spasm may end vomiting.	Isolate for 4 weeks from onset, or 3 weeks after coughing begins.	Quarantine for 14 days after exposure.	Shots (begun as part of 3-in-1, DPT shots). Early immunization important.
UPPER RESPIRATORY INFECTION (URI)	3 to 9 days.	Fever, chills, headache, general aching, upset stomach, cough, runny nose.	Until symptoms subside (usually 2 to 5 days).	None.	Keep away from large crowds and known infective individuals.
ROSEOLA INFECTION	10 days (usually 7 to 18 days).	Usually in children under 4 yrs. of age and commonly 1-yr.-old. Sudden intermittent fever for 3 to 5 days followed by generalized rash.	Until symptoms subside (2 to 5 days).	None.	None.

Source: American Baby, April 1980, p. 32, as prepared by Children's Memorial Hospital, Oklahoma City, OK.

CHAPTER 15

EMOTIONAL SELF-CARE

Life is filled with crises; no one can escape them, because they are part of being alive. As a result, each of us suffers a kind of stress that accompanies each crisis. We each inherit and develop abilities that enable us to deal with crisis and stress; the difference between healthy and unhealthy people is the ability to **manage** that stress. Continued physical health seems to depend on the ability to deal with—not simply evade—stress. You can take an active part in managing the stress and crises in your life; you can change your ability to adjust and cope.

In psychosocial terms, a crisis is a state of temporary disequilibrium brought on by unavoidable life changes. Crises are considered to be temporary, because in a healthy individual, the personality systems and defenses correct a crisis-induced imbalance within a few weeks or months. The steady, usual pattern of the individual's life is disrupted only until the body defenses have a chance to compensate.

The causes of some crises may be easy to identify, but in other cases the causes are underlying and elusive. A state of crisis may begin in anticipation before the event actually takes place—a college senior, for example, may anticipate his or her father's death from cancer and may enter a crisis state before the father dies. A crisis may also be precipitated by an event that seems mild but that reminds the individual of a past crisis. One seven-year-old girl did not cry at all when her mother died, but when her kitten was killed, she experienced the grief all over again and this time was able to cry and release her feelings.

Most of the life changes that bring crisis involve relationships with other people. If a crisis is to occur, the situation must be a "no exit" one; the situation must be one that cannot be changed or escaped. Once such a change occurs, the individual's mental and emotional health will determine the person's ability to cope.

Certain characteristics enable an individual to better cope with a crisis situation. The capacity to orient quickly to change is helpful, as is the ability to plan and make decisions in the face of change. An individual who can call on others for help and who can recognize his or her own need for help is better equipped to deal with crisis than an individual who becomes paralyzed or disoriented and does not recognize the need for a helping hand.

The result of an inability to cope with crisis and the change that it brings is often physical and/or emotional illness.

WHAT HAPPENS DURING CRISIS?

Four major phases describe what happens to an individual who faces crisis.

1. **Impact.** When the crisis first hits, the impact brings on a state of dazed shock that lasts for several hours. Because most crises involve a loss—loss of a job, loss of status, loss of a loved one—the impact phase consists of the individual's searching for the lost object and reminiscing about the lost object.
2. **Recoil/Turmoil.** Within several hours, the individual enters the recoil/turmoil phase, a period marked by depression, rage, anxiety, and guilt. The individual becomes detached and confused. This stage of ambiguity and uncertainty generally lasts for several days while the individual relives the past and tries to sort out the events of the crisis.
3. **Adjustment.** The adjustment phase begins as the individual explores alternatives to replace the loss. A man who was fired begins making positive plans for finding a new job. A couple whose freedom and sense of privacy were lost when their new baby was born searches for new ways of experiencing those lost senses while they enjoy their new baby. A college student who does not make the football team after a brilliant high school career begins to assess other activities in which he can excel at college. During the adjustment phase, the individual's thoughts are centered on the future, and he or she generally approaches the task with an attitude of hope and aggressive problem-solving.
4. **Reconstruction.** In this final phase, the individual tests alternatives

and reattaches himself or herself over a period of several months. A woman who was laid off and who then made positive plans for finding another corporate-level position now moves forward with new determination, making appointments with prospective employers and brushing up her resumé; once hired, she makes new attachments that will replace the ones at her previous job. Again, the individual's thoughts and efforts concentrate on the future, and her attitude is one of hope.

STRESS

Once the body is under stress, it reacts—physically as well as emotionally—to try to normalize things again. In other words, stress demands that the body adjust. That kind of wear and tear takes its toll: as many as 80 percent of all people who go to the doctor do so because of stress-related illnesses. Some doctors believe that all illnesses are at least partially caused by stress.

The trouble comes when the stress becomes long-term: there is no clear resolution of the crisis, no real return to equilibrium as one stressful situation follows another with no respite in between. In this kind of long-term stress, the body never returns to normal between periods of stress. Unrelieved, long-term stress cannot be tolerated, and it generally results in mental or physical illness.

What Causes Stress?

Each of us experiences stress as a result of different stimuli in our environment. Because of our individual biological heritage and our unique emotional and intellectual background, each of us reacts differently to the same situation.

The word **stress** is too often darkly colored with negative connotation —we almost always think of stress as a result of bad events in our lives, such as death, divorce, illness, bad luck, or the loss of a job. But it is important to realize that stress also comes from the positive, happy experiences in our lives—the birth of a new baby, marriage, a promotion at work, or being recognized for an outstanding achievement. Negative stress

(distress) produces a decrease in health and performance; positive stress **(eustress)** usually produces just the opposite. The problem is this: your mind can distinguish between the two, but your body cannot. Your body reacts the same whether the stress comes from a positive or negative event. In some cases, you develop anticipatory stress just thinking about an upcoming event; most of the time, the stress that you get from anticipating the event is worse than the stress that you would suffer from the actual event.

What Stress Does to the Body

Whenever you are threatened, your body gets ready to protect itself. As part of your general adaptation, you experience rapid pulse, increased perspiration, a pounding heart, a tightened stomach, tensing of the muscles in the arms and legs, shortness of breath, gritting of the teeth, clenching of the jaw, racing thoughts, and an inability to sit still.

When the stress becomes chronic—lasting for weeks, or months, or even years—the body systems literally break down. You lose your appetite, feel nauseated, and experience heartburn; you cannot seem to cry (or, on the other hand, you burst into tears for no obvious reason). You experience high blood pressure, frequent headaches, chronic diarrhea, and dizziness, to name only a few physical symptoms. Mentally, you feel anxious, irritable, frustrated, depressed, and, in the extreme, self-destructive.

Who Is Most Prone to Stress?

Researchers have stretched the human race along an axis from the poles of two general personality types: Type A and Type B. Many of us exhibit a combination of traits along the continuum between each personality extremity; studying the extremes, however, teaches us about stress and about the ways in which we can learn to cope with it.

Type A Personality

The Type A individual copes poorly with stress and is most likely to develop a stress-related illness. But there is an additional, more serious problem: a type A individual actually **creates** stress by the way in which he or she lives and through behavioral patterns.

The individual with a Type A personality exhibits the following traits:

- Is extremely competitive; likes to win
- Is schedule- and time-oriented
- Tries to cram too much work into too little time
- Is extremely concerned with success and social acceptance
- Is numbers-oriented (counts successes, possessions, achievements)
- Is a rapid talker
- Is not content with working on one project at a time
- Sets several goals at once (often unrealistic)
- Is punctual and is intolerant of those who are not
- Appears outwardly confident but is inwardly insecure
- Is impatient, hates to wait
- Has a tendency to tackle several activities at once (dictates into a tape recorder while driving, eats lunch while working at desk)
- Feels guilty while relaxing or slowing down
- Dominates or interrupts conversations
- Has nervous gestures or tics
- Is easily upset by others
- Is hostile and aggressive toward those whom he or she perceives as "competition"

These natural go-getters, with their overabundance of ambition, suffer. They pace themselves, rising quickly through the ranks, experiencing real success early in their careers. But then comes the tragedy: the Type A personality burns up from a high degree of involvement. This person literally crashes and flames out.

Why?

Because the mind and body simply cannot keep up with the pace; the stress that the individual has suffered has literally "torn up" the body. The person is exhausted and depressed; he or she loses interest in activities outside of work, but enjoyment on the job disappears, too. The individual tries harder but even then cannot achieve what he or she did before.

Soon the physical problems set in. The Type A personality often develops headaches, muscle spasms, lethargy, increase in appetite, sluggishness, fatigue, and an inability to relax. Because they tend to hurry to finish jobs more quickly, Type A individuals have also been isolated as those more likely to develop heart disease.

Type B Personality

The Type B personality is opposite the Type A personality: he or she copes better with stress, partly because the person does not create stress for himself or herself. Type B personalities have the following characteristics:

- Easygoing
- Seldom impatient
- Able to make decisions easily, without undue influence from others
- Realistic about what can be achieved
- Realistic about time schedules
- Does not worry much, especially about the future
- Much less critical of himself and others
- Not concerned with petty irritations
- Accepts the fact that everything cannot be achieved at once

The Type B person is not necessarily lazy or lacking in force—he or she simply moves ahead through a relaxed, patient, and methodical application of technique, while the Type A person moves ahead through sheer drive and energy. While the Type A person pushes frantically forward, working harder and harder and jamming in more assignments while giving up leisure time, the Type B person patiently plods toward achieving goals.

Neither personality type has a corner on intelligence or ambition. Each category includes company presidents, truck drivers, carpenters, fashion models, attorneys, beauticians, and college students. Some doctors believe that Type B individuals make the better executives: they do not rush decisions, make snap judgments, or antagonize subordinates. In short, they know their capabilities and limitations; Type A individuals often do not know their own limitations—and do not want to.

Because of the overload of stress that they take upon themselves, Type A individuals are much more prone to develop a stress-related disease, such as high blood pressure, heart disease, or diabetes.

COPING WITH STRESS AND CRISIS

Here are some simple steps that you can take when confronted with stress or a crisis.

1. **Decide what is causing the problem.** Look toward, not away from, your problems and feelings—you cannot begin to work out a solution until you identify a cause. This seems like a frightening step to take, but you will find that knowledge often kills fear. Once you find out more about what is causing your feelings, you can get a grip on them.

Try keeping a journal; as you write about your problems, you can isolate them and begin to think of how to solve your dilemma. Reviewing journals from the past allows you to relive other times of depression or tension when you mobilized your resources and pulled through. A father who had lost his son in a tragic accident pulled out an earlier journal and reread the entry that he had written after witnessing the boy's birth. The father wept afterward, but he appreciated the joy of his son's companionship for those short years more fully. This appreciation helped to start the healing process.

2. **Learn to relax.** The actual method of relaxation depends on what works best for the individual. Some things that may be very relaxing to one person may actually induce additional stress in another. Assess ways that you can relax during the day; try taking a short nap in the afternoon, taking a fifteen-minute walk during the morning break at work, finding a quiet place to be by yourself during the day, taking a hot bath when you get home from work, massaging your feet, reading a favorite book or magazine, or taking up a hobby (such as carpentry, sewing, quilting, writing, or hiking). The important thing is to regularly spend time doing something that you enjoy and that you do not feel pressure to succeed at. You should learn to take time out of your schedule to simply sit back and take a breather—to forget about the problems that are weighing on you as a result of your job, your family, or some social situation that concerns you.

   Don't choose something that you think will be good for you as a leisure-time activity: choose something that you **like.** Really enjoy yourself.
3. **Learn how to say no to things that you don't want to do.** Too many people feel guilty about saying no, but you are the master of your own self and you have the freedom to choose how you spend your time and energies. Don't get involved in something that you don't really want to do just because you couldn't say no.
4. **Treat those around you with respect.** It's easy to get suspicious and paranoid about people who are causing you stress. Instead of lashing out with hostility, try treating them with courtesy and respect. They'll probably return the favor, and you may find that they don't cause you that much stress after all.
5. **Learn to accept what you cannot change.** Realize that the only person who can change is yourself—you are the only person over whom you have total control. You have no control over most things and never will; you cannot right every injustice, nor can you make people over. You must come to the realization that you cannot change many situations—you can only learn to cope with them and adjust to them.
6. **Share your worries with someone else.** Verbalizing your problems and

BREAKING OUT OF THE TYPE-A RUT

Do you feel so tightly wound up that you're afraid you'll break under the pressure? Colorado State University psychologist Richard M. Suinn contends that you can take steps to eliminate most of your stress by changing your Type-A habits. Here's how:

1. **Learn to relax.** There are as many ways to relax as there are people who need to relax. You can do it almost anywhere — as long as it's quiet, free of interruption, and comfortable. Try listening to some soothing music. Or try deep breathing for ten minutes as you let the tension flow from your body. You might try deep muscle relaxation: alternately tense and then relax the muscles of your arms, legs, chest, stomach, feet, hands, shoulders, and face.

   Once you learn a method that works for you, use it when you feel stressed — retreat to a quiet place for a few minutes, and regain your equilibrium.
2. **Slow down.** You'll feel pressure if you're acting rushed. Make a conscious effort to slow down in every way — walk more slowly, talk at a more relaxed rate, eat more slowly — try putting your fork down between each bite. Be better organized, and allow yourself a few extra minutes to get to class or work. You'll find yourself relaxing when you stop rushing.
3. **Take control of your environment.** You'd be surprised at how much of your stress you create yourself: you set unrealistic goals, you try to please too many people, you schedule your time too tightly, you fail to accomplish what you want to. Allow yourself enough time during the day to get from one activity to another — don't commit to being at a play rehearsal across town ten minutes after your last class is dismissed, for example, or you'll just get upset in the traffic. When you wake up each morning, decide which activities are your priority ones — those things that *have* to be done — and then accomplish them first. Don't move on to other things until you have done what is necessary for the day. And learn how to say "no" — if you don't have time to reasonably accomplish something, don't commit to it. If you do commit, make clear how much you can do by when — in other words, let people know how much they can expect from you. And, perhaps most importantly, schedule some time during the day when you can have a quiet period of relaxation, free from telephone calls and interruptions.
4. **Learn to react differently.** We all face situations that make us tense — and most of us react with some degree of tension. Learn to retrain your reactions — you will need to start with a pencil and paper. Think of a situation that normally makes you tense — perhaps you always get stuck in traffic as you hurry to get to your part-time job downtown. Write down how you normally react; now, reevaluate. What could you do to make the situation better? How could you react differently to avoid getting so uptight? "Practice" this way with a number of situations until you have a definite set of plans for reducing your tension.

fears to someone whom you love, trust, or respect helps to relieve the stress and often helps you to discover alternatives that otherwise might have escaped your eye. A good confidante will listen empathetically and will often ask questions that will help you to explore your feelings honestly.

7. **Get enough exercise.** Exercise has all sorts of benefits: one of the greatest is that it provides a physical release for the pent-up rage and hostility that accompany a crisis. The physical changes that your body undergoes during a crisis are the same ones that it experiences in reaction to danger—and that physical and mental tension can be worked off physically. Choose any kind of exercise that will relieve your boredom, excite your senses, and provide you with fun and relaxation—jogging, tennis, swimming, handball, or walking are good ones to try. You will find that as you concentrate on your exercise, your mind will be diverted from your problems—and you will be refreshed enough later to tackle them with new vigor.
8. **Avoid self-medication.** Reaching for a bottle—whether it is filled with alcohol or pills—does not teach you to cope with a crisis. Your problems are still there when you come out of the stupor, and sometimes they have become worse because you did not act on them immediately. Your crisis may be causing you pain, but do not add the extra pain of dependence on alcohol or drugs.
9. **Serve others.** Do something for someone else, and you will find yourself thinking of them instead of your crisis. Learn to love people and use things, rather than love things and use people.
10. **Avoid loneliness.** You will undoubtedly need some time alone to collect your thoughts, but the difference between aloneness and loneliness is vast. Withdrawing will not solve the crisis.
11. **Try a temporary diversion.** If you have tried everything and are at the end of your rope—try a brief diversion to refresh yourself. Go see a funny movie, read a book that you have always been meaning to get around to, or go to a concert with a friend. You will be refreshed and will find an inner strength to tackle the problem afterward.
12. **Take active management steps.** Once you have identified your problem, create a plan of action for solving it. Try to remember the small details. Keep your options open, and be creative in solving your problems—your solution might not be the one that you originally thought of, but try it anyway.
13. **Assess your priorities.** During a time of confusion like a crisis, it is hard to decide what to do first. But take the few valuable minutes required to list on paper your priorities. Decide what is **the** most important thing that you need to do; write that down first. Order the

rest of your priorities the same way, listing the most important ones first. Then tackle them in that same order—and do not move on down the list to an easier task until you have completed all of the tasks before it.

14. **Have a physical checkup.** A crisis may precipitate a condition mimicking physical illness as a result of sheer stress; if the physical illness lingers, however, see your doctor. A woman who remained ill and depressed after a miscarriage finally consulted her doctor, who discovered that she had diabetes. With treatment, she was able to bounce back from the crisis of the miscarriage much more easily.
15. **Take care of yourself physically.** It is tempting to forget all about your normal health routines in a time of crisis—but good health and nutrition are even more important during times of stress and upset. Get plenty of sleep (consult your doctor if you simply are unable to fall asleep for more than a few nights), and eat well-balanced, nourishing meals.

Relaxation Exercises

There are many breathing exercises that will help you relax. The important thing is to breathe properly and not too hard. Avoid tight clothing and make yourself comfortable.

Exercise #1. Inhale through your nose. Try to take the air all the way down to your stomach. Expand your stomach so that you fill your lungs completely. Exhale slowly through your mouth. Try to completely empty your lungs and stomach. As you exhale, your stomach should contract. Relax, and then repeat.

Exercise #2. Inhale slowly through your nose to the count of 3. Hold your breath to the count of 3. Exhale through your nose to the count of 3. Relax to the count of 3. Repeat this pattern for several minutes. You may find that using a count of 4 or 5 may be best for you.

Exercise #3. After you've done one of the preceding exercises, try this one: lie down, get comfortable, and close your eyes. Think about your body. Imagine that you are transparent and filled to the top of your head with orange drink (or one of your favorite beverages). The liquid represents tension in your body. Imagine the liquid beginning to drain out through your finger tips and your toes. The level will begin to drop, from the top of your head, past your eyes, nose, etc. Feel the tension draining with it. Watch the level of the liquid drop. As it drains out of your body, so does the tension. Let the liquid drain down past your neck, shoulders, torso, thighs, knees, legs, right out the bottom of your toes. Are there any puddles of liquid (tension) left? Imagine you soak them up with a paper towel. Lie there and enjoy the feeling of total relaxation.

Source: American Hospital Association.

CHAPTER 16

SELF-CARE NUTRITION, DIET, AND FITNESS

Learning about nutrition, diet, and fitness makes sense, because together, these three elements can improve your health, expand your capabilities, keep you from developing a host of diseases, and increase your life span.

NUTRITION

Proteins

Protein, the chief tissue builder, is the basic substance of every cell in the body, including muscle, blood, and bone; protein supports growth and maintains healthy body cells. Antibodies that assist the body in resisting infection are protein, as are enzymes.

All protein is made up of smaller units called amino acids; during the process of digestion, proteins are broken down into the most simple amino acids. After absorption into the body, the amino acids are rearranged in the cells to form the many special and distinct proteins in the body. The proteins in food are usually composed of eighteen or more amino acids. The body can manufacture its own supply of more than half of them, but the others — essential amino acids — must be supplied through the intake of food.

The amino acid makeup of a food protein determines its nutritive value. Those proteins that supply all of the essential amino acids in about the same proportions as they are needed by the body are considered highest in value; most are foods of animal origin, and they include eggs, fish, poultry, meat, and milk.

While they do not supply as good an assortment of amino acids as animal proteins do, the proteins from cereal and grains, vegetables, and fruits still supply valuable amounts of many amino acids. Proteins from legumes — especially soybeans and chickpeas — are almost as good as the proteins derived from animal sources.

To improve the percentage of essential amino acids that you receive from your food, you should combine foods that do not provide optimum amino acids with those that do — for instance, have milk with cereal or macaroni with cheese. Foods of vegetable origin can also be combined to improve protein quality. Try combining beans and corn, beans and rice, and wheat bread with peanut butter. If meat is not included in a meal, you should try to eat a variety of vegetable proteins. Beans, peas, soybeans, grains, and nuts are good choices.

Carbohydrates

Foods supply carbohydrates chiefly in three forms — starch, sugar, and cellulose (fibrous material). Cellulose furnishes bulk in the diet, and starches and sugars are the major sources of energy.[1]

Glucose, commonly called blood sugar, is the form in which starches and sugars are used by cells to furnish energy for body processes. The energy cells derived from glucose (carbohydrates) allow protein to be used for building and rebuilding. Carbohydrates also assist the body in utilizing fat and in achieving normal and regular elimination.

Good sources of starches include grains (such as wheat, oats, corn, and rice), products made from grains (such as macaroni, flour, spaghetti, noodles, grits, breads, and breakfast cereals), potatoes, sweet potatoes, and dry beans and peas. Most vegetables contain some starch; most fruits contain some sugar. Cane and beet sugars, jellies, jams, candy and other sweets, honey, molasses, and syrups contain carbohydrates that are highly concentrated sugars.

Fruits, vegetables, and whole-grain cereals provide the most effective bulk for normal functioning and health of the digestive tract; you should eat some fruits and vegetables raw and avoid peeling as many as possible.

Dietary Guidelines

The U.S. Department of Agriculture has given the American public seven dietary guidelines that are based on the assumption that food alone cannot make you healthy, but good eating habits based on moderation and variety can help keep you healthy and even improve your health.

1. Eat a variety of foods. To assure yourself an adequate diet, eat a variety of foods daily, including selections of:
   - Fruits
   - Vegetables
   - Whole grains and enriched breads, cereals, and grain products
   - Milk, cheese, and yogurt
   - Meats, poultry, fish, and eggs
   - Legumes (dry peas and beans)

2. Maintain an ideal weight. To improve your eating habits that may contribute to weight:
   - Eat slowly
   - Prepare smaller portions
   - Avoid "seconds"

   To lose weight:
   - Increase physical activity
   - Eat less fat and fatty foods
   - Eat less sugar and sweets
   - Avoid too much alcohol

3. Avoid too much fat, saturated fat, and cholesterol. To accomplish this:
   - Choose lean meat, fish, poultry, dry beans and peas as your protein source
   - Moderate your use of eggs and organ meats (such as liver)
   - Limit your intake of butter, cream, hydrogenated margarines, shortenings and coconut oils, and foods made from such products
   - Trim excess fat off meats
   - Broil, bake or boil rather than fry
   - Read labels carefully to determine both amounts and types of fat contained in foods

4. Eat foods with adequate starch and fiber. To eat more complex carbohydrates daily:
   - Substitute starches for fats and sugars
   - Select foods which are good sources of fiber and starch, such as whole grain breads and cereals, fruits and vegetables, beans, peas, and nuts

5. Avoid too much sugar. To avoid excessive sugars:
   - Use less of all sugars including white sugar, brown sugar, raw sugar, honey, and syrups
   - Eat less of foods containing these sugars, such as candy, soft drinks, ice cream, cakes, and cookies
   - Select fresh fruits or fruits canned without sugar or light syrup rather than heavy syrup

(Continued)

Dietary Guidelines (Continued)

- Read food labels for clues on sugar content—if the names sucrose, glucose, maltose, dextrose, lactose, fructose, or syrups appear first, then there is a large amount of sugar
- Remember, how often you eat sugar is as important as how much sugar you eat

6. Avoid too much sodium. To accomplish this:
   - Learn to enjoy the unsalted flavors of foods
   - Cook with only small amounts of added salt
   - Add little or no salt to food at the table
   - Limit your intake of salty foods, such as potato chips, pretzels, salted nuts and popcorn, condiments (soy sauce, steak sauce, garlic salt, etc.), cheese, pickled foods, and cured meats
   - Read food labels carefully to determine the amounts of sodium in processed foods and snack items

7. If you drink alcohol, do so in moderation.

Fats

Concentrated sources of energy, fats give more than twice as much energy, weight for weight, as do either carbohydrates or protein. Fats make up part of the structure of every cell, they form a protective cushion around vital internal organs, they supply an essential fatty acid (linoleic acid), and they carry fat-soluble vitamins such as A, D, E, and K. Because the body does not manufacture its own linoleic acid, this substance must be provided by food. The best sources include oils that come from plants —particularly corn, cottonseed, safflower, sesame, soybean, and wheat germ. Many margarines, salad dressings, mayonnaise, and cooking oils are manufactured from plant oils and are referred to as polyunsaturated. Nuts contain less linoleic acid than do most vegetable oils; walnuts rank quite high among the nuts. Poultry and fish oils have more linoleic acid than other animal fats, which rank fairly low as sources of linoleic acid.

Because fats digest slowly, they delay feelings of hunger after a meal; used in cooking, they add flavor and variety to many foods. In planning meals, you should keep the total amount of fat at a moderate level, and you should include some foods that contain polyunsaturated fats.

FOOD AND NUTRITION BOARD, NATIONAL ACADEMY OF SCIENCES-NATIONAL RESEARCH COUNCIL

Recommended Daily Dietary Allowances,[a] Revised 1979

Designed for the maintenance of good nutrition of practically all healthy people in the USA

	Age (years)	Weight (kg)	Weight (lbs)	Height (cm)	Height (in)	Protein (g)	Fat-Soluble Vitamins: Vitamin A (μg R.E.)[b]	Vitamin D (μg)[c]	Vitamin E (mg α T.E.)[d]	Water-Soluble Vitamins: Vitamin C (mg)	Thiamin (mg)	Riboflavin (mg)	Niacin (mg N.E.)[e]	Vitamin B_6 (mg)	Folacin[f] (μg)	Vitamin B_{12} (μg)	Minerals: Calcium (mg)	Phosphorus (mg)	Magnesium (mg)	Iron (mg)	Zinc (mg)	Iodine (μg)
Infants	0.0-0.5	6	13	60	24	kg x 2.2	420	10	3	35	0.3	0.4	6	0.3	30	0.5[g]	360	240	50	10	3	40
	0.5-1.0	9	20	71	28	kg x 2.0	400	10	4	35	0.5	0.6	8	0.6	45	1.5	540	360	70	15	5	50
Children	1-3	13	29	90	35	23	400	10	5	45	0.7	0.8	9	0.9	100	2.0	800	800	150	15	10	70
	4-6	20	44	112	44	30	500	10	6	45	0.9	1.0	11	1.3	200	2.5	800	800	200	10	10	90
	7-10	28	62	132	52	34	700	10	7	45	1.2	1.4	16	1.6	300	3.0	800	800	250	10	10	120
Males	11-14	45	99	157	62	45	1000	10	8	50	1.4	1.6	18	1.8	400	3.0	1200	1200	350	18	15	150
	15-18	66	145	176	69	56	1000	10	10	60	1.4	1.7	18	2.0	400	3.0	1200	1200	400	18	15	150
	19-22	70	154	177	70	56	1000	7.5	10	60	1.5	1.7	19	2.2	400	3.0	800	800	350	10	15	150
	23-50	70	154	178	70	56	1000	5	10	60	1.4	1.6	18	2.2	400	3.0	800	800	350	10	15	150
	51+	70	154	178	70	56	1000	5	10	60	1.2	1.4	16	2.2	400	3.0	800	800	350	10	15	150
Females	11-14	46	101	157	62	46	800	10	8	50	1.1	1.3	15	1.8	400	3.0	1200	1200	300	18	15	150
	15-18	55	120	163	64	46	800	10	8	60	1.1	1.3	14	2.0	400	3.0	1200	1200	300	18	15	150
	19-22	55	120	163	64	44	800	7.5	8	60	1.1	1.3	14	2.0	400	3.0	800	800	300	18	15	150
	23-50	55	120	163	64	44	800	5	8	60	1.0	1.2	13	2.0	400	3.0	800	800	300	18	15	150
	51+	55	120	163	64	44	800	5	8	60	1.0	1.2	13	2.0	400	3.0	800	800	300	10	15	150
Pregnant						+30	+200	+5	+2	+20	+0.4	+0.3	+2	+0.6	+400	+1.0	+400	+400	+150	[h]	+5	+25
Lactating						+20	+400	+5	+3	+40	+0.5	+0.5	+5	+0.5	+100	+1.0	+400	+400	+150	[h]	+10	+50

a The allowances are intended to provide for individual variations among most normal persons as they live in the United States under usual environmental stresses. Diets should be based on a variety of common foods in order to provide other nutrients for which human requirements have been less well defined. See text for detailed discussion of allowances and of nutrients not tabulated.

b Retinol equivalents. 1 Retinol equivalent = 1 μg retinol or 6 μg carotene. See text for calculation of vitamin A activity of diets as retinol equivalents.

c As cholecalciferol. 10 μg cholecalciferol = 400 I.U. vitamin D.

d α tocopherol equivalents. 1 mg d-α-tocopherol = 1 α T.E. See text for variation in allowances and calculation of vitamin E activity of the diet as α tocopherol equivalents.

e 1 NE (niacin equivalent) is equal to 1 mg of niacin or 60 mg of dietary tryptophan.

f The folacin allowances refer to dietary sources as determined by Lactobacillus casei assay after treatment with enzymes ("conjugases") to make polyglutamyl forms of the vitamin available to the test organism.

g The RDA for vitamin B_{12} in infants is based on average concentration of the vitamin in human milk. The allowances after weaning are based on energy intake (as recommended by the American Academy of Pediatrics) and consideration of other factors such as intestinal absorption. see text.

h The increased requirement during pregnancy cannot be met by the iron content of habitual American diets nor by the existing iron stores of many women; therefore the use of 30-60 mg of supplemental iron is recommended. Iron needs during lactation are not substantially different from those of nonpregnant women, but continued supplementation of the mother for 2-3 months after parturition is advisable in order to replenish stores depleted by pregnancy.

Fats and Health

Of late, the cholesterol question has come to the forefront in relationship to heart disease. It has been found that saturated fats (or those found in animal fats) produce larger concentrations of cholesterol in the blood than unsaturated and polyunsaturated fats (or those found in vegetable fats). Cholesterol is used beneficially in the body to form sex and adrenal hormones, produce bile acids, form cell membranes, and provide Vitamin D. However, when cholesterol from dietary sources (such as animal fats) combines with already existing sources of cholesterol in the body, a high cholesterol blood level is produced in some people. Increased blood cholesterol can be deposited in blood vessel walls so that plaques are formed. These placques may in turn contribute to heart and blood vessel problems by the formation of clots or the closure of blood vessels.

Certain foods are high in animal fats and raise blood cholesterol levels in the body. Some of these foods are as follows:red meats (especially those that are marbled with fat), butter, egg yolk, cheese, chocolate, whole milk, and ice cream. It has been found that to protect the body from too much cholesterol in the blood, less than 10 percent of the fats found in the diet should be saturated. That means that **if you have a high risk of heart disease** you should eat less high-fat meats (and more low-fat meats such as fish and poultry). It also means that you should cut off all fat on meat before cooking, and you should bake, broil, roast, and stew your meat rather than fry it. You should substitute skim or low-fat milk for whole milk. You should consider using margarine rather than butter and eating fewer eggs. You should use polyunsaturated fats in cooking, such as vegetable oils. If you are not a high risk for heart or blood vessel diseases, then eating fats in moderation is recommended. You should, lastly, achieve and maintain an ideal body weight by eating more fruit, vegetables, and whole grains and less sugar-sweetened foods and foods that contain saturated fats.[2]

Minerals

A number of minerals are required by the body to give strength and rigidity to body tissues and to maintain basic body functions. Some are major minerals that are required by the body in large amounts, and others are metals that are required only in traces.

Vitamins

Vitamins are chemical substances that are essential for growth and maintenance of body tissue. Typically, vitamins are said to be used in conjunction with enzymes to promote growth, maintenance, repair, and coordination of cell and tissue functions.

Most nutritionists agree that individuals can get all of the vitamins that they need to fulfill the RDA (Recommended Daily Allowance) from the foods that they eat — provided they get the right kinds of foods. Eating the proper foods in the proper amounts from the basic four food groups (meat, milk and dairy products, fruits and vegetables, and breads and cereals) can insure adequate intake of the vitamins that can help you maintain a healthy body. It must be remembered, though, that even if you are taking in the right foods in the proper amounts, you may not be getting all of the vitamins that your body needs. Certain vitamins can be easily destroyed by several means. Exposure to air, light, heat, and multiple

---

SITUATIONS WHERE SUPPLEMENTS ARE USEFUL

The following are common conditions in which vitamin supplements are valuable — or an increased consumption of vitamin-rich foods.

1. **Pregnancy and breast-feeding** boost a woman's vitamin requirements. A multi-formula tablet with iron guarantees meeting these clearly-defined needs. In fact, *every* woman of child-bearing age needs extra iron, whether from foods or supplements.
2. **Oral contraceptives** lower bloodstream vitamin levels by disrupting the body's ability to utilize B vitamins (particularly niacin and B_6). Some physicians recommend a B-complex tablet to counter this.
3. **Smoking** cuts vitamin C supplies by as much as 30 percent, which can be harmful, depending upon dietary habits. A small supplement (100 mg.) will be enough to compensate.
4. **Dieting** reduces overall vitamin intake, at times dangerously, especially among the fad diets. Unless the diet is nutritionally balanced (an example is Weight Watchers), multivitamin tablets are needed.
5. **Alcohol** can disrupt diet. Multi-tablets (especially those high in B-complex vitamins, which absorb alcohol) may prevent serious physical damage.
6. **Caffeine,** taken in large quantities from coffee, tea, or cola drinks, causes the body to flush out the water-soluble vitamins more rapidly. Small daily supplements of the B-complex and C vitamins will replenish supplies.

NEEDLESS VITAMIN SUPPLEMENTS

The following are heavily-advertised vitamins you should never need to take.

Vitamin	General Sources
A	Dairy products, meat and vegetables; excessive dosage causes health damage, particularly to children
D	Potentially lethal in large doses; the body manufactures sufficient quantities from sunlight
K	Is produced internally as needed by the body
Pantothenic Acid	Present in almost all foods and cannot be destroyed by cooking — adequate supply is guaranteed by almost all people
Biotin	Useful in only small amounts, otherwise eliminated by the body, survives cooking and processing so is present in many foods

Reprinted with permission from: Consumers Digest, July/August 1981, p. 48.

handling can destroy the vitamin value of many of our foods. To insure that you get the most from your food in the way of vitamins, you should use fresh foods, use a minimum of water in cooking, and cook foods for the least possible time.

Although there are very few full-blown, clinical cases of vitamin deficiencies in the United States, nutritionists feel that there are many subclinical deficiencies where individuals do not manifest gross abnormalities or symptoms of the deficiency. If you notice abnormalities in body tissues, it could mean a vitamin deficiency. Check with your doctor to be sure.

Water

Water is essential for life. If you are not drinking enough, you may tire easily and find it hard to concentrate. Many people drink less water than is optimum for the best functioning of the body.

Your need for liquids depends on your size and weight. As a general guide, adults should drink between one and one-half and two quarts of

SUMMARY OF VITAMINS & MINERALS

Essential Nutrients	Function in the Body	Good Food Sources	Comments
Pantothenic acid	Necessary for the body's use of carbohydrates, fats, and protein in conjunction with other substances.	Almost universally present in plant and animal tissue. Loss of fifty percent in milling of flour; thirty-three percent lost in cooking meat.	Water soluble; destroyed easily by dry heat and alkaline.
Niacin	Active in normal functioning of tissues, particularly of the skin, gastrointestinal tract, and nervous system; with other vitamins, used in converting carbohydrates to energy.	Lean meat, liver, kidney, whole-grain and enriched cereals and breads, green vegetables, peanuts, yeast.	Water soluble; stable to heat, air, light.
Biotin	Essential for the functioning of many body systems and use of food for energy.	Liver, kidney, molasses, milk, yeast, egg yolk, and green vegetables.	Water soluble; quite stable in heat, air, and light.
Vitamin C (Ascorbic acid)	Essential for the formation of collagen, a protein which supports the body structures; needed for the absorption of iron, some proteins, and folic acid.	Citrus fruits, strawberries, cantaloupe, tomatoes, cabbage, potatoes, green peppers, and broccoli.	Water soluble; destroyed by heat, air, and light, as well as by aging, drying, and copper contact.
Vitamin D	Promotes normal bone and tooth development; necessary for absorption and stabilization of calcium and phosphorus.	Fish-liver oils, fortified milk, exposure to sunlight; very small amounts in butter, liver, and egg yolks.	Fat soluble: stable to heat and air.
Vitamin E (Tocopherol)	Protects the body's store of vitamin A and the tissue fat from destructive oxidation; also prevents breakdown of red blood corpuscles.	Oils of wheat germ, cottonseed, and the germs of other seeds; green leafy vegetables, nuts, and legumes.	Fat soluble: breaks down in presence of lead and iron salts, alkalies, and ultraviolet light.
Sodium	Protects body against excessive fluid loss, regulates muscle and nerve irritability, and maintains water balance.	Table salt, meat, fish, fowl, milk, eggs, and sodium compounds.	Excessive salt intake dangerous for persons subject to hypertension and kidney disorders.

Fluorine	In small quantities, protects the teeth against cavities. In larger quantities, fluorine causes mottling of the teeth.	Milk, eggs, and fish; many communities add low concentrations of fluorine to drinking water.	Prolonged high intake of fluorine may cause skeletal abnormalities.
Vitamin A	Important for skeletal growth and normal tooth structure; necessary for health mucus membranes in mouth, nose, throat, digestive and urinary tracts; and essential for night vision.	Fish-liver oils, liver, butter, cream, milk, cheese, egg yolk, dark green and yellow vegetables, yellow fruits, and fortified margarine.	Fat soluble; destroyed by oxidation and very high temperatures.
Vitamin B_1 (Thiamine)	Necessary to help convert sugar and starches into energy.	Pork, liver, heart, kidney, milk, yeast, whole-grain and enriched cereals and breads, soybeans, legumes, peanuts, and wheat germ.	Quickly destroyed by heat in neutral or alkaline solutions.
Vitamin B_2 (Riboflavin)	Essential link in the body's use of protein, carbohydrates, and fats for energy.	Milk, powdered whey, liver, kidney, heart, meats, eggs, green leafy vegetables, dried yeast.	Decomposes quickly in light or in alkaline solutions.
Vitamin B_6 (Pyridoxine, pyridoxal, pyridoxamine)	Important for the body's use of protein, carbohydrates, and fat; aids in formation of hemoglobin.	Wheat germ, meat, liver, kidney, whole-grain cereals, soybeans, peanuts, corn; some in milk and green vegetables.	Water soluble; destroyed by ultraviolet light and heat.
Vitamin B_{12} (Cobalamin)	Essential for forming red blood cells; helps in forming all cells in body and in functioning of nervous system.	Milk, eggs, cheese, liver, kidney, muscle meats contain small amounts needed for normal body functioning.	Inactivated by air or light; water soluble.
Folic acid	Needed for use of protein in body and for regeneration of blood cells.	Green leafy vegetables, liver, kidney, yeast, and — in lesser quantities — many foods.	Easily inactivated in sunlight and acid solutions.
Vitamin K	Essential for blood clotting.	Green leafy vegetables such as alfalfa, spinach, cabbage; liver.	Fat soluble: unstable to light.
Minerals Calcium	Builds bones and teeth; aids in proper functioning of muscles, heart, and nerves; helps in blood coagulation.	Milk, hard cheese, and in kale, mustard, turnip, and collard greens. Also some in oysters, shrimp, salmon, clams, and in other dairy products.	Calcium is the most abundant mineral in the body.

Iron	One of the constituents of hemoglobin, which carries oxygen to the tissues by blood circulation. Iron is present in all body cells.	All kinds of liver are the best source of iron; also, meat, egg yolk, legumes, molasses, dark green leafy vegetables, peaches, prunes, apricots, raisins, and food made with enriched flour or cereal.	Iron deficiency is most common in growing children, adolescent girls, and pregnant or nursing women.
Magnesium	Most of the body's magnesium is in bones; the remainder is inside body cells taking part in many enzyme reactions. Important for nerve and muscle function.	Dried peas and beans, nuts, whole-grain cereals, cocoa, and chocolate are the best food sources. Green, leafy vegetables are good sources.	Deficiency causes muscle tremors, convulsions, hyperexcitability, weakness, behavioral disturbances, Usually seen only in disease conditions, e.g., alcoholism, kidney disease, malabsorption syndromes.
Phosphorus	Builds bones and teeth (with other minerals): important in a number of body systems involving fats, carbohydrates, salts, and enzymes.	Milk, cheese, egg yolk, meat, fish, fowl, legumes, nuts, whole-grain cereals.	Some forms of phosphorus are not utilized if the vitamin D level is inadequate in the diet.
Iodine	Required to regulate the exchange of food for energy.	Iodized salt best protection: also, salt water fish.	The need for iodine is increased in adolescence and during pregnancy.
Potassium	Needed to maintain fluid balance within the cell; regulates muscular and nervous irritability; necessary for regular heart rhythm.	Meat, fish, fowl, cereals, fruits, vegetables.	Deficiency in diet is uncommon, but may occur in connection with some diseases.
Zinc	Constituent of many important enzymes; necessary for normal growth and sexual maturity; appears to be involved in wound healing.	Seafoods, especially oysters, are rich in zinc. Red meats and some cheeses are good sources. Whole-grain foods, nuts, dried peas and beans furnish good amounts. Chicken, vegetables.	Conditions in humans related to zinc deficiency include: growth failure, sexual immaturity, impaired wound healing, and reduced taste sensation, poor appetite.

fluid a day. Children, of course, need proportionately less. Water, which makes up more than half your body weight, is constantly being lost and must be replaced. Not all of this water is lost through urination. It is also lost through perspiration and unseen and unfelt evaporation through the skin. Some water comes from your lungs; you can see this moisture by breathing on a mirror.

It is very important that you drink enough. If you drink too little, the salts and minerals excreted by your kidneys may not be flushed completely from your system. These minerals are the building blocks for kidney stones. Also, many doctors believe that bacteria, which cause infections, can grow more easily when urine flow is low. However, very large amounts of urine may weaken certain protective mechanisms that suppress the growth of bacteria.

Planning

At Each Meal

1. **One serving of a protein.** You could try eggs, meat, fish, poultry, cheese, seafood, or lentils. Peanut butter counts as a protein. So do certain combinations, such as whole-grain cereal with milk or macaroni with cheese.
2. **At least one grain food.** Depending on your protein, you can try bread, rice, noodles, macaroni, or cereal. If you choose rice, cereal, macaroni, noodles, or similar products, they should be enriched. If you can, eat whole-grain cereals. Whole-grain or whole-wheat bread is best, but make sure that you eat it enriched if you choose white bread.
3. **At least one fruit or vegetable.** Raw is best; frozen is second best. The canning process sometimes removes nutrients, so cook your vegetables as little as possible if you are using canned items out of season. Use fresh fruit if it is in season. Once a day you should have a deep yellow or a dark green vegetable; once each day you should have a citrus fruit (or its juice).
4. **A beverage.** You need eight to twelve cups of fluid a day; you can drink coffee, tea, juice, or water. If you want to use a milk serving here, you could have a glass of milk. You should try to drink at least one cup of beverage so that you can begin to fulfill your daily requirement. If you do not drink milk, you need to plan cheese, cottage cheese, or yogurt into two of your meals for the day, or you need to have two milk group snacks during the day.

At One Meal

At one meal, or with a snack sometime during the day, you need to include the following:

1. A food high in fiber (try bran muffins, whole-grain bread, raw carrots, sunflower seeds, and so on).
2. Iodized salt (this may be contraindicated for those with severe acne or for those who are on salt-free diets).
3. A food high in vitamin C (try tomato juice if you are tired of citrus fruit juice).
4. An unsaturated oil (you can get it in cooking, in salad dressings, and in margarines).

OVERWEIGHT

One of the nation's leading health problems, obesity affects more than one-fourth of all American adults. It has been implicated as the leading or contributing cause in a number of diseases and disorders[3].

The Calorie

If you are overweight, you are probably well acquainted with the word *calorie.* However, many do not understand what a calorie is and how it functions in weight loss and control. A calorie is one unit of energy that is used to measure the "fuel value" contained in food; the body requires a certain amount of this energy (or fuel) to carry on the basic functions of living (such as standing, which uses almost two calories a minute, and sleeping, which uses one calorie a minute) and to enable the body to work and exercise. It takes three and one-half calories per minute to shower and the same to dress or undress. Brushing teeth and hair, washing your face and hands, or shaving require about two calories per minute. Even eating itself requires an energy level of one and one-half calories a minute.

As long as the caloric intake remains equal to the body's energy needs, current weight will be maintained. If too little fuel is taken in — as happens when you cut calories on a reducing diet — the body turns to its stored fat, breaks down fat tissue, and reclaims the energy that is stored there. The result is lost weight and tissue. When you take in more calories than your body's energy requires — as happens when you eat too much or exercise too little — the body stores the excess energy in the tissues in the form of fat. The result is extra tissue and added weight.

It takes 3,500 calories to form one pound of fat. It is an insidious process: eating only 100 excess calories daily — the equivalent of one banana or one glazed doughnut — can make you gain ten pounds of fat in one year and more than fifty pounds of fat in just five years!

Protein and Calories at Fast Food Chains

RESTAURANTS (In alphabetical order)	**MENU ITEMS** (Main dish, side dish and beverage)	**PROTEIN**	**CALORIES**
		(in grams)	
A&W	Super Papa Burger	19	448
	Small fries	3	249
	Root Beer Float	3	200
	TOTAL	25	897
BURGER CHEF	Super Chef	23	423
	Small fries	4	285
	Large Chocolate Shake	9	361
	TOTAL	36	1069
BURGER KING	Whopper	29	563
	Small fries	2	218
	Large Chocolate Shake	7	407
	TOTAL	38	1188
DAIRY QUEEN	Super Brazier	43	732
	Small fries	3	239
	Large Chocolate Shake	10	376
	TOTAL	56	1347
HARDEE'S	Deluxe Huskee	32	635
	Small fries	4	283
	Large Chocolate Shake	10	328
	TOTAL	46	1246
JACK-IN-THE-BOX	Jumbo Jack	28	558
	Small fries	2	226
	Large Chocolate Shake	13	540
	TOTAL	43	1324

(All data compiled by Jacobs-Winston Laboratories Inc., New York, N.Y.)

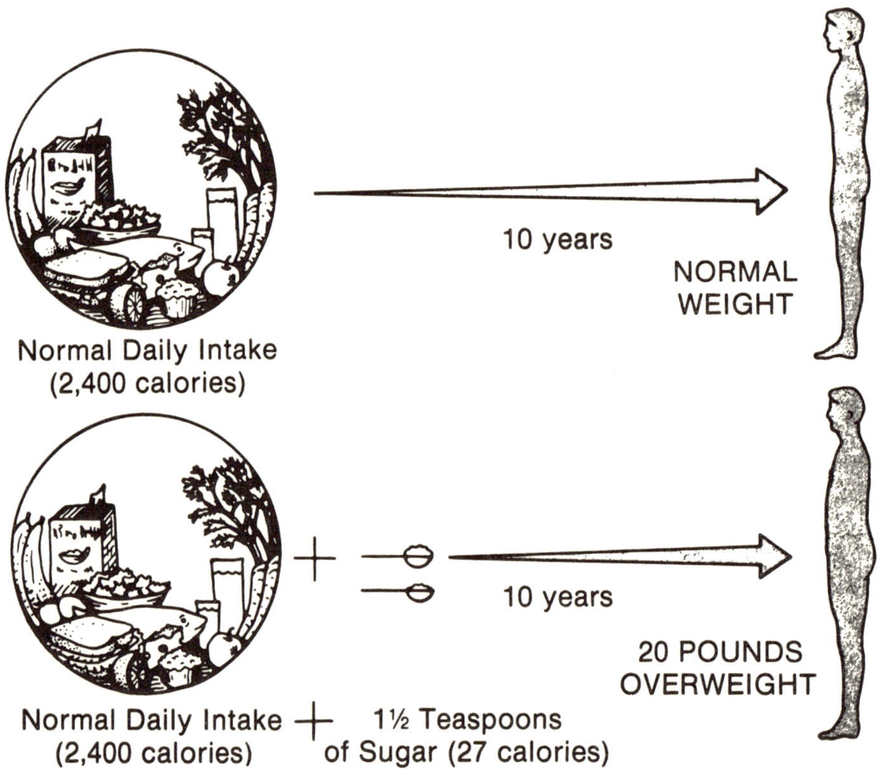

Figure 16-1

Recognizing Good and Fad Diets

Despite the abundance of fad reducing regimens, you can locate a sound diet and exercise program if you are willing to spend a little time and effort. Consider the following characteristics of reduction programs when evaluating a new diet or exercise gadget:

Earmarks of a Sound Diet

1. Based on a negative caloric balance.
2. Is a long-term program. Once ideal weight is achieved, the diet can be adjusted slightly to maintain the weight for life.
3. Limits calories but maintains balance of daily nutrient requirements.
4. Based on slow, regular weight loss.
5. Emphasizes self-control. There is no guaranteed success.
6. Includes an exercise program.

7. Is an exaggeration of proper eating habits with food that you normally eat.
8. Provides for social, cultural, and psychological needs relating to overeating.
9. Is adjusted to the individual's percent of body fat and metabolism.

Earmarks of a Fad or Fraudulent Diet

1. Claims that calories do not count.
2. Promises quick, easy weight loss but does not provide a permanent program for maintenance of ideal weight.
3. Alters proportions or omits certain nutrients. Claims that some foods are naturally more fattening than others.
4. Guarantees sudden weight loss or spot reduction.
5. Promises weight control without effort.
6. Recommends diet or exercise but not both.
7. Recommends drastic change in the types of foods that you are used to eating.
8. Ignores emotional and psychological factors involved in overeating.
9. Promises cures for disease through diet.
10. Carries spectacular advertising appealing to the emotions.
11. Guarantees success for everyone.

Sensible Procedures of Weight Control

Behavior Modification

Too many people regard a diet as a short-term tool by which to lose weight; they figure that they can exist on cottage cheese and clear broth and green salad for a month or two, because after the torture is over they can once again enjoy pizza and chocolate doughnuts and french fries with their hamburgers.

Diet is not temporary; diet — the kind of diet that allows you to maintain your ideal weight and your optimum health — is a continual pattern of eating habits. Every day, every month, every year you need to eat in a way in which you can maintain healthy weight and fulfill your nutritional needs. It is a permanent, gradual process.

Behavior therapy, or modification, is a new concept in weight control that focuses on helping change habits and life-style on a long-term basis. Behavior control tries to guide people away from the all-or-nothing

CALORIC VALUES FOR COMMON SNACKS

Food	Amount or Average Serving	Calories
"Just a Little Sandwich"		
Hamburger on bun	3-in. patty	330
Peanut butter	1 tbsp. p.b.	330
Cheese	1-oz.	280
Ham	1-oz.	320
Pizza, cheese	⅛ pie	180
Beverages		
Carbonated drinks, soda, root beer, etc.	6-oz. glass	80
Pepsi-Cola	12-oz. glass	150
Club soda	8-oz. glass	5
Chocolate malted milk	10-oz. glass	500
Ginger ale	6-oz. glass	60
Tea or coffee, straight	1 cup	0
Tea or coffee, with 2 tbsp. cream and 2 t. sugar	1 cup	90
Alcoholic Drinks		
Ale	8-oz. glass	155
Beer	8-oz. glass	110
Highball (with ginger ale)	8-oz. glass	185
Manhattan	average	165
Martini	average	140
Wine, muscatel or port	2-oz. glass	95
Sherry	2-oz. glass	75
Scotch, bourbon, rye	1½-oz. jigger	130
Fruits		
Apple	1 medium	70
Banana	1 small	85
Grapes	30 medium	75
Orange	1 medium	70
Pear	1	65
Salted Nutes and Potato Chips		
Almonds, filberts, hazelnuts	12-15	95
Cashews	6-8	90
Peanuts	15-17	85
Pecans, walnuts	10-15 halves	100
Potato chips	1 serving	108
Candies		
Chocolate bars		
Plain, sweet milk	1 bar (1 oz.)	155
With almonds	1 bar (1 oz.)	140

CALORIC VALUES FOR COMMON SNACKS (continued)

Food	Amount or Average Serving	Calories
Candies (continued)		
Chocolate-covered bar	1 bar	270
Chocolate cream, bonbon, fudge	1 piece 1-in. sq.	90-120
Caramels, plain	2 medium	85
Hard candies, Lifesaver type	1 roll	95
Peanut brittle	1 piece 2½ × 2½ × ⅜ in.	110
Desserts		
Pie		
Fruit	1/6 pie	375
Custard	1/6 pie	265
Mince	1/6 pie	400
Pumpkin with whipped cream	1/6 pie	460
Cake		
Chocolate layer	3-in. section	350
Doughnut, sugared	1 average	150
Sweets		
Ice cream		
Plain vanilla	1/6 qt.	200
Chocolate and other flavors	1/6 qt.	260
Orange sherbet	½ cup	120
Sundaes, small chocolate nut with whipped cream	average	400
Ice-cream sodas, chocolate	10-oz. glass	270
Midnight Snacks for Icebox Raiders		
Cold potato	½ medium	65
Chicken leg	1 average	88
Milk	7-oz. glass	140
Roast beef	½ in. × 2 in. × 3 in. piece	130
Cheese	¼ × 2 in. × 3 in. piece	120
Leftover beans	½ cup	105
Brownie	¾ in. × 1¾ in. × 2¼ in.	140
Cream puff	4-in. diam.	450

Source: Adapted from Helen S. Mitchell et al., *Cooper's Nutrition in Health and Disease*, 15th ed. (Philadelphia: J. B. Lippincott Co., 1968), pp. 232-83. Data provided by Smith, Kline and French Laboratories.

approach to losing weight. Modifying eating habits is not necessarily a drastic procedure. The focus is not solely on eating, but also on the person's knowledge, misconceptions, activity, time management, and life stresses. The program stresses control of the hows, whys, and whens of eating.

Many physicians utilize a behavior assessment evaluation to identify specific behavior patterns and what influences these patterns, and to help the person recognize and control cues or make them less tempting. Here is an outline of one program:

1. **Keep a Food Intake Sheet.** Keep track of what you eat for two weeks. Your record should be very detailed, including a remark on where you ate, when, your emotional state while eating, etc.
2. **Try to Pinpoint Your Eating Problems.** Check your eating speed. This may prove vital. Also check places where you ate, how you felt when you ate, and when.
3. **Make Eating a Pure Experience.** Learn to eat just for the joy of eating. Sit in the same place each time that you eat, and just eat. No television, no newspaper, nothing else. Eat more slowly by beginning after others or cutting your food into smaller pieces or putting your fork down after every third bite; for snacking problems, create an alternative set of activities at the time that you usually snack, i.e., walking, hobbies.
4. **Reduce Temptations.** Make a shopping list, and purchase only those items that are on your list. Snacking is much less likely if you have to spend fifteen to twenty minutes preparing the snack.
5. **Enlist Your Family's Support.** Explain your plans to them, and ask for their moral support. Requesting that they have fewer snack foods around would also help.
6. **Cope with Emotions.** Do not eat when you get upset or angry; try jogging instead.
7. **Take It Slowly.** Aim at a gradual weight loss; keep a record, but do not starve yourself.
8. **Get More Exercise.** You are more likely to do this (jogging, calisthenics, etc.) if you have a partner to do it with.
9. **Special Situations.** If you are going to a wedding, party, or church social, eat something substantial before you leave the house so that you will not arrive at the function hungry. To avoid temptation while you are there, dance a lot, engage in conversation. In short, keep yourself busy.[4]

These general rules apply to everyone, but authorities emphasize that habit changes should be individually worked out and applied. For

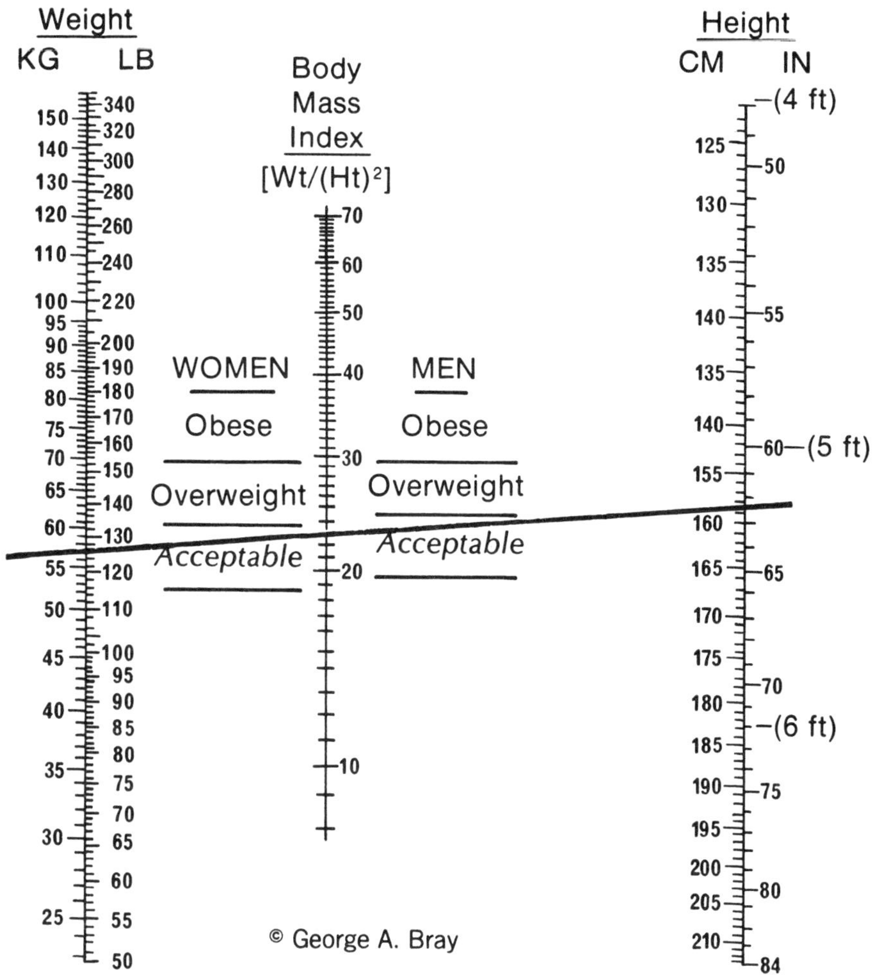

Figure 16-2
This chart was devised by Dr. George A. Bray of the University of California at Los Angeles Medical School. Find your weight in the left column; find your height in the right column. Using a ruler, draw a straight line between the two. The line will intersect the middle column at what is called your "body mass index," and will indicate whether your weight is normal for your height.

example, some persons can easily eliminate all between-meal snacking, while others cannot.

The constant eater should be advised to satisfy his or her need with a handy, plentiful supply of high-bulk, low-calorie foods (celery, carrots, cucumber sticks, lettuce, raw cauliflower, radishes, green peppers, apples, fruit sticks, etc.). This person will not be very hungry at mealtime and can round out meals with leafy salads to get a filled feeling without eating lots of high-calorie foods.

Changing Eating Habits

Many of us overeat because we eat too fast. The feeling of fullness comes on slowly.

1. Eat in slow motion.
2. Sip your beverages, do not gulp.
3. After each mouthful, place your utensils on the plate until you have swallowed that mouthful.
4. Before your main meal, drink a low-calorie drink or a cup of boullion to help to take the edge off your appetite.
5. If invited out, eat a few low-calorie snacks before going.
6. Eat the salad before the rest of the meal.
7. Get in the habit of leaving at least two forkfuls of food on the plate at the end of the meal.
8. Eat foods that take time to eat — such as an orange that has to be peeled instead of an apple.
9. Put scraps of food directly in the garbage.
10. If sweets must be kept around the house, put them in a seldom-used cupboard or in an unlikely place, e.g., broom closet, and let others get their own sweets.
11. When the meal is over, do not linger at the table unless all food has been cleared.
12. Make small portions of food appear larger on the plate by using smaller plates and spreading your food on the plate.
13. Put your own portions on your plate — preferably in the kitchen.
14. Resist the temptation to eat what others have left when you are cleaning up after a meal.
15. If you envy a food that someone else is eating, take one small bite of it to satisfy yourself.
16. Reduce or eliminate use of salt at the table.

FITNESS

Physical fitness — the ability to carry out daily tasks with vigor and alertness, without undue fatigue, and with ample energy to enjoy leisure-time pursuits — is composed of three major elements:

1. **Muscular strength.** The strength of the muscles has to do with their contraction power. This is important not only to your ability to perform manual labor or participate in your favorite sports activity: the body is dependent for survival on the strength of the muscles in the heart, respiratory system, digestive system, and organs of elimination.
2. **Muscular endurance.** The ability of the muscles to perform work is an indication of their endurance; how quickly you tire out is directly related to the amount of endurance that you have. When you have endurance, you probably also have muscular strength, but the two are not dependent on each other and are separate phenomena.
3. **Circulatory-respiratory endurance.** The heart is the best gauge of physical fitness: how quickly does it adapt to stress, working with the respiratory system to pump fresh oxygen to the body tissues during time of physical labor and activity?

A good key to fitness is to measure your resting pulse rate and compare it against your pulse rate after you engage in several different kinds of activities — a measurement of how well your heart is adapting, and how fit your cardiovascular system is.

Measuring the Resting Pulse Rate

To measure your resting pulse rate, use the artery in your wrist (the best place), at the crook of your elbow, or in your neck just next to the Adam's apple. Your pulse is slowest after you have been asleep for six hours — so take your pulse in the morning when you first wake up, before you get out of bed, eat, or perform any kind of movement (even the act of walking across the room will increase your pulse rate and give a false reading). Count the pulsations for one full minute to obtain your resting pulse rate. According to the American Heart Association, a normal resting heart rate is between sixty and eighty beats per minute — and the "normal" for you is dependent on your age, weight, and level of fitness.

Once you have obtained a resting heart rate, measure it against your pulse after you perform different kinds of activities. Choose a specific kind of exercise or activity, and perform it for a few minutes. Take your pulse immediately after you stop: measure your pulse for ten seconds, and multiply the number by six to obtain an accurate measurement. (The heart rate slows rapidly once you stop exercising, and to count the pulsations for

Figure 16-3

HOW TO READ AND RECORD YOUR HEART RATE

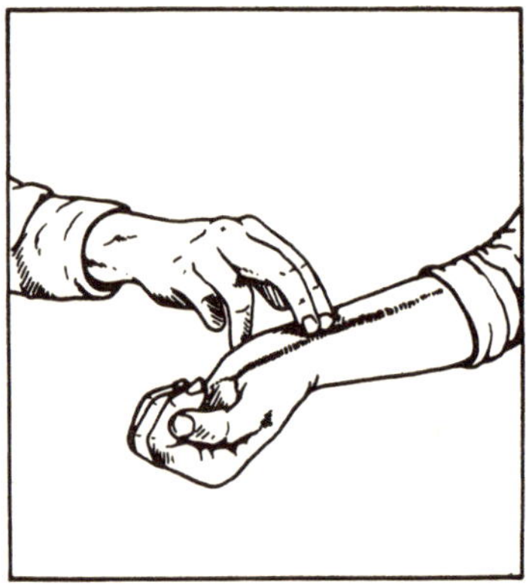

The action of your heart is the best gauge of your physical fitness. An accurate record of your heart rate (beats per minute) under various conditions over a period of time will enable your physician to gauge your progress. Accordingly, you'll need to learn to take your pulse under these conditions:

- At rest; for example, when you first awaken in the morning, before rising or exercising.
- After a specific period of exercise, as directed by your physician.
- After you have performed your regular work for a specific period, as directed by your physician.

Taking your pulse is, for these purposes, the same as counting the number of times your heart beats per minute. Don't be concerned that your heart rate seems fast at one reading or slow at another, many factors, including sex and age, affect the heart rate under various circumstances. To get an accurate measurement for your physical fitness program, follow the simple steps below:

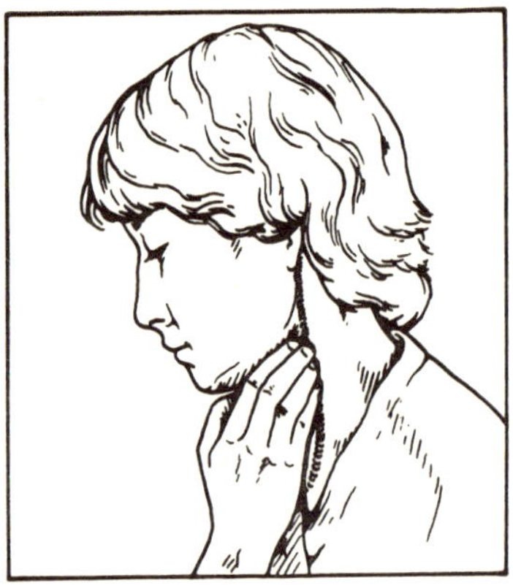

1. Experiment a bit and select the best body site to take your pulse. In some sites the pulse is prominent at rest; in others, after exercise. The best locations are typically at the wrist, just below the base of the thumb; at the neck, just over the collar line and to the right or left of the windpipe; and at the inside of the elbow, just above the skin crease.
2. When taking your pulse at rest, simply count the number of pulsations for a full minute, using a watch with a second hand for accuracy.
3. *Immediately* after exercise count the beats for the first 10 seconds *only*; then mutiply this number by six to get a per minute reading. Don't try to take your pulse during exercise, but start *immediately* after the prescribed exercise. The reason for this is that the heart rate rapidly slows after the stress of exercise; in fact, the faster it slows the more fit you are, as a rule. If you do take a full minute's count, you'll notice a significant difference in the number of heartbeats during the first 10 seconds of the minute and the last 10 seconds.
4. One of the reasons for testing your heart rate is to find out what normal work activity does to your heart. Select an activity that is ordinary and usual — both in the stress it creates and the muscular power it requires. Take a resting pulse count just before doing the activity, then take a post-activity count for 10 seconds and multiply by six.
5. Write down the count of your pulse immediately after taking it. Keep a small notebook for the purpose, and enter the date, time, and kind of reading (resting, postexercise, postwork) for each count.

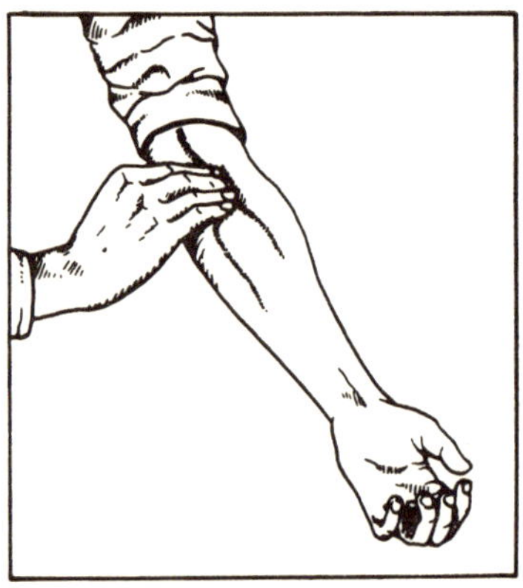

a full minute would give a false reading.) Then take your pulse every minute after you stop exercising — how long does it take your heart to return to normal rate?

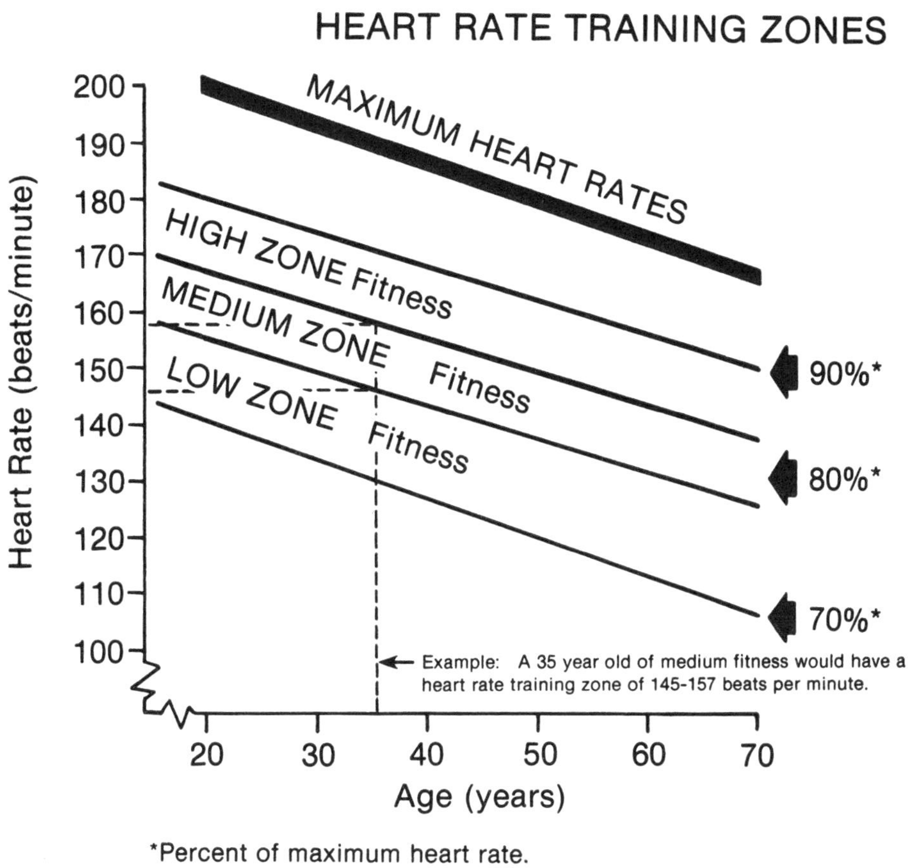

Figure 16-4
This chart illustrates average maximum heart rates as well as heart rate training zones for those in low, medium, and high fitness categories. The heart rate training zone tells you how intense your exercise must be to gain a training effect.

Benefits of Exercise

Exercise, in a word, improves the overall condition of your body. Simply, it improves your health. Some of the specific benefits of exercise include the following:

Figure 16-5

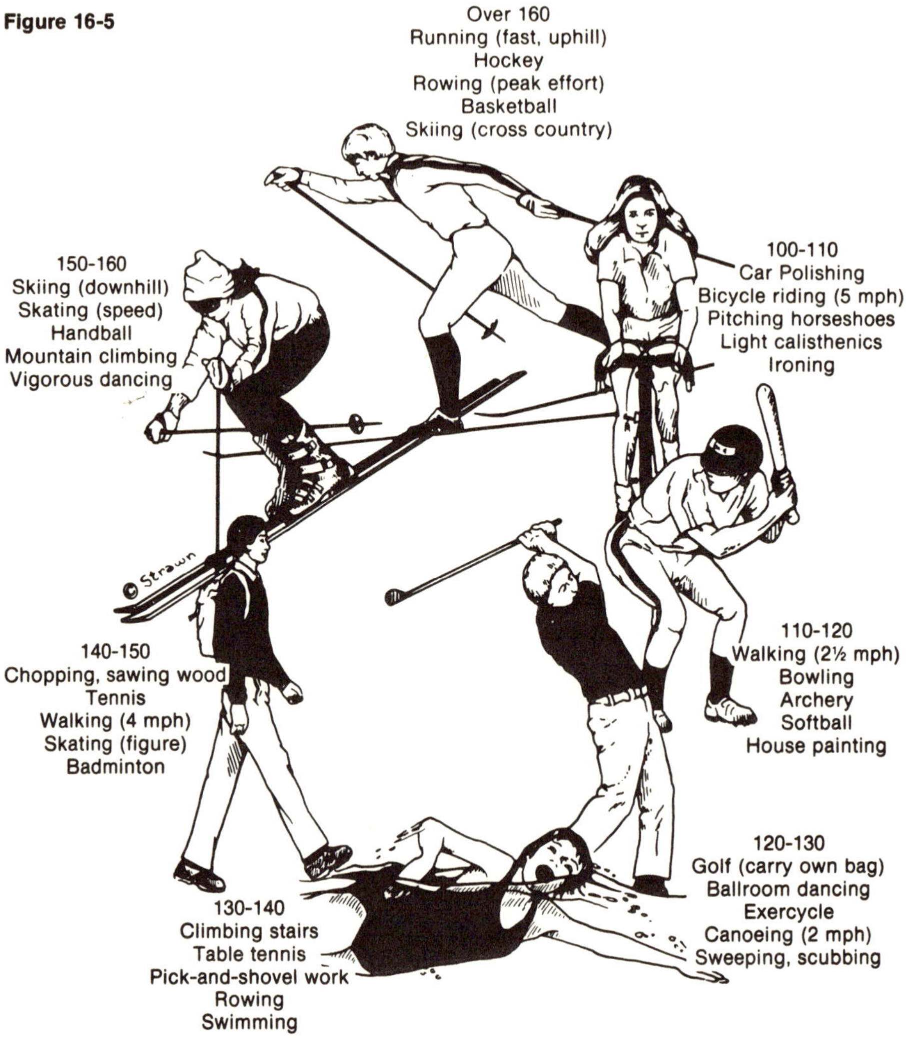

ACTIVITIES AND HEARTBEATS —
CHOOSE THE ONE FOR YOU

1. **Body posture is improved.** As you exercise, the muscles, tendons, and ligaments that support your skeleton are strengthened, and your ability to stand erect with ease is improved. Good posture is important for reasons other than physical attraction, too — it guarantees a better blood supply to the brain and eases the process of returning venous blood to the heart.
2. **Stress is reduced.** As little exercise as walking for fifteen minutes has a more tranquilizing effect than even powerful drugs for relieving anxiety and muscle tension and stress. In addition, exercise improves your ability to deal with stress, provides an outlet for your hostilities, and improves your alertness. Researchers do not know exactly why exercise relieves stress, but several theories cite that exercise reduces the level of salts in the brain, promotes sound sleep, raises hormonal levels critical to the thinking process, sends more oxygen to the brain, and gives people a sense of accomplishment — something that simply makes them feel better about themselves and less prone to suffer from stress.

Figure 16-6

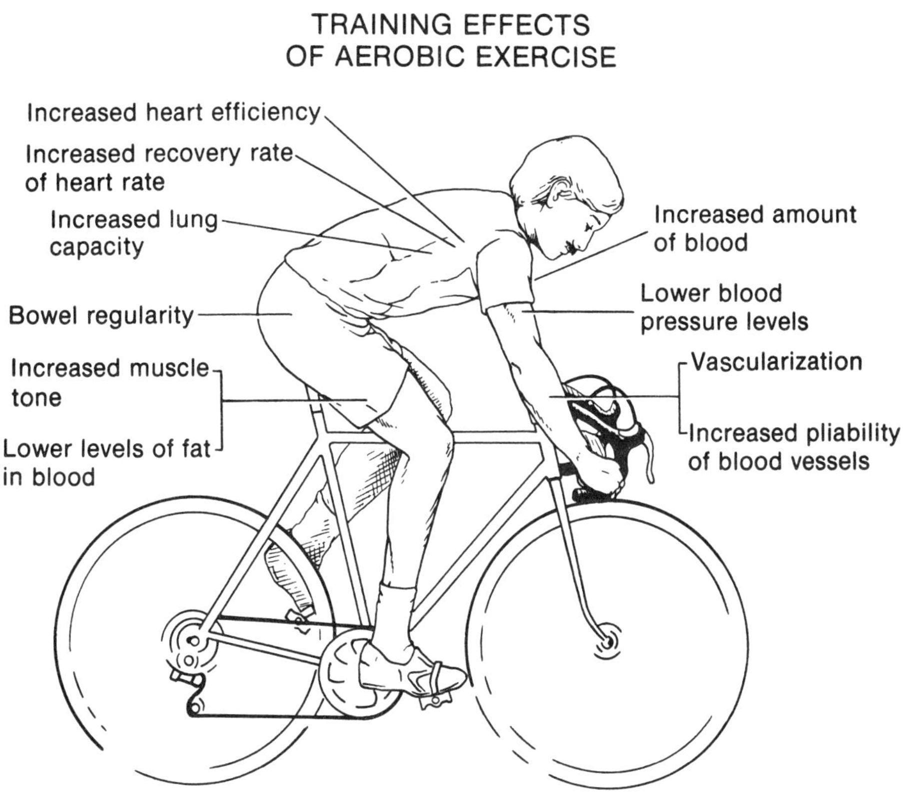

3. **Exercise increases bone mass.** Among those who do not exercise, the bones undergo an actual physical change — they get brittle and frail, more prone to injury, and they lose vital minerals, which requires more healing time if a break does occur. An hour of exercise three times a week is generally sufficient to promote bone mass and insure the health of the bones.
4. **Exercise improves the condition of the heart and the blood vessels,** contributing greatly to the health of the entire cardiovascular system. Regular exercise increases the strength of the heart, enabling it to be more effective in pumping blood and causing it to pump more slowly while at rest (which means that it will wear out less quickly!). Because the heart muscle is strengthened, it returns to normal more quickly after exertion, lessening the danger of damage to the heart muscle resulting from participation in sports or other activities. And because the heart muscle is stronger, circulation is improved throughout the entire body. With a stronger heart, you run less of a risk of heart attack, but if you do suffer an attack, you will recover more fully and more quickly if you are in good condition.
5. **Exercise lowers the blood pressure.**
6. **Exercise enhances the production of red blood cells in the bone marrow,** expanding the ability of the blood to effectively circulate nutrients throughout the system.
7. **The lungs and the respiratory system are strengthened and improved.** During aerobic exercise, the lungs are expanded, and the muscles that cause the lungs to expand and contract are strengthened, making it easier for you to breathe. With regular exercise and its effects, you take in more oxygen and slough off more carbon dioxide. The blood itself becomes richer in oxygen content, which means that the heart has to pump more slowly to circulate the same amount of oxygen throughout the body.
8. **Exercise increases the efficiency of the digestive system.** The peristaltic motion of the system is speeded up, digestion is improved, and food is absorbed more completely and more quickly. For some, exercise results in a natural urge to eat better, more balanced foods. And there is another digestive benefit to exercise: the strengthening of all of the body's muscles tends to eliminate the problem of constipation.
9. **Regular exercise makes the degenerative process of aging less devastating to the body.** People who have exercised continuously throughout their lives maintain better muscle strength and flexibility into old age and have less of a tendency to develop arthritis or other afflictions involving the joints. Both physical and mental health are prolonged as a result of regular exercise.

10. **Regular exercise is one of the most effective ways of maintaining normal weight.** Exercise burns off calories and increases metabolism — which means that you will continue to burn more calories throughout the day, long after you have stopped exercising. Exercise should always be added to a program of calorie control — it speeds the process of weight loss and firms and tones the body as the pounds are shed.

Developing an Exercise Program

There are many aspects of your health over which you do not have much control — your hereditary tendency to cancer of the colon, your body's rate of metabolism, the amount of air pollution in your city — but you have optimum control over how physically fit you are[5]. Even those with severe physical disabilities can do some activities to make themselves as physically fit as possible. Those without disability can take the initiative to exercise and bring their weight into control: and that includes the majority of us.

Think about your own program of physical fitness — if you have one. If you think that you are too busy to exercise every day, reassess your values: physical fitness needs to be part of your life. Think about the reasons why you want to be physically fit — there are health reasons, appearance reasons, and personal reasons, and all of them are compelling reasons!

Do not think of physical fitness as being a short-term, crash program to correct or reverse years of inactivity. Go slowly at first, without stress; take the time and energy required to find a program that is just right for you — one you can stick with for the rest of your life with only a few modifications to accommodate aging and changes in environment.

Have fun with physical fitness. There are many ways to exercise: you can jog on a treadmill for an hour, staring into a full-length mirror, or you can play a rigorous game of tennis at the park, or swim for an hour at the community pool, or choose to do your jogging along a country road. And do not take yourself so seriously that the whole experience becomes grim — slow, steady improvement is what you are after. Do not get discouraged and quit your exercise program if you have not reached a certain self-set level of fitness in the first four weeks.

Try not to concentrate on what is going on inside your body while you exercise — forget how much you are huffing and puffing, forget how hard your heart is pounding, and just concentrate on slamming that racquetball across the court. There are certain warning and danger signs from your

Calories Burned in Various Physical Activities*

Activity **Work Tasks**	*Calories per minute*	Activity **Recreation**	*Calories per minute*
Carpentry	3.8	Archery	5.2
Chopping wood	7.5	Badminton	5.2-10.0
Cleaning windows	3.7	(recreation-competition)	
Clerical work	1.2-1.6	Baseball (except pitcher)	4.7
Dressing	3.4	Basketball - Half-full court	6.0-9.0
Driving car	2.8	(more for fastbreak)	
Driving motorcycle	3.4	Bowling (while active)	7.0
Farming		Calisthenics	5.0
Chores	3.8	Canoeing (2.5-4.0 mph)	3.0-7.0
Haying, plowing		Cycling (5-15 mph -	5.0-12.0
with horse	6.7	10-speed bicycle)	
Planting, hoeing, raking	4.7	Dancing	
Gardening		Modern: moderate-vigorous	4.2-5.7
Digging	8.6	Ballroom: waltz-rumba	5.7-7.0
Weeding	5.6	Square	7.7
Hiking		Football (while active)	13.3
Road-field (3.5 mph)	5.6-7.0	Golf (foursome-twosome)	3.7-5.0
Snow: hard-soft		Handball and squash	10.0
(3.5-2.5 mph)	10.0-20.0	Horseshoes	3.8
Downhill: 5-10% grade		Judo and karate	13.0
(2.5 mph)	3.5-3.6	Mountain climbing	10.0
Downhill: 15-20% grade		Pool or billiards	1.8
2.5 mph)	3.7-4.3	Rowing (pleasure-vigorous)	5.0-15.0
Uphill: 5-15% grade		Running	
(3.5 mph)	8.0-15.0	12-min mile (5 mph)	10.0
40-lb. pack: (3.0 mph)	5.0	8-min mile (7.5 mph)	15.0
40-lb. pack: 36% slope		6-min mile (10 mph)	20.0
(1.5 mph)	16.0	5-min mile (12 mph)	25.0
House painting	3.5	Skating	5.0-15.0
Ironing clothes	4.2	(recreation-vigorous)	
Making beds	3.4	Skiing	
Metal working	3.5	Moderate to steep	8.0-12.0
Mixing cement	4.7	Downhill racing	16.5
Mopping floors	4.9	Cross-country (3-8 mph)	9.0-17.0
Pick-and-shovel work	6.7	Snowshoeing (2.5 mph)	9.0
Plastering walls	4.1	Soccer	9.0
Pulaski (depends on rate	7.8	Swimming	
of work and other factors)		Pleasure	6.0

*Calories burned depends on efficiency and body size. Add 10 percent for each 15 pounds above 150; subtract 10 percent for each 15 pounds under 150.

Calories Burned in Various Physical Activities (continued)

Activity **Work Tasks**	Calories per minute	Activity **Recreation**	Calories per minute
Repaving roads	5.0	Swimming (cont.)	
Sawing		Crawl (25-50 yd/min)	6.0-12.5
Chain saw	6.2	Butterfly (50 yd/min)	14.0
Crosscut saw	7.5-10.5	Backstroke (25-50 yd/min)	6.0-12.5
Shining shoes	3.2	Breaststroke (25-50 yd/min)	6.0-12.5
Shoveling (depends on weight of load, rate of work, height of lift)	5.4-10.5	Sidestroke (40 yd/min)	11.0
Forest Service data (average)	8.0	Skipping rope	10.0-15.0
Showering	3.4	Table tennis	4.9-7.0
Stacking lumber	5.8	Tennis (recreation-competition)	7.0-11.0
Standing, light activity	2.6	Volleyball (recreation-competition)	3.5-8.0
Stone masonry	6.3	Water skiing	8.0
Sweeping floors	3.9	Wrestling	14.4
Tree felling (ax)	8.4-12.7		
Truck and auto repair	4.2		
Walking			
Downstairs	7.1		
Indoors	3.1		
Upstairs	10.0-18.0		
Washing clothes	3.1		
Washing and dressing	2.6		
Washing and shaving	2.6		

body that signal overexertion, and you need to be aware of those. Beyond that, have fun, and forget all the mechanics.

Get outside and into your environment as much as you can. The sunshine, fresh air, and change of scenery are good for your mind as well as your body. Try riding your bicycle, playing a game of golf (no carts!), walking briskly to the library, or some other form of activity that enables you to take advantage of the outdoors. If you dress for the weather, you will be comfortable and rejuvenated.

Do not stick to just one activity. Get some variety into your fitness regime. Variety cannot only alleviate boredom, but it helps guarantee that your fitness program is a well-rounded one that tones and conditions your entire body.

Part of becoming fit is changing your life-style — learning new habits. You will probably need to force yourself at first, so try writing yourself a contract. Make it cover a three-month period for starters. Agree with yourself to do a certain number of activities and to make a certain amount of progress within that time. Every week or so, review your contract. See how you re doing, how far you have come toward reaching your eventual goals. It will help you get into the habit of fitness, and it will provide you with positive reinforcement and a sense of achievement.

Perhaps most important, be sensible. If you are really out of shape, get a physical exam and talk your plans over with your doctor. Sudden exertion could shock your cardiovascular system and lead to serious complications. The goal of a fitness program is to help you — not hurt you. Pay attention to your body's warning signs, get your doctor's approval, and work into your program steadily but gradually. Avoiding illness and injury will make it easier to stick with any fitness program that you choose for yourself.

Warming Up

Whatever you decide to do, make sure that every time you exercise, you take a few minutes for "warming-up" exercises: exercises that slowly stretch your muscles and prepare them for the upcoming workout. Warming up helps prevent injury from exercising — and if you do not warm up, you can suffer heart irregularities, muscle cramps, and serious leg injurius.

Warming up is especially critical for those over the age of thirty, who may have lost some of the flexibility of the muscles. The key to any kind of warm-up exercise is to *stretch* — do not jerk. There are plenty of warm-up exercises available, and you can choose whichever ones work best for you. Take about ten minutes to warm up. Then begin your main exercise slowly, working up to regular pitch over the period of a few minutes. Taking these precautions can help you avoid serious injury from exercising.

Cooling Down

Many people remember to do warm-up exercises, but too many forget that it is just as important to take ten minutes to cool down once you have finished exercising. Do not just stop abruptly — it can be too stressful to the body. If you have been jogging or running, walk slowly and leisurely for about ten minutes. If you have been swimming vigorously, swim slowly. You can even repeat the exercises that you used for warming up.

Cooling down is important for several reasons. First, it prevents muscle stiffness because it allows time for the metabolic wastes to be worked out of your muscles. Second, it redistributes the blood that may be pooled in the extremities from a vigorous workout.

Cool down for about ten minutes, then take a lukewarm bath or shower to promote circulation and relaxation. Steer away from hot water — it reduces circulation and causes fatigue.

Exercise Warning Signs

Any of these warning signs can be indicative of danger. If any of these occur **even once**, stop exercising immediately and call your physician.[6]

1. **Abnormal heart action** — pulse irregular, fluttering, pumping, or palpitations in chest or throat; sudden burst of rapid heartbeats; very slow pulse when a moment earlier it had been high.
2. **Pain or pressure** in the middle chest or in the arm or throat, either during exercise or after exercise.
3. **Dizziness,** lightheadedness, sudden loss of coordination, confusion, cold sweat, glassy stare, pallor, blueness, or fainting. Stop exercise immediately, lie down with your legs and feet elevated, and rest until symptoms stop. Then call your doctor.

If any of the following occur, try the suggested remedy first; if, after a brief period of time, the symptom does not clear up, call your doctor.

1. **Persistent rapid heart action** five to ten minutes after you have stopped exercising. Keep your heart rate lower during exercise (monitor with pulse), and cool down after exercising.
2. **Flare-up arthritis.** Rest, and do not resume exercising until the symptoms of arthritis have disappeared. If you cannot get relief with your usual remedies, call your doctor.

The following can usually be remedied without medical attention, but if they are a persistent problem, you should call your doctor.

1. **Nausea or vomiting after exercise.** Exercise less vigorously, and take a more gradual cool-down period.
2. **Extreme breathlessness** lasting more than ten minutes after you stop exercising. Do not exercise so vigorously; never become so breathless during exercise that you cannot speak while exercising.

3. **Prolonged fatigue** even twenty-four hours after exercising or **insomnia** that was not present before starting the exercise program. Exercise less vigorously, and increase your level gradually.
4. **Side stitch.** A spasm in the diaphragm, the side stitch can be relieved by leaning forward while sitting, attempting to push the abdominal organs up against the diaphragm.

Health Clubs

The kind of exercise that you can get at health clubs is generally not the kind that improves lung and heart function. There are a few exceptions: some offer swimming or cardiovascular exercise such as the exercycle or jogging on a treadmill. If your main exercise needs are for cardiovascular exercise, and if you are on a limited budget, you will probably not be wise to consider joining a health club. If you do, you should look for some factors that indicate the quality of the club.[7]

Ask for the qualifications of the staff. Former athletes or sportsmen who have little or no training are not qualified to run a health club, where staff members are catering to people who have usually been unfit for a period of time and now desire to get fit or lose weight. Good qualifications would include training as a physiotherapist, a gymnast gymanist, or an academically qualified teacher of physical education.

The health club should have a variety of good-quality equipment, including leg-exercising machines, a selection of barbell and dumbbell weights, horizontal and sloping benches, wall pulleys, and, most important, a pulsometer.

The health club personnel should require that they check your pulse before they allow you to start exercising. Any health club whose staff gives you the go-ahead to start exercising without giving you any kind of a stress test or pulse test should be viewed with caution.

Good health clubs strictly monitor the progress of their patrons; a club whose staff members allow you to choose your own weights, program your own exercising, or pedal too long on the exercycle is not properly monitoring your progress, and you may not benefit from the gradual buildup of exercise.

You should not join a health club unless you are sure that you have the time to go at least once each week; any less, and you are missing the benefits besides losing money. If you have unused exercise books or equipment at home, you are probably a poor candidate for a health club, most of which require long-term contracts. The classified ads in newspapers in most major cities are full of ads pleading for buyers to relieve owners of their health club memberships.

Watch out for health clubs that try to lure members with special introductory offers; most of the time they are no bargain, and in some cases, the "special" price offered is actually higher than the membership cost.[8]

Ask a health club staff member if you can have two or three trial visits before signing a contract; that way, you can see if you can really utilize the equipment and if you have time to visit the club. If the staff refuses to let you try the facilities two or three times, steer clear!

Take the time to make exercise a regular part of your life — and you will reap the benefits of a longer, happier life that is free from many diseases and afflictions.

REFERENCES

1. Lawrence E. Lamb, ed. *The Health Letter* (San Antonio, Texas: Communications, Inc., September 26, 1975), vol. 6, no. 6.

2. Adapted from Donald B. Ardell, *High Level Wellness* (Emmaus, Pennsylvania: Rodale Press, 1977), pp. 151-158.

3. List of tips compiled and adapted from Laurence E. Morehouse, "You and Your Heart," *Reader's Digest*, October 1971, p. 79; Charles T. Kuntzleman and the editors of *Consumer's Guide, Rating the Exercises* (New York: William Morrow and Company, 1978), pp. 65-77; "The Fitness Mania, "*U.S. News and World Report*, February 27, 1978, p. 38; "Are You Getting the Right Kind of Exercise?" *Changing Times*, January 1978, p. 35; and the President's Council on Physical Fitness and Sports, *Cureton's Basic Principles of Physical Fitness Work*, 1973.

4. Morehouse, "You and Your Heart," p. 79.

5. Mary Carpenter, "See Dick Run! See Jane Run! Everybody's Doing It Now!" *SCI/DI*, August 1978, p. 12; and Brian J. Sharkey, *Fitness and Work Capacity* (U.S. Department of Agriculture, Forest Service, Washington, D.C.: U.S. Government Printing Office, May 1977), pp. 55-56.

6. Adapted from Lenore Zohman, *Exercise Your Way to Fitness and Health*, 1974, as reprinted in Sharkey, p. 57.

7. "What To Look for in a Health Club," pp. 152-153 in *Feel Younger, Live Longer* (New York: Rand McNally, 1976).

8. "Thinking of Joining a Health Club? Exercise Caution!" *Family Health*, February, pp. 34, 36.

CHAPTER 17

SEEKING PROFESSIONAL HELP

With the recent interest in self-care, consumers have recognized a personal responsibility for their own health and are taking a more direct role in the decision-making process. Decisions relating to consumer health range in importance from selecting a toothbrush to selecting a physician in whose hands you may place your life. With the abundance of sometimes conflicting information, these decisions are not always easy.

SELECTING A PHYSICIAN

The ideal physician is one who is adequately trained to provide direct assistance to the patient. To locate a physician who will serve you best, begin by calling your county medical society and asking for the names of two or three family physicians, general practitioners, or family internists in your neighborhood. Ask the same question of the local medical exchange answering service and the administrator's office of your local hospital. When you call, describe the kind of medical service that you require (your age, how many children you have, or any special problems that you may have). Membership on the staff of an accredited hospital is essential. If hospital care is required, your physician is helpless if he has no hospital privileges. Seek the advice of people in the community whom you respect and who have lived there for a number of years. Check with related professionals, such as dentists, nurses, and pharmacists. Select a physician who is available to your neighborhood or town, thus making medical care more readily accessible.

As a patient, you have certain rights:[1]

1. **The right to choose a physician.**
2. **The right to change physicians.**
3. **The right to privacy.** No one who is not involved directly in your health care should have access to any information about your medical condition or history unless you give specific permission.
4. **The right to full information.** You not only have the right to ask questions, but you have the right to complete, truthful answers.
5. **The right to know medical costs and fees, before you submit to treatment.**
6. **The right to a second opinion.** One prominent West Coast surgeon estimated that obtaining second and third opinions reduces the amount of unnecessary surgery as much as 60 percent.

Most physicians are of sufficient integrity to refer a patient to other personnel when the health problems are beyond the scope of their professional expertise. Although medicine today is highly specialized, the average patient is usually best served by the general practitioner or doctor of family medicine. Such physicians are generalists with a wide scope of training that enables them to deal effectively with 80 percent of the ailments commonly found in the population. When the general practitioner encounters a patient with problems demanding additional training, the patient is referred to the appropriate specialist.

DO YOU NEED AN ANNUAL CHECKUP?

Recent medical developments have caused doctors to question the need for an annual checkup of active, healthy people. You should certainly have an annual checkup (and sometimes one at more frequent intervals) if you or your doctor determine that you are a member of a high-risk group and that you have a good possibility of developing a medical problem.

If you do not run the risk of developing specific medical problems,

A Glossary of Common Medical Specialists

Administrative Medicine. Those in administrative medicine are the physicians who have administrative positions that require the particular services of a physician.

Allergy. The physician who specializes in allergy deals primarily with allergies that commonly occur in the respiratory tract, in the gastrointestinal tract, and on the skin.

Anesthesiology. The physician who specializes in anesthesiology deals with the administration of various forms of anesthetic drugs before surgical operations. He is further responsible for helping to support the life functions under the stress of anesthesia and surgery.

Colon and Rectal Surgery. Those pursuing the specialty of colon and rectal surgery are concerned with the diagnosis and treatment of diseases that affect the lower digestive tract.

Dermatology. The dermatologist specializes in the diagnosis and treatment of skin and scalp diseases.

Family Physician or General Practitioner. A family physician or general practitioner is trained to take care of general medical problems that occur from birth to death. In most cases, he or she can handle diagnosis and treatment; in some cases, referral to a specialist must be made.

General Surgery. Surgeons deal with the treatment of disease, injury, or deformity by manual or operative means. Usually in the practice of general surgery, there is a heavy concentration of abdominal and vascular surgery. Many surgeons often further specialize within the field of surgery—for example, some surgeons prefer colon and rectal surgery while others specialize in thoracic surgery.

Internal Medicine. The internist is primarily concerned with the diagnosis and treatment of diseases of the internal organs—especially the cardiovascular system, the organs of respiration, and the digestive system. The internist most commonly deals with chronic illnesses such as arthritis, heart disease, and diabetes.

Neurological Surgery. Those in neurological surgery are concerned with the diagnosis and surgical treatment of the brain, the spinal cord, and disorders that involve the nerves.

Obstetrics and Gynecology. The Ob-Gyn deals with the diagnosis and treatment of diseases and disorders of the female reproductive system. It is also concerned with the care of women during and immediately following pregnancy.

Ophthalmology. This physician specializes in the medical and surgical treatment of diseases of the eye and all its related structures.

Orthopedic Surgery. The orthopedic surgeon diagnoses and treats diseases of the bones and joints as well as fractures and other deformities.

Continued

A Glossary of Common Medical Specialists (Continued)

Otolaryngology. The otolaryngologist is a specialist of the ears, nose, and throat. He diagnoses and treats diseases and disorders of these organs.

Pathology. One who specializes in pathology analyzes body fluids and tissue specimens so that he is able to interpret changes in organs, tissue, and cells as well as alterations in other aspects of body chemistry.

Pediatrics. Pediatrics is concerned with the prevention, diagnosis, and treatment of children's diseases. The pediatrician is especially interested in the growth and development monitoring of healthy youngsters.

Physical Medicine and Rehabilitation. Those in physical medicine and rehabilitation are concerned with the diagnosis of disease or injury in the various systems of the body. In addition, they institute treatment of disease by means of physical procedures as well as treatment and restoration of the convalescent and physically handicapped.

Plastic Surgery. The plastic surgeon specializes in corrective or reparative surgery to improve physical appearance, correct inherited and acquired deformities, and minimize scarring.

Preventive Medicine. Preventive medicine deals with the prevention of disease and the promotion of health through such means as epidemiological studies and other public health measures.

Psychiatry and Neurology. Those trained in psychiatry and neurology are concerned with the diagnosis and treatment of emotional disturbances, mental disorders, and organic diseases affecting the nervous system.

Radiology. Radiology deals with the diagnosis and treatment of disease by the use of radiant energy.

Thoracic Surgery. Thoracic surgery deals with the operative treatment of diseases of the chest.

Urology. The urologist specializes in the diagnosis and treatment of disease of the kidneys, bladder, prostate, male reproductive organs, and other related structures.

---

you probably do not need a **complete** physical checkup every year. If you or your family have a high risk in any of the following areas, you may want to schedule an annual checkup:

1. If you have been exposed to tuberculosis or if you live in an area where tuberculosis is common, you should be tested regularly for the disease. While chest x-rays used to be the most common method of testing, you should ask for a tuberculin skin test instead to avoid unnecessary exposure to x-ray.

2. If you are a female over the age of twenty-five, you should have a Pap smear every year. Women over twenty-five should also conduct breast self-examination each month and should have their breasts examined annually by a physician (this can be accomplished at the same time that the Pap smear is taken).
3. After the age of forty, you should be examined annually for glaucoma.
4. After the age of thirty, you should have an annual examination that includes urine cultures, urinalysis, and tests for blood in the stools (to detect cancer of the digestive tract, kidneys, or bladder).
5. Your blood pressure should be checked at least once a year regardless of your sex or age.

The following represents a schedule that may be used to determine when physical exams are necessary. Note that this schedule applies only if you are well, not on regular medication, have no complaints or symptoms, or have had tests to determine your state of health.[3]

- Infant: within twenty-four hours of birth, between the ages of two to four weeks, and at the age of one year
- Toddler: every three to six months during the second year of life
- Children from three to thirteen years: every two to three years
- Teenagers: every four to five years
- Young adults, ages twenty to thirty-four years: every five to seven years
- Adults, ages thirty-four to forty years: every five years
- Adults, ages forty to fifty years: every three years
- Adults, ages fifty to sixty years: every two years
- Adults, ages sixty to seventy years: every two years
- Adults over age seventy-five: every year

X-RAY EXAMINATION

Probably the most valuable and the most widely used tool for diagnosis is the x-ray—high energy electromagnetic impulses that cannot be seen or felt as they pass through the body.[4] In extremely high doses, x-rays are capable of severely damaging or destroying human tissue. The low doses required for most diagnostic tests will not damage normal tissue unless certain precautions are not taken or unless a patient receives too many x-rays.[5]

While the benefits of diagnostic x-rays outweigh the disadvantages, recent findings indicate that overexposure to x-ray radiation may trigger serious disease or tissue destruction, including cancer. As an x-ray passes through the body, some of the radiation is absorbed—more is absorbed by the dense body parts. The radiation, which is instantly dissipated into other forms of energy, can result in damage or destruction of cells from the transfer of energy. Most such damage is repaired by natural body processes, but some damaged cells can remain and cause serious problems as long as thirty years after exposure.

You can take measures to protect yourself against the potential harms of x-ray by doing the following:[6]

1. Keep accurate records of each x-ray that you have—the type of x-ray, the reason for the x-ray, the name of the dentist or physician that gave you the x-ray, and the date. Record the location of the facility where you received the x-ray so that you can obtain the x-rays if necessary.
2. Whenever your physician or dentist orders an x-ray, find out why the x-ray is necessary. If you are not satisfied with the reason, say that you feel that the x-ray is unnecessary. Find out if an alternate diagnostic method will work as well. Be sure to tell your doctor if you have had similar x-ray tests performed before.
3. If you are changing communities or physicians, ask for your x-rays. Some doctors or hospitals will release your x-ray file to you, and such files should be given to your new physician; they may prevent the need for further x-rays.
4. Chest x-ray screening programs for the diagnosis of tuberculosis are no longer recommended. If your employer requires that you be tested for tuberculosis prior to accepting employment, ask the doctor to give you a tuberculin skin test instead of a chest x-ray.
5. Dental x-rays are no longer recommended on a regular basis but should only be used in specific instances to diagnose a suspected problem that the dentist cannot diagnose in any other way. The American Dental Association has ruled that dental x-rays should **not** be a standard part of every dental examination.
6. If it does not interfere with the diagnostic procedure, insist that a lead shield be placed around your reproductive organs if you are having x-rays of the lower stomach, lower back, abdomen, or any area near the reproductive organs. In addition to causing sterility in some rare cases, exposure to x-ray may cause chromosomal damage that is then passed on to subsequent generations. Because the male's reproductive organs are located outside the body, it is particularly critical that a man request a gonadal shield if he is to receive x-rays of the abdomen or lower back.

7. If you are a woman and have any suspicion that you might be pregnant, tell your doctor. Because x-rays are damaging to a fetus, you should not receive x-rays during pregnancy unless the x-rays are vital to saving your life. Even if you do not think you are pregnant, you should limit x-ray exposure to the first fourteen days of the menstrual cycle to prevent exposure to a fetus.
8. Never demand an x-ray if your physician seems reluctant. Some physicians have resorted to unnecessary x-ray to protect themselves against charges of malpractice.

UNNECESSARY SURGERY

It is estimated that 2 million unnecessary operations are performed in the United States annually. Some physicians, through poor judgment or greed, perform needless operations on uninformed patients. However, many operations are done because **patients** insist upon them. Surgery has become so common and successful in the minds of the patients that they find it hard to believe that it would not remedy their medical problem.

Regardless of the reasons, it is apparent that patients need to become more informed concerning surgical matters. Every patient should ask the following when confronted with a surgical decision:

1. Is the surgery the only way to treat the medical problem?
2. Does the disease necessitate any treatment at all?
3. Is the surgeon qualified to perform this type of surgery?
4. Is the **individual** considered when the diagnosis is made?
5. Upon evaluation, do you feel that the surgery was recommended because **you** applied so much pressure to have it done?

If you still have questions or doubts, a second opinion from another physician often is in order. Many times, your own physician will encourage you to do this, or your insurance will require you to seek a second opinion. Studies have shown that second opinions have reduced the number of operations, but the long-term results are being questioned. Studies are now being done to determine whether patients who do not have surgery end up having it done later and if they require more extensive surgery.

MEDICAL INSURANCE

To determine whether you are adequately covered by health insurance, check the coverage of your policy. It should include the following as a standard of minimum coverage.[7]

1. **Hospital insurance.** For a maximum deductible fee of $100, you should have hospital expense coverage that includes hospital room and board, the cost of general nursing care, and special diets for at least twenty-one days of continuous confinement. Your hospital policy should cover at least 80 percent of a semiprivate room charge (in some areas, insurance pays a flat rate per day, such as fifty dollars; this may not come close to covering the costs considering the rapidly increasing hospitalization expenses).

   Your policy should also cover at least 80 percent of the costs for surgery, recovery room fees, equipment (such as wheelchairs), intensive care, drugs, vaccines, intravenous preparations, dressings, plaster casts, oxygen, anesthesia, physiotherapy, chemotherapy, x-rays, electrocardiograms, radiation, or other customary hospital services rendered in connection with your hospitalization. Your hospital policy should also cover outpatient services on the day surgery is performed or for a period of up to twenty-four hours following an accident, and should cover at least 80 percent of the emergency room charges.
2. **Medical insurance.** Your policy should cover at least 80 percent of all surgical charges (including pre- and postoperative care by a physician), at least 80 percent of anesthetic charges, and at least 80 percent of all in-hospital medical services (including the physician's fee for a bed patient).
3. **Major-medical insurance.** Your policy should include maximum benefits of at least $10,000. You should have coverage for laboratory tests, x-rays, drugs, radiation therapy, artificial limbs, treatment, and therapy performed outside a hospital. If you are at risk of developing a critical disease and your risk is extremely high, you may want to consider taking out a catastrophic illness policy in addition to your regular health insurance (such a policy, for example, would cover expenses incurred from cancer).

SELECTING A DENTIST

In general, a patient must look for a dentist who will provide the following services:

1. Provides a thorough examination.
2. Is concerned about and relieves pain.
3. Is concerned about the proper care and maintenance of baby teeth. The child's first visit to the dentist should occur around two years of age. Subsequent regular dental care should be directed at saving teeth, be they baby or permanent.
4. Puts in fillings that will last. Temporary fillings are occasionally appropriate but may be a gimmick for setting up another visit and collecting another fee. If permanent fillings crack or are lost, the dentistry was inadequate.

Glossary of Dental Specialties

Pedodontics. Pedodontics deals with the care of children's teeth.

Periodontics. This specialty treats the supportive tissues of the mouth such as the gums and the bones.

Orthodontics. This area of dentistry deals with the prevention and correction of irregularities of the teeth.

Prosthodontics. Prosthodontics specializes in the mechanics of making and fitting artificial teeth.

Oral surgery. Oral surgeons deal with the treatment of dental problems by operative means.

Oral pathology. Oral pathology is a specialty which is concerned with the analysis of fluids and tissue specimens from the mouth and related structures. By use of the laboratory, the oral pathologist is able to help in diagnosis of oral disease.

Dental public health. The major emphasis of a public health dentist is on prevention and control of dental diseases through community heath education.

Endodontics. Endodontics is concerned with treating problems connected with the tooth pulp or nervous structure of the mouth.

5. Helps prevent periodontal disease. The dentist's major contributions to preventing this problem are meticulous scaling and cleaning of the teeth and advice or counsel on plaque control and on what the patient can do to prevent and alleviate the condition.
6. Applies advanced techniques. Appropriate use of high-speed drills (risky for deep decay close to the pulp cavity), use of new resin adhesives for inlays, repair of broken teeth, replacement of teeth that have come out, and application of sealants for cracks and fissures, which are the sisters of decay, are all new approaches to effective dentistry.
7. Educates the patient concerning proper nutrition and its effects on good dental health. Explains the role of excessive sugar in promoting dental caries and gum disease and elaborates upon the importance of proper cleaning of the teeth by flossing and brushing.

THE CHIROPRACTIC PHYSICIAN

One controversial area in health services today concerns chiropractic. According to the Chiropractic Fact Sheet prepared by the National College of Chiropractic, chiropractic may be defined as the diagnosis and treatment of human ailments without the use of drugs, medicine, or incisive surgery. It is a nonmedical, nonsurgical form of therapy utilizing manipulation of the spine and other articulations, clinical nutrition, physical therapy, psychological counseling, hygiene, and sanitation in the prevention and treatment of disease.

Chiropractic is **not** a branch of medicine. Chiropractics are not licensed medical doctors; by law they cannot prescribe drugs or perform surgery. They are not allowed to practice in any hospital accredited by the Joint Commission of Accreditation of Hospitals. Their treatment is usually confined to spinal and soft tissue manipulation. The limitations of chiropractic training would seem to cast doubt on its potential for delivering adequate health care.

Physicians maintain that the idea of illness being derived from a malposition of spinal bones is ridiculous; that chiropractors have not done scientific research for eighty-five years to support its claims; and that chiropractic is potentially dangerous because it may well aggravate some serious conditions and delay urgent medical attention to others. Chiropractors accuse the medical profession of economic and professional jealousy, of operating out of conservatism. They claim that chiropractic is clinically, if not scientifically, proven and point to many years and hundreds of thousands of satisfied patients.

For those who choose to use the services of a chiropractor, read the following advice:

1. Avoid any practitioner who makes claims about cures, either orally or in advertising. Anyone who implies or promises guaranteed results from treatment should be held suspect.
2. Beware of chiropractors who ask you to sign a contract for services. A written agreement is not customary practice.
3. Reject anyone advertising free x-rays. Radiation should not be used as a lure.
4. Do not make advance payments.
5. Do not be pressured by scare tactics, such as threats of "irreversible damage" if treatment is not begun promptly.
6. See a physician as well and find out what he or she has to say about the problem.
7. Only go to a chiropractor for back ailments or muscle pain, not for organic or visceral disorders.
8. Be wary if the chiropractor is involved in anything other than muscles or bones.
9. Do not give up any medication that you are already taking just on a chiropractor's say-so.
10. Determine whether the chiropractor whom you are considering has ACA (American Chiropractic Association) membership.

RECOGNIZING "QUACKERY"

Most "quacks" are friendly, well-dressed, attractive people who approach you in a most sympathetic and kind way. Some have offices in reputable buildings. Many hire nurses and receptionists. So how can you recognize a "quack?" Some of the following characteristics are common:

1. **Secret remedies.** They claim to know of the latest discoveries and have access to their use. Secret remedies are usually worthless.
2. **Quick cure.**

3. **Guarantee of cure.** Science has not progressed to the point where it can guarantee results—there are simply too many unpredictables and individual variables. Even with the guarantee, the "quack" seldom refunds any money.
4. **Testimonials.** Testimonials may be fakes, may be bought, or may be given by people who only thought that they had a disease and were cured.
5. **Claims persecution.** They claim that the medical association, government agencies, and research institutions are persecuting them. They clamor for medical recognition but avoid scientific evaluation of the products and methods that they claim are superior.
6. **Discredits accepted procedures.** Since "quacks" may not be able to legally use drugs, surgery, laboratory, or other proven procedures, they try to discredit them.
7. **Low-cost diagnosis.** They may invite patients to mail in a description of their symptoms, and they will make the diagnosis and prescribe the proper medication or food supplement. Not even the most skilled physician can make an accurate diagnosis by mail or phone.
8. **Questionable degrees.** They may display diplomas in a conspicuous manner in order to create an illusion of credibility. Certificates can be obtained for a price, and degrees are granted from schools that are nothing more than a "diploma mill." The so-called "school" may be a short course workshop, a correspondence course, or merely a post office box.

EVALUATING MEDICAL INFORMATION[8]

One of the problems of modern society is how to evaluate the mass of information that pours out of the media. And when health information is involved, that problem becomes more personal and pertinent. In order to provide guidance through the maze of health information, use the following guidelines when evaluating medical information:

1. In general, the kind of medical information that deserves attention comes from studies published in reputable journals for scrutiny by other scientists. The purpose of a study—versus a story—is to remove personal bias from the conclusions. Personal bias rarely takes the form

of intentional distortion resulting from financial or ego involvement. More often, bias stems from honest errors of observation, undue optimism, or limited evidence. Proper studies attempt to remove these and other sources of error. When you encounter new information, **ask yourself if it goes beyond personal observation and whether it has stood the test of criticism by other scientists.**

2. A major theme of medical information is the **effectiveness** of new treatments. Proof of effectiveness must depend on more than individual, anecdotal "stories" about how someone (or even many) got better doing this or that. **Proof of effectiveness requires controlled studies that compare the treatment under discussion to other treatment —or to no treatment.** As described above, such studies must be done with proper controls to remove bias, in large enough numbers to be statistically valid, and in a manner that makes the results available for examination. When you encounter a claim of effectiveness, **ask yourself if the treatment in question was compared either to other treatments or to "doing nothing."**
3. Another major issue in medical information is the **safety** of new (or old) treatments. The question, in our complex and technological age, is not **absolute** safety (even staying in bed is risky) but **relative** safety. All of life—including medical treatment—involves some risk. The question becomes whether the risk is justified when compared to alternatives. Studies to determine risk usually require large numbers of observations over long periods of time, though occasionally an intolerable danger becomes apparent very early in a study. When you encounter information about "safety," **ask yourself—"safe compared to what?"**
4. Be especially wary of enthusiastic claims for unusual remedies for chronic or incurable diseases—such as crippling arthritis or terminal cancer. There are, unfortunately, some people who deliberately profit from the understandable desperation of others.

In short, when evaluating medical information, remember that **the burden of proof rests with those who recommended doing or giving something**—especially if it involves a remedy or procedure not well established in medical practice.

Excerpted from the November 1981 issue of *The Harvard Medical School Health Letter*,

Self-Care Medicine Chest

It's a good idea to have useful medical supplies on hand for emergencies and to treat minor ills, but the family medicine chest does not have to be a mini drug store. What should be kept in the average household will depend on the makeup of the family. For instance, when there are young children, the medicine chest might include baby aspirin, anti-bacterial topical ointments and medicine to treat symptoms of diarrhea. For that family, syrup of ipecac to induce vomiting and activated charcoal are important for emergency treatment for some accidental poisonings. Persons who are likely to use or administer them, however, should understand the types of poisoning for which they should not be used, as when a caustic agent has been swallowed, for instance.

If there are teenagers, the medicine chest might include acne preparations. An older family member might have a special need for liniment. An adult in reasonably good health may have little use for most over-the-counter medicines.

Generally, medicine chests should include only those health care products likely to be used on a regular basis. A person rarely bothered by constipation, for instance, would have little need for a laxative.

Overstocking drugs in the household should be avoided. Some drug products lose their potency on the shelf in time, especially after they are opened. Other drugs change in consistency. Milk of magnesia, for instance, dries out if it remains on the shelf for a while after opening. Buying the large "family size" of a product not used frequently may seem like a bargain, but it's poor economy if it has to be thrown out before the contents are used up. Ideally, supplies in the medicine chest should be bought to last over a period of no more than six to 12 months.

Obviously, selecting health care items for the family medicine chest is a matter of common sense. Here are some suggested items that will meet the needs of most families:

Non-drug products

Adhesive bandages of assorted sizes
Sterile gauze in pads and a roll
Absorbent cotton
Adhesive tape
Elastic bandage
Small blunt-end scissors
Tweezers
Fever thermometer including rectal type for a young child
Hot water bottle
Heating pad
Eye cup for flushing objects out of the eye
Ice bag
Dosage spoon (common household teaspoons are rarely the correct dosage size)
Vaporizer or humidifier
First aid manual

Self-Care Medicine Chest

Drug items

Analgesic — Aspirin and/or acetaminophen. Both reduce fever and relieve pain, but only aspirin can reduce inflammation.

Emetic — syrup of ipecac to induce vomiting and activated charcoal. Read the instructions on how to use these products.

Antacid

Antiseptic solution

Hydrocortisone creams for skin problems

Calamine for poison ivy and other skin irritations

Petroleum jelly as a lubricant

Anti-diarrhetic

Cough syrup — non-suppressant type

Decongestant

Burn ointment

Anti-bacterial topical ointment

The medicine chest might also include anti-nausea medication if any family member is prone to motion sickness, a laxative and some liniment. Seasonal items, such as insect repellents and sunscreens round out the list.

When it comes to storing these health care items the cardinal rule is to keep all medicines out of the reach of children. In addition, be sure all medicatons have child-resistant caps. Elderly people who have difficulty opening such caps can ask the druggist for regular closure. However, they should be extra careful to see that young visitors can't get to these drugs.

Both prescription and non-prescription drugs should be kept in a cool, dry place away from foods and other household products. Some drugs may need to be kept in the refrigerator. This should be indicated on the label. If in doubt, ask the pharmacist.

Many people keep medicines on a high shelf in a hall or bedroom closet. Some experts suggest using a locking box. A tackle box might do. A word of warning, however: Be sure all responsible adults in the family know where the key is kept.

To avoid confusion keep prescription and non-prescription drugs in separate boxes clearly labeled to distinguish one type of drug from the other. A list of what's in each box, attached to the outside if possible, will make it easier to find specific items, particularly in an emergency.

The medicine chest should be checked periodically to be sure supplies haven't run low and to get rid of drugs that may have gone bad or become outdated. Many drug labels have an expiration date beyond which the product should not be used. If there isn't a date, put a label on the container with the date of purchase and the date it was first opened. Then, if there are any questions in the future, a pharmacist can tell whether the product is safe to use.

Tablets that have become crumbly, medicines that have changed color, odor or consistency, or are outdated, should be destroyed. Empty the bottle of medicine into the toilet, flush it down, and rinse out the bottle. Don't put leftover drugs in the trash basket where they can be dug out by inquisitive youngsters. Newly purchased drug products that don't look right should be returned to the pharmacy. Drug products that have lost their labels also should be destroyed.

Keep the telephone numbers of the local poison control center, physician, hospital, rescue squad, fire and police departments near every phone in the house. Tape the emergency phone list inside the bathroom medicine cabinet door and also keep it with the emergency supplies.

From Annabel Hecht, *FDA Consumer,* April 1982, p. 12, 13

USE YOUR DRUGS SAFELY

There are many things that you can do to make better use of prescription drugs by using them safely. Consider the following suggestions:

1. Do not pressure your physician into prescribing a drug if you do not really need it.
2. Never take prescription drugs on your own.
3. Do not take a friend's prescription drug just because your symptoms are just like his.
4. Do not give anyone else — even a family member — your prescription drug unless your physician tells you to. It is against the law.
5. Do not change the dose or timing of your drug unless your physician tells you to.
6. If you start to suffer serious side effects that your physician warned you about, get in touch with the physician as quickly as you can. Or, if a drug is not doing what it is expected to, notify your physician.
7. Do not stop taking a prescription drug without letting your doctor know.
8. Do not take *any* drug while you are pregnant or nursing a child unless your doctor specifically tells you to. Make sure that your doctor knows that you are pregnant or nursing before he prescribes a drug for you.
9. Do not take more medications than you have to.
10. Never take any drug in the dark. If you get up in the middle of the night to take your medicine, turn on the light and make sure that you have the right bottle.
11. Do not mix medications in the same container. Potency may be destroyed—and if the medications look alike, you may take the same drug twice.
12. Learn the name and correct spelling of each drug that you are using.
13. Ask your doctor what dietary adjustments you can make to help your drug work better. Some drugs, for instance, are neutralized by milk—if you know that, stay away from dairy products.
14. If you are scheduled for surgery, tell your dentist, surgeon, or anesthesiologist about *all* of the drugs that you have taken in the last several weeks.
15. If you get pregnant while you are taking any kind of a drug, inform your doctor immediately.
16. Keep a written record of all drugs that you take and all vaccines you receive during the entire nine months you are pregnant. Include the name of the drug, how much you took, the dates you took it, and what you took it for.
17. Keep the same kind of written record for all drugs to which you are allergic. Do the same for members of your family.
18. Tell your doctor about *any* allergy you have—not just allergies to drugs.
19. Call your doctor immediately if you think that you have taken an overdose.
20. Clarify with your doctor whether it is safe to drive a car or operate machinery while you are taking your prescription drug.
21. Ask the doctor if you can safely drink alcoholic beverages while you are taking the drug.

NOTES

1. Jean E. Laird, "Know Your Rights as a Patient," *Family Weekly*, November 13, 1977, p. 32.

2. Donald M. Vickery and James F. Fries, *Take Care Of Yourself: a Consumer's Guide to Medical Care*. (Reading, Massachusetts: Addison-Wesley Publishing Company, 1976), p. 12.

3. Lewis Miller, *The Life You Save*, (New York: William Morrow and Company, 1979), pp. 56-57.

4. "X-Ray Hazards—Real and Imagined," *Sci/Di*, March 1979, p. 82.

5. "The New Worry Over X-Rays and What You Can Do About It," *Good Housekeeping*, July 1979, p. 221.

6. "Growing Debate Over Dangers of Radiation," *U.S. News and World Report*, May 14, 1979, p. 26; Public Health Service, *We Want You to Know About Diagnostic X-Rays* (Rockville, Maryland: U.S. Department of Health, Education, and Welfare, DHEW Publication No. (FDA) 73-8048, 1973).

7. "Health Insurance Policies: Why It's Hard to Pick a Good One," *Changing Times*, December 1978, p. 8.

8. From "Evaluating Medical Information," *Harvard Medical School Health Letter*, November 1981, p. 6.

Appendix

The following "Health Action Plan," originally published by Preventive Medicine Institute - Strang Clinic is provided as a self-assessment for cancer, stroke, and heart attack. It is intended to help you determine if you are at risk for any of the above-listed conditions. The assessment covers the skin and lymph nodes, the head and neck, the respiratory system, the cardiovascular system, the urinary tract, the gastrointestinal tract, the male reproductive system, the female reproductive system, and the breasts. You will also be able to use this insert as your personal health record.

HEALTH ACTION PLAN

PAGE 1. Skin and Lymph Nodes

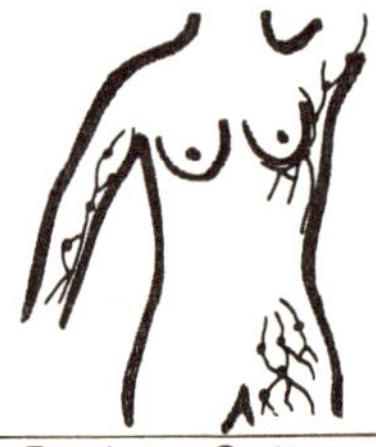

PAGE 2. Head and Neck

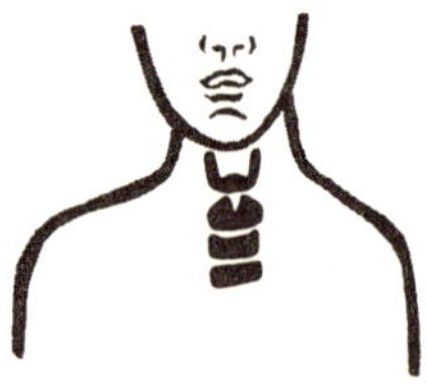

PAGE 3. Respiratory System

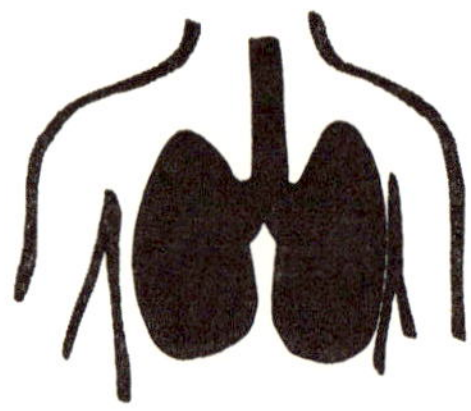

PAGE 4. Cardiovascular System

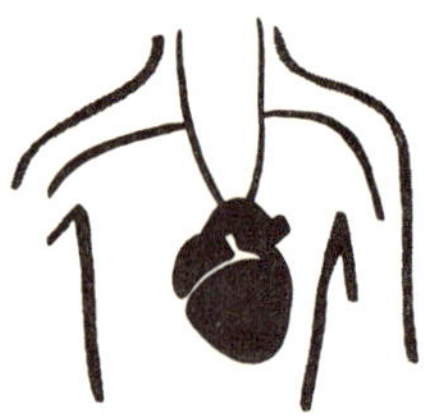

PAGE 5. Urinary Tract

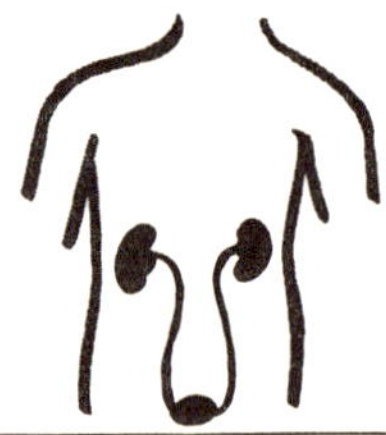

PAGE 6. Gastrointestinal Tract

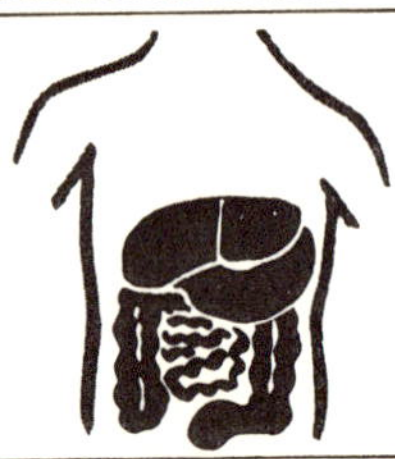

PAGE 7. Male Reproductive System

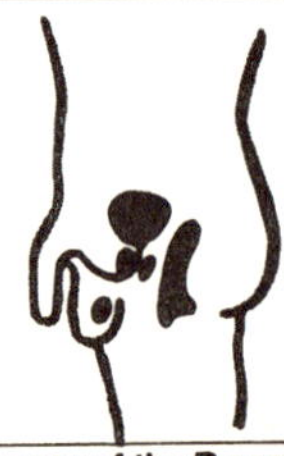

PAGE 8. Female Reproductive System

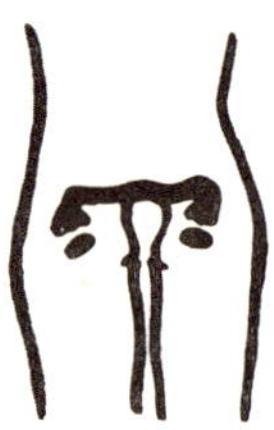

PAGE 9. Cancer of the Breast (For Women)

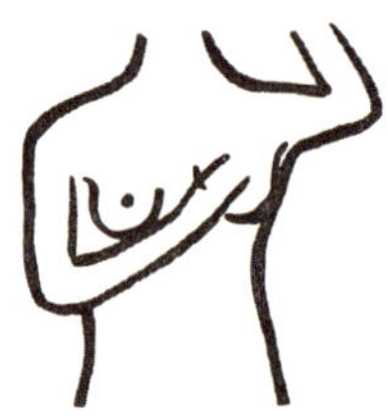

The ***HEALTH ACTION PLAN*** consists of 9 topics — one per page.

Each page is divided into 3 parts:

Questions:

The Questions to be answered under each topic heading are separated into 4 Categories — A, B, C, D.

A CATEGORY refers to symptoms which may indicate some thing is wrong. A "yes" answer in this category does not necessarily mean there is a problem, but that these symptoms should be brought to the attention of a physician as soon as possible. You can be alert to the symptoms, but only a trained person can evaluate them.

B CATEGORY is a family history your physician should have. If you are not sure about some of these, check with other family members.

C CATEGORY is important medical history your physician should have.

D CATEGORY is to alert you to preventive measures which can help you to protect yourself from certain health hazards. There is additional information available from the Preventive Medicine Institute to help you control some of these health hazards.

Drawings:

The drawings illustrate those areas of the body that relate to the diseases we are discussing. They are to assist you to place the organs and sites in the body.

Risk Factors:

A risk factor indicates whether you are more likely to get a particular disease than someone who does not have that risk factor. Having any of the risk factors does NOT mean that you will get the disease. Even though some risk factors cannot be changed, such as family history, some are up to you. Controlling smoking, drinking, and weight can reduce some risks.

TEAR OFF THIS FOLDER. IT WILL BE YOUR *PERSONAL HEALTH RECORD*

Instructions:

Keep the record next to each page as you answer the questions in **The Health Action Plan.** The **Personal Health Record** is divided into the same topics and categories as the **Health Action Plan.** Under each topic heading (see example below) there are categories A, B, C, and D. Check "yes" or "no" in the circle to the right of the questions.

All "yes" answers should then be written down under the appropriate category in this record. Continue answering the questions until all nine topics from Skin and Lymph Nodes to Breast Cancer have been completed and all "yes" answers are written on this record.

FOR EXAMPLE, the following illustration shows how you might fill in the "yes" answers for topic 1. Skin and Lymph Nodes.

1. Skin and Lymph Nodes Copy the "yes" answers from topic 1 of the test under the letters A, B, C, D shown here

FOR PHYSICIAN EVALUATION **A.** Do you now have . . . ?	FOR PHYSICIAN ATTENTION **B.** Has a member of your family ever had . . . ?	FOR PHYSICIAN RECORD **C.** Have you ever had . . . ?	FOR PERSONAL ACTION **D.** Do you . . . ?
. . . Unexplained sweating or fever during the night which has lasted for more than two weeks	. . . Cancer of the skin	. . . Cancer of the skin	. . . Have skin that sunburns more easily than others
. . . Swelling or enlargement (painful or not) of lymph glands	. . . Hodgkins disease	. . . A skin growth removed	

A "YES" ANSWER IN A Category: These current symptoms need physician evaluation. See physician within two weeks for their evaluation; do not attempt to evaluate these yourself.

A "YES" ANSWER IN B Category: These items of family history should be brought to the attention of your physician at the time of your next physical examination. These are risk factors to be aware of.

A "YES" ANSWER IN C Category: Your physician should have a record of this important medical history. At the time of your next physical examination make sure that he knows about it.

A "YES" ANSWER IN D Category: There are preventive measures which can help you protect yourself and reduce your risks from these health hazards. You may wish to have additional information about these. If you write to the Community Service Division of the Preventive Medicine Institute at 55 East 34th Street, N.Y., N.Y. 10016, you may obtain health action material for: obesity, smoking, alcohol abuse, breast self-examination, occupational safety and health, and hypertension.

To Use the Completed *HEALTH ACTION PLAN*

1. If all the answers in A Category are "no", you may wish to keep this booklet as a personal record of your health status and repeat the questions again to see if there is any change in your status over time.
2. You may wish to take this plan with you to your physician at the time of your next examination as a reference.
3. You may wish to suggest that other members of your family develop a personal health plan to refer to.

NAME ______ SEX ______ AGE ______ DATE ______

Self-Evaluation for Cancer, Heart Disease, Stroke

1. Skin and Lymph Nodes

PERSONAL HEALTH RECORD

FOR PHYSICIAN EVALUATION	FOR PHYSICIAN ATTENTION	FOR PHYSICIAN RECORD	
A. Do you now have . . . ?	**B.** Has a member of your family ever had . . . ?	**C.** Have you ever had . . . ?	

2. Head and Neck

Copy the "yes" answers from the second page of the test under the letters A, B, C, D shown here

FOR PHYSICIAN EVALUATION	FOR PHYSICIAN ATTENTION	FOR PHYSICIAN RECORD	FOR PERSONAL ACTION
A. Do you now have . . . ?	**B.** Has a member of your family ever had . . . ?	**C.** Have you ever had . . . ?	**D.** Do you . . . ?

3. Respiratory System

Copy the "yes" answers from the third page of the test under the letters A, B, C, D shown here

FOR PHYSICIAN EVALUATION	FOR PHYSICIAN ATTENTION	FOR PHYSICIAN RECORD	
A. Do you now have . . . ?	**B.** Has a member of your family ever had . . . ?	**C.** Have you ever had . . . ?	

4. Cardiovascular System

Copy the "yes" answers from page 4 of the booklet under the letters A, B, C, D shown here

FOR PHYSICIAN EVALUATION	FOR PHYSICIAN ATTENTION	FOR PHYSICIAN RECORD	FOR PERSONAL ACTION
A. Do you now have . . . ?	**B.** Has a member of your family ever had . . . ?	**C.** Have you ever had . . . ?	**D.** Are you . . . ?

5. Urinary Tract

Copy the "yes" answers from page 5 of the booklet under the letters A, B, C, D shown here

FOR PHYSICIAN EVALUATION	FOR PHYSICIAN ATTENTION	FOR PHYSICIAN RECORD	FOR PERSONAL ACTION
A. Do you now have . . . ?	**B.** Has a member of your family ever had . . . ?	**C.** Have you ever had . . . ?	**D.** Do you . . . ?

6. Gastrointestinal Tract

Copy the "yes" answers from page 6 of the booklet under the letters A, B, C, D shown here

FOR PHYSICIAN EVALUATION	FOR PHYSICIAN ATTENTION	FOR PHYSICIAN RECORD	FOR PERSONAL ACTION
A. Do you now have . . . ?	**B.** Has a member of your family ever had . . . ?	**C.** Have you ever had . . . ?	**D.** Do you . . . ?

7. Male Reproductive System

Copy the "yes" answers from the seventh page of the test under the letters A & C shown here

PERSONAL HEALTH RECORD

FOR PHYSICIAN EVALUATION		FOR PHYSICIAN RECORD	FOR PERSONAL ACTION
A. Do you now have . . . ?	**B.** DOES NOT APPLY	**C.** Have you ever had . . . ?	**D.** Do you . . . ?

8. Female Reproductive System

Copy the "yes" answers from page 8 of the booklet under the letters A, B, C, D shown here

FOR PHYSICIAN EVALUATION	FOR PHYSICIAN ATTENTION	FOR PHYSICIAN RECORD	FOR PERSONAL ACTION
A. Do you now have . . . ?	**B.** Has a member of your mother's side of the family ever had . . . ?	**C.** Have you ever had . . . ?	**D.** Do you . . . ?

9. Cancer of the Breast

Copy the "yes" answers from page 9 of the booklet under the letters A, B, C, and D shown here

FOR PHYSICIAN EVALUATION	FOR PHYSICIAN ATTENTION	FOR PHYSICIAN RECORD	FOR PERSONAL ACTION
A. Do you now have . . . ?	**B.** Has a member of your mother's side of the family ever had . . . ?	**C.** Have you ever had . . . ?	**D.** Do you . . . ?

Self-Evaluation for Cancer, Heart Disease, Stroke

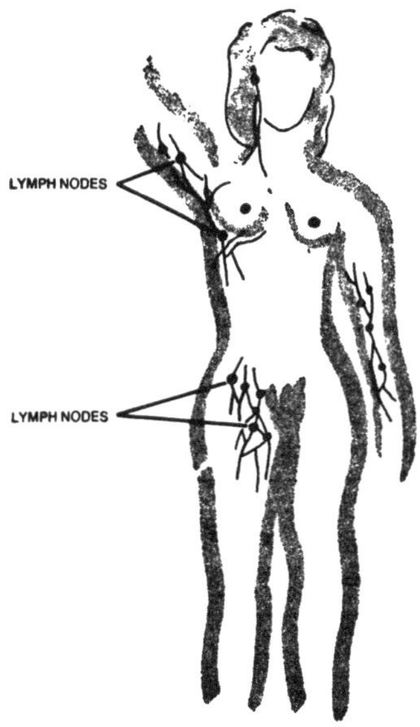

Both skin and lymph nodes cover the entire body. Lymph nodes are located at strategic points in the body to fight infection.

An enlarged lymph node will appear as a single firm swelling under the skin. It is often confused with a hernia, infection or cyst.

1. Skin and Lymph Nodes

A. Do you now have . . . ?	YES	NO
. . . Any unexplained itching	○	○
. . . Unexplained sweating or fever during the night which has lasted for more than two weeks	○	○
. . . Swelling or enlargement (painful or not) of lymph glands	○	○
. . . Non-healing ulcers, sores, or growths which have lasted for more than a month	○	○
. . . Red scaling patches of skin which do not heal	○	○
. . . Any moles which have changed color, changed size, become ulcerated (sore) or bleed	○	○
B. Has a member of your family ever had . . . ?		
. . . Cancer of the skin	○	○
. . . Leukemia	○	○
. . . Lymphosarcoma	○	○
. . . Hodgkin's disease	○	○
C. Have you ever had . . . ?		
. . . Cancer of the skin	○	○
. . . A mole removed	○	○
. . . A skin growth removed	○	○
. . . Treatment with X-rays (radiation therapy)	○	○
. . . A burn with scarring	○	○
D. Do you . . . ?		
. . . Have frequent boils or other skin infections	○	○
. . . Have skin that sunburns more easily than others	○	○
. . . Have an outdoor occupation (example: farmer, fisherman, etc.)	○	○

IF YOU HAVE ANSWERED "YES" TO ANY OF THESE QUESTIONS, ENTER THAT QUESTION ON YOUR *PERSONAL HEALTH RECORD.*

CANCER OF THE SKIN

RISK FACTORS:

- Extremely fair skin
- Prolonged exposure to the sun (more than 4 hours a day for 4 months out of the year)
- A history of skin cancer or malignant moles
- Moles on the soles of your feet or in areas irritated by tight clothing or shaving
- Scars from severe burns
- A non-healing scaling sore on your skin

AWARENESS COUNTS:

You can reduce your risks for skin cancer by wearing protective clothing, such as sun hats, or by lightly covering the over-exposed parts of your body when out in the sun for long periods.

Avoid excess sun-bathing if you are fair-skinned; apply *sun-screening ointment* (different from regular suntan lotion) to filter out harmful rays.

Avoid contact with arsenic (found in some insecticides) and coal tar derivatives since these agents play a role in the development of skin cancer.

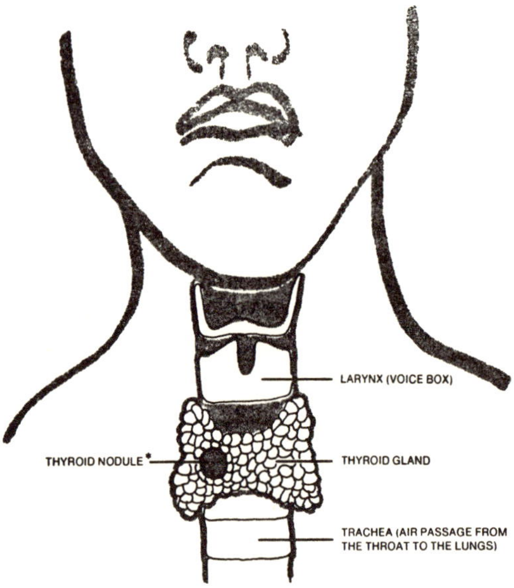

*Lumpiness or swelling of the thyroid are most often benign goiters (enlargement of the thyroid gland), while a single solid swelling (nodule) is more likely to be serious.

2. Head and Neck

	YES	NO
A. Do you now have . . . ?		
. . . Sores or white spots in the mouth or lip lasting for one month or more	○	○
. . . Fullness, soareness, or swelling in the lower front of the neck	○	○
. . . Hoarseness or changes in the voice	○	○
. . . Difficulty or pain in swalloing lasting one month or more	○	○
. . . Any irritation in the mouth due to poor-fitting dentures or sharp teeth	○	○
. . . Any small solid lump in the neck area	○	○
B. Has a member of your family ever had . . . ?		
. . . Cancer of the head and neck	○	○
C. Have you ever had . . . ?		
. . . A tumor in the throat or neck	○	○
. . . A thyroid disorder	○	○
. . . X-ray treatments to the head or neck in youth	○	○
D. Do you . . . ?		
. . . Smoke cigarettes, cigars or a pipe	○	○
. . . Drink beer, wine, or hard liquor daily	○	○
. . . If yes, is it more than 5 beers, 5 glasses of wine, or 3 hard liquor drinks per day?	○	○
. . . Fail to check inside your mouth and cheek monthly for signs of oral cancer (spots or irritations)	○	○
. . . Fail to have regular dental checkups	○	○

IF YOU HAVE ANSWERED "YES" TO ANY OF THESE QUESTIONS, ENTER THAT QUESTION ON YOUR *PERSONAL HEALTH RECORD.*

CANCER OF THE LARYNX

RISK FACTORS:
- Heavy smoking
- Heavy drinking
- Cancer of the oral cavity or lung

AWARENESS COUNTS:
WHEN DETECTED EARLY, CANCER OF THE LARYNX CAN BE CURED. The preventive measure you can take is to cut down on your drinking and smoking. Alcohol and smoke are irritants to the lining of your mouth and throat. Any reduction of this kind of irritation to your mouth and throat decreases your risk.

CANCER OF THE MOUTH AND THROAT

RISK FACTORS:
- A broken tooth which irritates the inside of your mouth
- Broken or ill-fitting dentures
- Heavy smoking or drinking
- A non-healing sore or white patch in your mouth

AWARENESS COUNTS:
Any sores of the mouth, throat or gums which do not heal properly should be brought to the attention of a physician or dentist.

Cutting down on alcohol consumption and smoking is an important preventive measure and can reduce your risks.

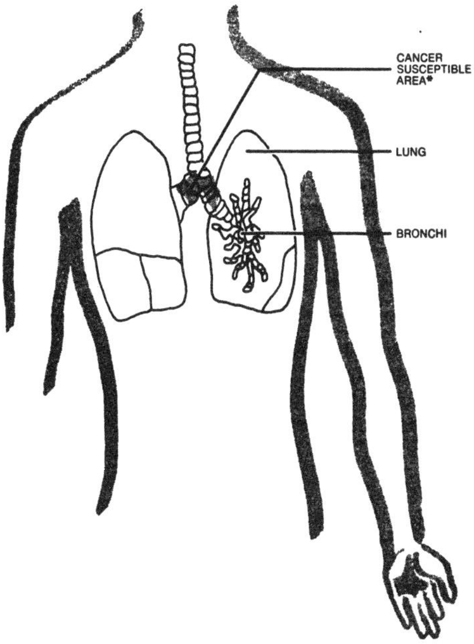

*Cancer of the lung most often starts in this area, which is continuously bathed in cigarette smoke.

3. Respiratory System

	YES	NO
A. Do you now have . . . ?		
. . . A cough, producing sputum (mucus from the lungs), which has lasted more than one month	○	○
. . . Sputum which is streaked with blood	○	○
. . . Chest colds more than 3 times a year	○	○
. . . Chest pain in the same area which has lasted more than one month	○	○
B. Has a member of your family ever had . . . ?		
. . . Tuberculosis (TB)	○	○
C. Have you ever had . . . ?		
. . . Tuberculosis	○	○
. . . Chronic bronchitis	○	○
. . . Asthma	○	○
. . . Emphysema	○	○
. . . Pneumonia, more than once	○	○
D. Do you . . . ?		
. . . Smoke cigarettes, cigars or a pipe	○	○
. . . Smoke more than one pack of cigarettes a day	○	○
. . . Work with or have you ever worked with: radioactive materials, asbestos, dust of coal, stone or other mineral, nickel or chromates	○	○

IF YOU HAVE ANSWERED "YES" TO ANY OF THESE QUESTIONS, ENTER THAT QUESTION ON YOUR *PERSONAL HEALTH RECORD.*

CANCER OF THE LUNG

RISK FACTORS:

- Cigarette smoking — the smoker's risk of developing lung cancer is proportional to the number of cigarettes smoked, number of years smoking, age at which smoking started, and how deeply smoke is inhaled.
- Working in an occupation which brings you into contact with asbestos, nickel, chromates or radioactive material
- A history of tuberculosis
- A chronic cough

AWARENESS COUNTS:

Your risk for lung cancer can be reduced if you avoid cigarette smoking. This is an effective preventive measure. Cigarette smoking can not only lead to death from lung cancer, but can also increase the chances of dying from other lung diseases (asthma, emphysema, pneumonia) or heart disease.

Occupational exposure to the cancer causing agents mentioned should be avoided or carefully controlled. Be aware of the materials you work with.

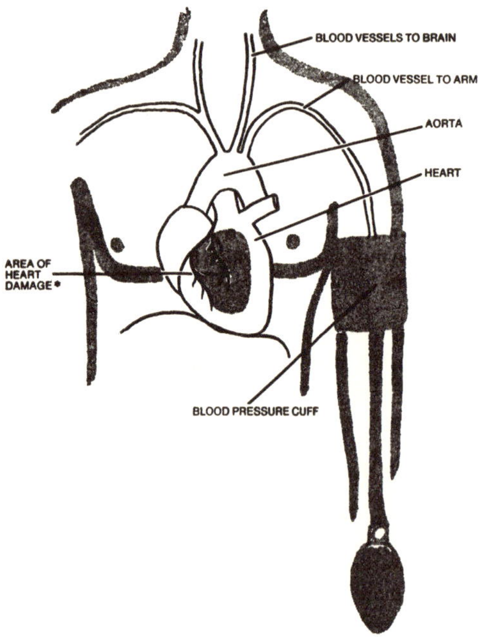

*A myocardial infarction, or heart attack, cuts off the supply of blood and causes damage to the muscle of the heart. This weakens the ability of the heart to circulate the blood.

4. Cardiovascular System

	YES	NO
A. Do you now have . . . ?		
. . . Shortness of breath for no apparent reason	○	○
. . . Palpitations of the heart	○	○
. . . A squeezing or pressing feeling in the mid-portion of your chest	○	○
. . . Swelling of both ankles	○	○
. . . Phlebitis (inflammation of the veins) more than once	○	○
. . . Unexplained dizzy spells	○	○
B. Has a member of your family ever had . . . ?		
. . . Hypertension (high blood pressure)	○	○
. . . Heart disease under age 60	○	○
. . . Stroke	○	○
C. Have you ever had . . . ?		
. . . Rheumatic fever, scarlet fever, heart murmur	○	○
. . . Hypertension (high blood pressure)	○	○
. . . Stroke	○	○
. . . An abnormal electrocardiogram (EKG)	○	○
. . . Abnormal blood cholesterol	○	○
. . . Diabetes	○	○
D. Are you . . . ?		
. . . A cigarette smoker	○	○
. . . Obese? (More than 20 pounds overweight)	○	○
. . . Eating eggs, butter and red meat daily	○	○
. . . A person who does not exercise regularly (at least 20 minutes a day, 3 days a week)	○	○

IF YOU HAVE ANSWERED "YES" TO ANY OF THESE QUESTIONS, ENTER THAT QUESTION ON YOUR *PERSONAL HEALTH RECORD.*

HEART DISEASE AND STROKE

RISK FACTORS:

- A history of cardiovascular disease
- Hypertension (high blood pressure)
- Phlebitis (inflammation of the veins)
- Heavy smoking
- Overweight
- An elevated level of cholesterol in your blood
- Diabetes
- Any of the symptoms listed under A

AWARENESS COUNTS:

You can reduce your risk for hypertension by weight control, low fat diet, avoiding cigarettes, and reduction of tension. Rest and regular exercise is recommended.

If you already have cardiovascular disease, you must have regular examinations by your physician.

WEIGHT CHART			
FEMALE		MALE	
HEIGHT	NORMAL	HEIGHT	NORMAL
4'9"	92 — 119	5'1"	112 — 141
4'10"	94 — 122	5'2"	115 — 144
4'11"	96 — 125	5'3"	118 — 148
5'0"	99 — 128	5'4"	121 — 152
5'1"	102 — 131	5'5"	124 — 156
5'2"	105 — 134	5'6"	128 — 161
5'3"	108 — 138	5'7"	132 — 166
5'4"	111 — 142	5'8"	136 — 170
5'5"	114 — 146	5'9"	140 — 174
5'6"	118 — 150	5'10"	144 — 179
5'7"	122 — 154	5'11"	148 — 184
5'8"	126 — 158	6'0"	152 — 189
5'9"	130 — 163	6'1"	156 — 194
5'10"	134 — 168	6'2"	160 — 199
5'11"	138 — 173	6'3"	164 — 204
		6'4"	168 — 209
		6'5"	172 — 214

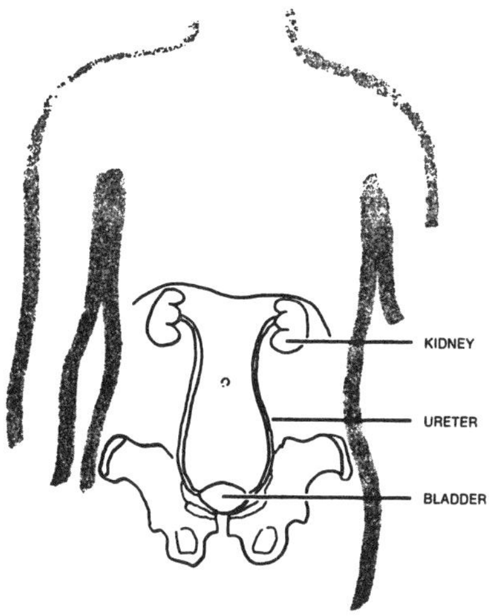

Kidney stones or urinary infections will cause bleeding and pain, but tumors in the kidney or bladder usually cause painless bleeding.

5. Urinary Tract

	YES	NO
A. Do you now have . . . ?		
. . . An urge to urinate more frequently than usual	○	○
. . . Pain or burning upon urination	○	○
. . . Narrowing stream of urine	○	○
. . . Blood in the urine	○	○
B. Has a member of your family ever had . . . ?		
. . . Cancer of the kidney or bladder	○	○
. . . Any congenital (present from birth) urinary tract disease	○	○
C. Have you ever had . . . ?		
. . . A urinary tract infection	○	○
. . . Blood in the urine	○	○
. . . Kidney stones	○	○
. . . Any chronic (long-lasting) kidney disease	○	○
D. Do you . . . ?		
. . Work daily with cleaning fluids, paints, dyes or in factories which manufacture these substances	○	○
. . . Smoke cigarettes	○	○

IF YOU HAVE ANSWERED "YES" TO ANY OF THESE QUESTIONS, ENTER THAT QUESTION ON YOUR *PERSONAL HEALTH RECORD*

CANCER OF THE KIDNEY AND BLADDER

RISK FACTORS:

- Congenital abnormalities of the kidney or bladder (your physician should have informed you if these conditions exist)
- Exposure to certain chemicals such as naphthalines, aniline dyes, or benzidine (be sure to read labels)
- Blood in the urine
- Frequent urinary tract infections, especially after age 50
- A history of schistosomiasis (a tropical disease)
- Heavy cigarette smoking — smoking leads to the presence of chemicals in the urine which may contribute to the development of cancer of the urinary tract

AWARENESS COUNTS:

You can prevent urinary tract cancer by avoiding occupational exposure to cancer-causing chemicals and by seeking medical attention when any symptoms exist.

Blood in the urine is always an important sign and requires *immediate* medical evaluation.

These symptoms are not specific for cancer; more commonly, they are found with bladder infection. However, a physician should be consulted. Frequent urinary tract infections may be due to underlying cancer.

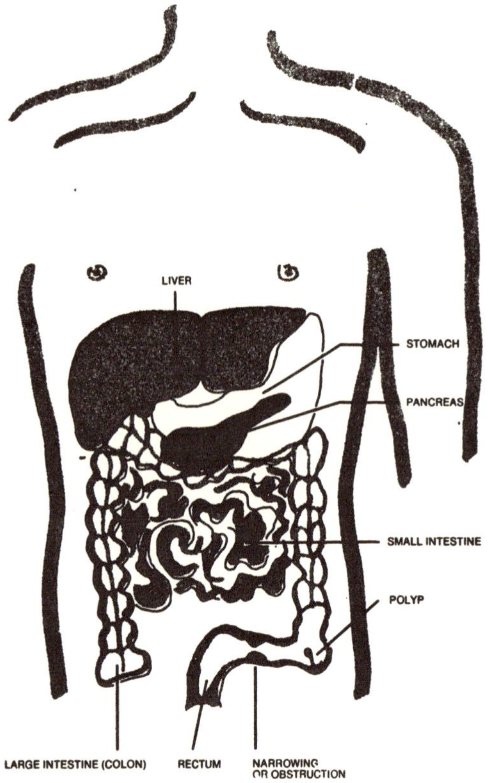

If the growth is removed early the chances of cancer of the colon spreading to other organs, especially the liver, is reduced.

6. Gastrointestinal Tract

A. Do you now have . . . ?	YES	NO
. . . Heartburn, indigestion or abdominal pain which has lasted for more than one month	○	○
. . . Nausea or vomiting which has lasted more than one week	○	○
. . . Fullness after eating small amounts	○	○
. . . Unexplained weight loss, more than 10 lbs. in three months or less	○	○
. . . Any vomiting of blood	○	○
. . . Bowel movements more frequently or less frequently than usual	○	○
. . . Increasing narrowness of stool (ribbon-like)	○	○
. . . Pain in rectum with bowel movements	○	○
. . . Blood in stool, or tarry-black stool	○	○
. . . Passage of mucus alone or with stool	○	○
B. Has a member of your family ever had . . . ?		
. . . Cancer of the stomach	○	○
. . . Stomach or duodenal ulcer	○	○
. . . Pernicious anemia	○	○
. . . Polyps of the colon	○	○
. . . Cancer of the colon or rectum	○	○
C. Have you ever had . . . ?		
. . . Gall bladder disorder	○	○
. . . Stomach or duodenal ulcer	○	○
. . . Pernicious anemia	○	○
. . . Jaundice, hepatitis, cirrhosis of the liver	○	○
. . . Polyps of the stomach or colon	○	○
. . . Ulcerative colitis or other chronic bowel problems	○	○
D. Do you . . . ?		
. . . Have more than 5 beers, 5 glasses of wine, or 3 hard liquor drinks a day	○	○

IF YOU HAVE ANSWERED "YES" TO ANY OF THESE QUESTIONS, ENTER THAT QUESTION ON YOUR *PERSONAL HEALTH RECORD.*

CANCER OF THE STOMACH

RISK FACTORS:

- A lack of normal stomach acid
- Pernicious anemia (a special kind of anemia treated by vitamin B_{12} injections)
- Chronic gastritis or stomach polyps

AWARENESS COUNTS:

Ulcers and ulcer symptoms may be mistaken for stomach cancer and vice versa. If any symptoms listed above last for more than one month, consult a physician.

CANCER OF THE COLON

RISK FACTORS:

- Polyps in the colon
- A family history of cancer of the colon or rectum

AWARENESS COUNTS:

Any changes in your regular bowel habits should be reported to your physician promptly.

Cancer of the colon is infrequent in countries where the diet is high in fruits, vegetables and fish and low in meat.

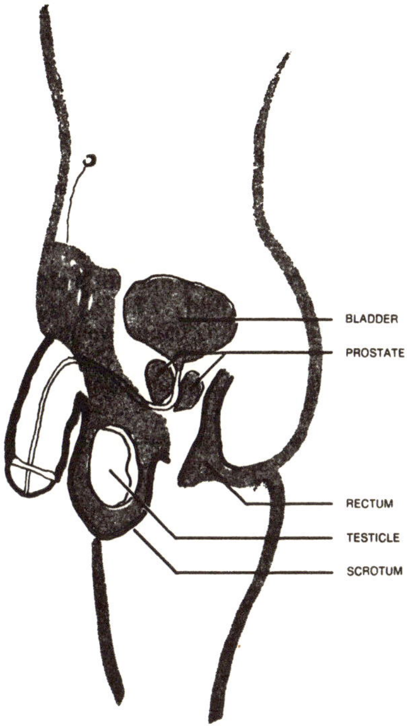

Cancer of the prostate changes the way the prostate feels when it is examined rectally. The usual rubbery firm consistency hardens to a wood-like firmness.

7. Male Reproductive System

	YES	NO
A. Do you now have . . . ?		
. . . A lump in the testicle or pain that has lasted for more than two weeks	○	○
. . . Swelling of either testicle	○	○
. . . Difficulty in starting to urinate	○	○
. . . Pain or uncomfortable pressure deep in the pelvis or between the legs	○	○
. . . Recent problems with sexual function, such as difficulty or pain with ejaculation	○	○
B. DOES NOT APPLY		
C. Have you ever had . . . ?		
. . . Undescended testicle (only one testicle in the scrotum)	○	○
. . . Inflammation of the prostate	○	○
. . . Cancer of the prostate or testicles	○	○
. . . Venereal disease	○	○
D. Do you . . . ?		
. . . Forget to have your prostate examined every three years, or every year if you are over 45	○	○
. . . Forget to examine your testicles for lumps or tenderness, especially if you are under 40	○	○

IF YOU HAVE ANSWERED "YES" TO ANY OF THESE QUESTIONS, ENTER THAT QUESTION ON YOUR *PERSONAL HEALTH RECORD.*

CANCER OF THE PROSTATE

RISK FACTORS:

- A history of venereal disease
- A history of prostate infections (more than 2)
- Risk increases after the age of 50

AWARENESS COUNTS:
The occurrence of cancer of the prostate cannot be controlled since the causes are not known. However, the death rate can be greatly lowered if men, especially those over age 50, are familiar with the above symptoms of the disease and if the prostate is examined regularly. Ask your physician to examine the prostate.

CANCER OF THE TESTES

RISK FACTOR:

- Undescended testicle not corrected before age 6

AWARENESS COUNTS:
There is a high incidence of cancer of the testicle in persons born with an undescended testicle, so this condition should be corrected early. Cancer of the testicle is most common in men under 40. Perform testicular self-exam once a month after a warm bath or shower, when the scrotal skin is most relaxed. Examine each testicle gently by rolling it between the thumb and fingers. Feel for a firm lump about the size of a pea. Most lumps are non-cancerous.

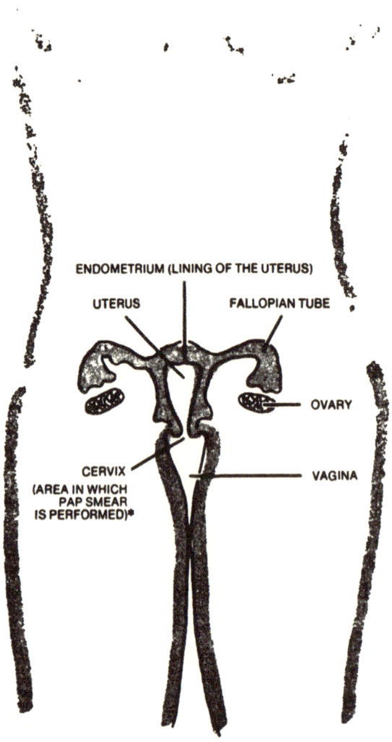

*A Pap smear is done by placing a cotton swab in the vagina and wiping cells off the surface of the cervix. The cells are then examined under a microscope for evidence of cancer. Having a Pap smear is a painless procedure.

8. Female Reproductive System

	YES	NO
A. Do you now have . . . ?		
. . . Bleeding between menstrual periods	○	○
. . . Bloody discharge unrelated to menstrual periods	○	○
. . . Bleeding after sexual intercourse	○	○
. . . Having completed the menopause, any bleeding or spotting	○	○
B. Has a member of your mother's side of the family ever had . . . ?		
. . . Cancer of the cervix, vagina, uterus (womb), or ovary	○	○
Did your mother take female hormones when she was pregnant with you?	○	○
C. Have you ever had . . . ?		
. . . Abnormal cervical (Pap) smear	○	○
. . . Ovarian cyst or tumor	○	○
. . . Fibroid tumor of the uterus	○	○
. . . A Dilatation and Curettage operation ("D & C" or scraping)	○	○
. . . Cauterization of the cervix	○	○
. . . Other surgery of female organs	○	○
Do you use birth control pills?	○	○
Do you use female hormones (estrogens)?	○	○
D. Do you . . . ?		
. . . Forget to have a Pap smear . . .		
. . . Every 3 years (if between 25-35 years of age)	○	○
. . . Every 2 years (if between 35-45 years of age)	○	○
. . . Every year (if over age 45)	○	○

IF YOU HAVE ANSWERED "YES" TO ANY OF THESE QUESTIONS, ENTER THAT QUESTION ON YOUR *PERSONAL HEALTH RECORD.*

CANCER OF THE CERVIX

RISK FACTORS:
- Completed pregnancies (more than 5)
- Marriage at an early age (intercourse before age 18)
- A history of syphilis or gonorrhea
- Any of the symptoms listed under A

AWARENESS COUNTS:
Cancer of the cervix is usually slow-growing and can be detected early by the Pap smear and cured. Examination of any adult female should include a Pap smear and pelvic examination as well as an examination of the breasts.

CANCER OF THE ENDOMETRIUM

RISK FACTORS:
- Having completed the menopause
- Never having been pregnant
- A family history of cancer of the endometrium (lining of the uterus)
- Being a diabetic
- Having hypertension
- Being obese
- Any of the symptoms listed under A

CANCER OF THE OVARY

AWARENESS COUNTS:
In most cases, a woman is unaware of the presence of tumors in the ovaries. There are seldom early symptoms. The ovaries are examined at the time of a Pap and pelvic examination. These examinations should be done on a regular basis (see **D.** above).

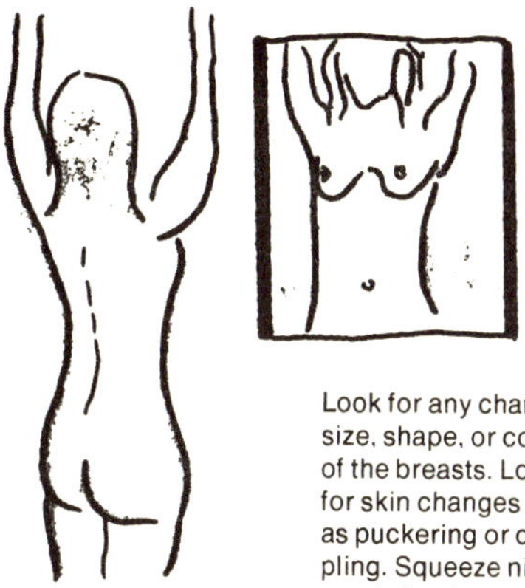

Look for any changes in size, shape, or contour of the breasts. Look for skin changes such as puckering or dimpling. Squeeze nipples gently for discharge. *(Remember it is perfectly normal to have one breast which is larger than the other.)*

Lying down, examine the breasts one at a time with one hand behind your head and the other hand crossed over to examine the opposite breast.

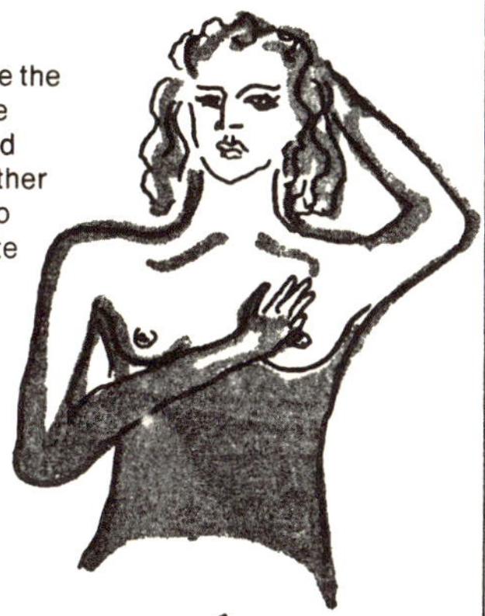

Still lying down, hold your fingers closely together; use gentle pressure and small circular motions. Start at the outer margins, proceed in the same way in smaller circles until you have covered the entire breast.

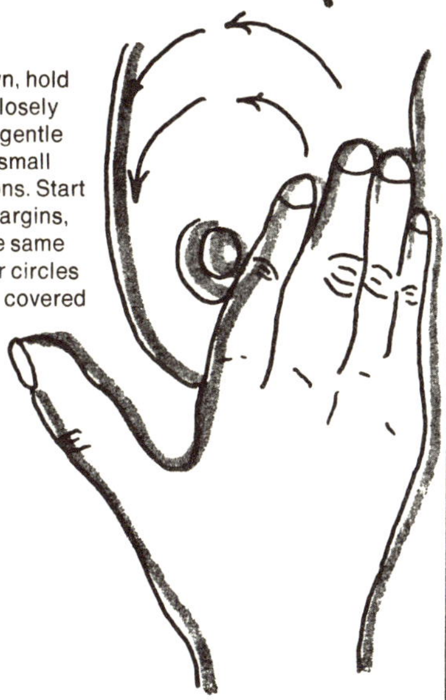

9. Cancer of the Breast (For Women)

	YES	NO
A. Do you now have . . . ?		
. . . Breast pain not related to menstrual periods	○	○
. . . A lump in either breast	○	○
. . . Any discharge from the nipples	○	○
. . . Ulceration (sores), puckering or scaling of breast or any unusual color change of skin or scaling or peeling of nipples	○	○
B. Has a member of your mother's side of the family ever had . . . ?		
. . . Cancer of the breast	○	○
. . . Cysts or tumors of the breast (which were not cancer)	○	○
. . . Any surgery of the breast	○	○
C. Have you ever had . . . ?		
. . . Cancer of the breast	○	○
D. Do you . . . ?		
. . . Forget to examine your breasts each month after your period?	○	○

IF YOU HAVE ANSWERED "YES" TO ANY OF THESE QUESTIONS, ENTER THAT QUESTION ON YOUR *PERSONAL HEALTH RECORD.*

CANCER OF THE BREAST

RISK FACTORS:

- A family or personal history of breast cancer
- Never having had a baby, if you are over age 45
- Having a first pregnancy after age 35
- Any of the symptoms under **A.**

If you have any of the above risks and are over 45, X-ray examination of the breasts (a mammography) is recommended.

AWARENESS COUNTS:

Breast cancer is curable if detected early. Breast examinations should be performed regularly and each time a Pap smear is done. Ask the doctor or nurse to teach you to do breast self-examination. Practice this yourself once a month 2 or 3 days after your menstrual period is over. Many women have cystic breasts. When cysts are present it is advisable to have breast examinations more frequently. This is not a premalignant condition, it just makes the breasts more difficult to examine. Most lumps are found by women themselves; therefore, regular self-examination is necessary. If you find any of the above symptoms, take immediate action. Remember, breast cancer is curable if identified at any early stage.

Index

Index

Index

Index

Index

Index